BASIC CONCEPTS IN DOPPLER ECHOCARDIOGRAPHY

DEVELOPMENTS IN CARDIOVASCULAR MEDICINE

Recent volumes

Hanrath P, Bleifeld W, Souquet, J. eds: Cardiovascular diagnosis by ultrasound. Transesophageal, computerized, contrast, Doppler echocardiography. 1982. ISBN 90-247-2692-1.
Roelandt J, ed: The practice of M-mode and two-dimensional echocardiography. 1983. ISBN 90-247-2745-6.
Meyer J, Schweizer P, Erbel R, eds: Advances in noninvasive cardiology. 1983. ISBN 0-89838-576-8.
Morganroth J, Moore EN, eds: Sudden cardiac death and congestive heart failure: Diagnosis and treatment. 1983. ISBN 0-89838-580-6.
Perry HM, ed: Lifelong management of hypertension. 1983. ISBN 0-89838-582-2.
Jaffe EA, ed: Biology of endothelial cells. 1984. ISBN 0-89838-587-3.
Surawicz B, Reddy CP, Prystowsky EN, eds: Tachycardias. 1984. ISBN 0-89838-588-1.
Spencer MP, ed: Cardiac Doppler diagnosis. 1983. ISBN 0-89838-591-1.
Villarreal H, Sambhi MP, eds: Topics in pathophysiology of hypertension. 1984. ISBN 0-89838-595-4.
Messerli FH, ed: Cardiovascular disease in the elderly. 1984. ISBN 0-89838-596-2.
Simoons ML, Reiber JHC, eds: Nuclear imaging in clinical cardiology. 1984. ISBN 0-89838-599-7.
Ter Keurs HEDJ, Schipperheyn JJ, eds: Cardiac left ventricular hypertrophy. 1983. ISBN 0-89838-612-8.
Sperelakis N, ed: Physiology and pathophysiology of the heart. 1984. ISBN 0-89838-615-2.
Messerli FH, ed: Kidney in essential hypertension. 1984. ISBN 0-89838-616-0.
Sambhi MP, ed: Fundamental fault in hypertension. 1984. ISBN 0-89838-638-1.
Marchesi C, ed: Ambulatory monitoring: Cardiovascular system and allied applications. 1984. ISBN 0-89838-642-X.
Kupper W, MacAlpin RN, Bleifeld W, eds: Coronary tone in ischemic heart disease. 1984. ISBN 0-89838-646-2.
Sperelakis N, Caulfield JB, eds: Calcium antagonists: Mechanisms of action on cardiac muscle and vascular smooth muscle. 1984. ISBN 0-89838-655-1.
Godfraind T, Herman AS, Wellens D, eds: Calcium entry blockers in cardiovascular and cerebral dysfunctions. 1984. ISBN 0-89838-658-6.
Morganroth J, Moore EN, eds: Interventions in the acute phase of myocardial infarction. 1984. ISBN 0-89838-659-4.
Abel FL, Newman WH, eds: Functional aspects of the normal, hypertrophied, and failing heart. 1984. ISBN 0-89838-665-9.
Sideman S, Beyar R, eds: Simulation and imaging of the cardiac system. 1985. ISBN 0-89838-687-X.
Van der Wall E, Lie KI, eds: Recent views on hypertrophic cardiomyopathy. 1985. ISBN 0-89838-694-2.
Beamish RE, Singal PK, Dhalla NS, eds: Stress and heart disease. 1985. ISBN 0-89838-709-4.
Beamish RE, Panagio V, Dhalla NS, eds: Pathogenesis of stress-induced heart disease. 1985. ISBN 0-89838-710-8.
Morganroth J, Moore EN, eds: Cardiac arrhythmias. 1985. ISBN 0-89838-716-7.
Mathes E, ed: Secondary prevention in coronary artery disease and myocardial infarction. 1985. ISBN 0-89838-736-1.
Lowell Stone H, Weglicki WB, eds: Pathology of cardiovascular injury. 1985. ISBN 0-89838-743-4.
Meyer J, Erbel R, Rupprecht HJ, eds: Improvement of myocardial perfusion. 1985. ISBN 0-89838-748-5.
Reiber JHC, Serruys PW, Slager CJ: Quantitative coronary and left ventricular cineangiography. 1986. ISBN 0-89838-760-4.
Fagard RH, Bekaert IE, eds: Sports cardiology. 1986. ISBN 0-89838-782-5.
Reiber JHC, Serruys PW, eds: State of the art in quantitative coronary arteriography. 1986. ISBN 0-89838-804-X.
Roelandt J, ed: Color Doppler Flow Imaging. 1986. ISBN 0-89838-806-6.
Van der Wall EE, ed: Noninvasive imaging of cardiac metabolism. 1986. ISBN 0-89838-812-0.
Liebman J, Plonsey R, Rudy Y, eds: Pediatric and fundamental electrocardiography. 1986. ISBN 0-89838-815-5.
Hilger HH, Hombach V, Rashkind WJ, eds: Invasive cardiovascular therapy. 1987. ISBN 0-89838-818-X
Serruys PW, Meester GT, eds: Coronary angioplasty: a controlled model for ischemia. 1986. ISBN 0-89838-819-8.
Tooke JE, Smaje LH: Clinical investigation of the microcirculation. 1986. ISBN 0-89838-819-8.
Van Dam RTh, Van Oosterom A, eds: Electrocardiographic body surface mapping. 1986. ISBN 0-89838-834-1.
Spencer MP, ed: Ultrasonic diagnosis of cerebrovascular disease. 1987. ISBN 0-89838-836-8.
Legato MJ, ed: The stressed heart. 1987. ISBN 0-89838-849-X.
Safar ME, ed: Arterial and venow systems in essential hypertension. 1987. ISBN 0-89838-857-0.
Roelandt J, ed: Digital techniques in echocardiography. 1987. ISBN 0-89838-861-9.
Dhalla NS et al., eds: Pathophysiology of heart disease. 1987. ISBN 0-89838-864-3.
Dhalla NS et al., eds: Heart function and metabolism. 1987. ISBN 0-89838-865-1.
Dhalla NS et al., eds: Myocardial Ischemia. 1987. ISBN 0-89838-866-X.
Beamish RE et al., eds: Pharmacological aspects of heart disease. 1987. ISBN 0-89838-867-8.
Ter Keurs HEDJ, Tyberg JV, eds: Mechanics of the circulation. 1987. ISBN 0-89838-870-8
Sideman S, Beyar R, eds: Activation, metabolism and perfusion of the heart. 1987. ISBN 0-89838-871-6.
Aliot E, Lazzara R, eds: Ventricular tachycardias. 1987. ISBN 0-89838-881-3.
Schneeweiss A et al., eds: Cardiovascular drug therapy in the elderly. 1987. ISBN 0-89838-883-X.
Chapman JV, Sgalambro A, eds: Basic concepts in Doppler echocardiography. 1987. ISBN 0-89838-888-0
Chien S et al., eds: Clinical hemocheology. 1987. ISBN 0-89838-807-4.
Morganroth J, ed: Congestive heart failure. 1987. ISBN 0-89838-955-0.

BASIC CONCEPTS IN DOPPLER ECHOCARDIOGRAPHY

Methods of clinical applications based on a multi-modality Doppler approach

edited by

J.V. CHAPMAN
Sonotron/Diasonics, Rotterdam, The Netherlands, and Department of Ultrasonology, University Medical Center, Henri Mondor, Paris, France

A. SGALAMBRO
Department of Non-Invasive Cardiology, Civic Hospital of Codogno, Milano, Italy

1988 **MARTINUS NIJHOFF PUBLISHERS**
a member of the KLUWER ACADEMIC PUBLISHERS GROUP
DORDRECHT / BOSTON / LANCASTER

Distributors

for the United States and Canada: Kluwer Academic Publishers, P.O. Box 358, Accord Station, Hingham, MA 02018-0358, USA
for the UK and Ireland: Kluwer Academic Publishers, MTP Press Limited, Falcon House, Queen Square, Lancaster LA1 1RN, UK
for all other countries: Kluwer Academic Publishers Group, Distribution Center, P.O. Box 322, 3300 AH Dordrecht, The Netherlands

Library of Congress Cataloging in Publication Data

```
Basic concepts in Doppler echocardiography.

    (Developments in cardiovascular medicine)
    Includes index.
    1. Doppler echocardiography.  I. Chapman, J.V.
II. Sgalambro, A.  III. Series.  [DNLM: 1. Echocardi-
ography--methods.  W1 DE997VME / WG 141.5.E2 B306]
RC683.5.U5B36  1987   616.1'207543    87-20423
```

ISBN 978-94-010-7995-2   ISBN 978-94-009-3329-3 (eBook)

DOI 10.1007/978-94-009-3329-3

Copyright

PREFACE

Basic Concepts in Doppler Echocardiography

The objective of this textbook is to offer a detailed yet concise overview of the various applications of Doppler echocardiography. The fundamental principles of pulsed mode, continuous mode, and color flow mapping are fully explained as well as the clinical applications of each modality in the evaluation of various cardiac pathologies . A copious amount of figures and illustrations is included so that the reader is able to follow the discussions in the text by referring to the appropriate case studies. The emphasis of this book is focused upon the practical Doppler examination. The sections on theoretical considerations are therefore brief but comprehensive, while the didactic sections concentrate upon how to perform and interpret the clinical examination. The instrumentation of the Doppler system is also discussed so that the physician or technologist can acquire a basic understanding of how the Doppler system actually functions.

CONTRIBUTORS

Bjorn A.J.Angelsen Dr.Tech.
Professor of Biomedical Engineering
University of Trondheim
Trondheim , Norway

Phillip Brun M.D.
Director of Research
Department of Ultrasonology
University Medical Center , Henri Mondor
Paris , France

Albert Meguira M.Sc.
Biomedical Engineer
Sonotron / Diasonics
Paris , France
and the
Department of Ultrasonology
University Medical Center , Henri Mondor
Paris , France

Andreas Strauss M.D.
Department of Ultrasonology
University Medical Center, Henri Mondor
Paris France

Sandra Yanushka B.Sc.
Clinical Specialist
Clinical Applications Department
Sonotron / Diasonics
Rotterdam , The Netherlands

ACKNOWLEDGMENTS

We are indebted to several persons who offered their time and expertise , making this book possible . The implementation of Doppler ultrasound encompasses many disciplines , and these people represent a great storehouse of technical and clinical knowledge. We would like to extend our thanks to **Terje Skjaerpe M.D.** , University of Trondheim, for his contribution in the sections on aortic valve area and right ventricular pressures . **David T. Linker M.D.** , also from the University of Trondheim , was a constant source of clinical and technical insight, especially in the area of pediatric Doppler echocardiography . Part of this book was based on an instruction manual prepared with **Ben Delemarre M.D.** from the Academic Medical Center , Amsterdam. And finally we would like to thank **Kjell Kristoffersen Dr.Tech.** ,head of research and development for Vingmed Inc.,Norway, whose ability to explain technically difficult issues was always appreciated.

I would like to acknowledge that case studies and clinical data where obtained at the following institutions:

Department of Ultrasound
C.H.U. Henri Mondor
University of Paris,
France

Department of Cardiology
Civic Hospital of Codogno, Milano,
Italy

Section of Cardiology Regional Hospital and
Institution of Biomedical Engineering
University of Trondheim,
Norway

Department of Cardiology
Academic Hospital Leiden,
The Netherlands

Department of Cardiology
Academic Medical Center Amsterdam,
The Netherlands

CONTENTS

CONTENTS

CHAPTER 1

BASIC PRINCIPLES
James V. Chapman

Ultrasound is a term used to describe acoustic waves of higher frequency than audible sound. The best known traditional application of ultrasound in cardiology is two-dimensional echocardiography. In this modality, reflected sound from tissue interfaces is used to construct an image of the cardiac structures under investigation. Doppler ultrasound uses the backscattered signals from moving red blood cells to measure blood flow velocity.

The use of Doppler ultrasound to measure flow velocity began at approximately the same time as the use of ultrasound for diagnostic imaging. Continuous wave Doppler instruments were initially used for the qualitative assessment of peripheral vascular blood flow. Pulsed Doppler instruments were later developed in order to study flow in a localized region. These devices were employed in the study of intra-cardiac blood flow, since flow in a specific chamber or vessel could be investigated.

This introductory chapter will explain the basic principles of pulsed and continuous wave Doppler ultrasound. A brief review of ultrasound physics and terminology is also included. Several ultrasound terms may be used interchangeably in the current medical literature, and a common vocabulary is established in this chapter in order to avoid ambiguity.

Sound Wave Propagation

In the Doppler ultrasound examination, a piezoelectric crystal is used to transmit and receive the acoustic signal as in imaging modalities. The piezoelectric crystal is said to function as a transducer, because it converts variations of one quantity to those of another quantity. For imaging applications, the piezoelectric crystal or element converts the electrical energy of a sinusoidal waveform to mechanical energy, and vice versa. The crystal is composed of a synthetic mixture of lead titanate and lead zirconate. In response to an applied voltage, the crystal is rapidly deformed. Such rapid deformation results in the production of an alternating pressure in the surrounding medium which propagates as a sound wave.

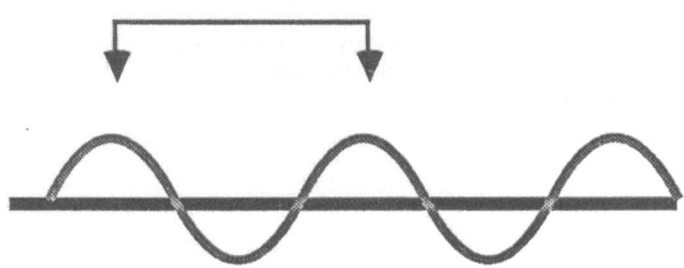

Fig. 1-1. Wavelength. The wavelength is defined as the length of space over which consecutive pressure maxima or pressure minima occur.

1

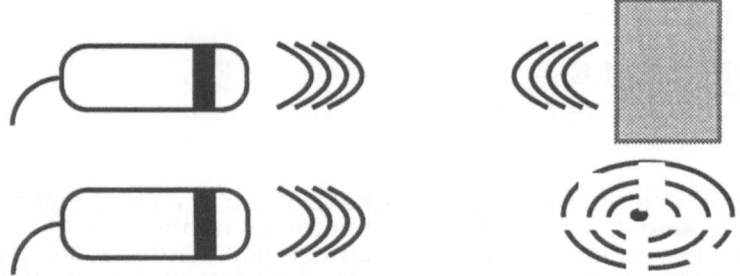

Fig. 1-2. Specular reflection (A) occurs when the wavelength is small in comparison with the boundry surface. Backscattering occurs when the reflector area is small in comparison with the ultrasonic wave length.

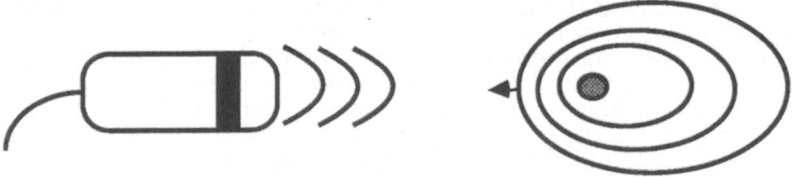

Fig. 1-3 The Doppler shift.

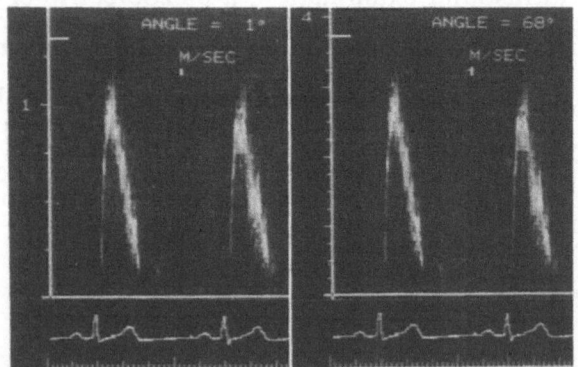

Fig. 1- 4. Effect of angle correction. A represents the true peak velocity recorded in the ascending aorta; B demonstrates the introduced error in the estimation of the flow velocity by overestimation of the beam-to-flow angle.

2

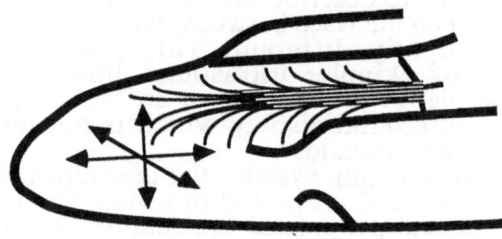

Fig 1- 5. The sample volume is three-dimensional, and blood flow is interrogated in the axial, lateral, and elevational planes. The elevational or Z plane is not visualized in the two-dimensional image.

Sound wave propagation through a medium occurs as a series of compression and rarefactions of the particles in the medium. The time between consecutive pressure minima or presssure maxima is called a cycle, and the number of cycles taking place in one second is termed the frequency. The frequency of the emitted sound is equal to the frequency of the applied voltage. This operating frequency is also known as the resonant frequency of the transducer. The propagation velocity of the sound in a particular medium is determined by the density and the stiffness of the medium. In biological soft tissue, the average propagation velocity is approximately 1540 m/s.

Since the ultrasonic wave is traveling at a relatively constant velocity, there is a small but measureable distance between the successive pressure maxima or pressure minima. This distance is defined as the acoustic wavelength. The formula relating wavelength (λ), propagation velocity and frequency is:

Wavelength (λ) = c/f

$$(1\text{-}1)$$

where c is the propagational velocity of sound in tissue and f is the transducer frequency.

When a transmitted signal traveling through a homogeneous medium encounters an interface, a portion of that signal is reflected, a portion is attenuated (scattered or absorbed), and a portion is refracted. The angle of reflection is determined by the angle of incidence between the signal and the interface. If the incident angle is 90 degrees, the path of the reflected portion of the signal is essentially parallel to that of the transmitted signal provided that the dimensions of the reflecting surface are greater than the ultrasonic wavelength and beamwidth. The surface may then be described as a specular reflector. When the reflecting interface dimensions are smaller then the wavelength or beamwidth, specular reflection no longer takes place. Instead the sound is scattered in many directions. This phenomenon is known as backscattering and is encountered when interrogating blood flow. The red cell diameter is approximately 8 microns (8 millionths of a meter) and is much smaller than the ultrasonic wavelength or beamwidth. Backscattering will also occur when a large but uneven interface is encountered.

Refraction is a term used to describe the bending of the incident ultrasound beam as it passes through an interface between two adjacent media in which the acoustic velocity is slightly different. This phenomenon is of minor importance in tissue or Doppler ultrasound imaging although it may infrequently be reponsible for the creation of artifacts. An artifact is a piece of information in the ultrasound display which is not representative of the structure or flow under interrogation.

In a pulsed Doppler or imaging system, the piezoelectric crystal is excited only at certain intervals for a short period of time. The number of electrical pulses deforming the crystal per second is equal to the number of ultrasonic pulses emitted per second. This number is called the pulse repetition frequency and is expressed in cycles per second or Hertz. Ther pulse or burst duration is the length of time needed for one ultrsonic pulse to occur. The spatial pulse length is the distance taken up by a single ultrasonic burst.

The Ultrasound Beam

The sound emitted by the transducer propagates as a beam. Close to the transducer surface, the beam is shaped like a cylinder with a diameter approximately equal to the transducer diameter. The acoustic energy is not uniformly distributed throughout a given beam cross-section. The beam dimensions increase with distance, and this divergence causes the beam to assume a conical shape (Fig6). A considerable amount of sound may travel outside the beam boundaries; these additional small beams are known as side lobes and can generate artifacts.

The well-defined central portion of the beam which has a cylindrical shape is called the near field or Fresnel zone. The near field length can be calculated if the transducer radius (r) and the ultrasonic wavelength are known;

Near Field Length = [(r)(r)]/wavelength
(1-2)

From this equation, one can deduce that an increase in transducer frequency (decrease in wavelength) or an increase in transducer radius will result in a longer near field. The beam diameter is determined by the ultrasonic wavelength, transducer radius, and the distance from the transducer.

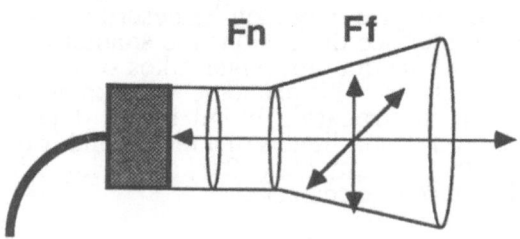

Fig 1- 6. Beam geometry. The ultrasonic beam tends to diverge as the signal travels further from the transducer. The effects of beam divergence are more pronounced in the far field (Ff) than in the near field (Fn). Beam divergence occurs in both the lateral and elevational planes.

The region beyond the near field is termed the far field or Fraunhofer zone. In this region, the beam has a conical configuration. The distribution of acoustic energy at a given beam cross-section is more diffuse in the far field due to attenuation effects and the widening of the beam. Weaker ultrasonic signals will be reflected by structures lying in a wide beam cross-section when compared to the signals produced by the same structures lying in narrow beam cross-section at the same imaging depth.

Resolution and Penetration

The selection of transducer frequency is clinically relevant because it determines the resolution and penetration of an ultrasound system to a large extent. Resolution may be defined as the ability to separate two neighboring reflectors in close proximity to each other. Since the ultrasonic beam is three-dimensional, resolution may be described in the axial, lateral or elevational planes. Generally, the axial and lateral resolution are the most frequently discussed parameters.

Axial or range resolution is defined as the minimum distance between two structures lying along the beam path which will produce two distinct reflections. The axial resolution of a system can be no less than the signal wavelength. Using equation 1-1, the wavelenght of a 1.0 MHz transducer and a 3.5 MHz transducer can be calculated:

f = 1.0 MHz   Wavelength(λ) = 1.5 mm

f = 3.5 MHz   Wavelength(λ) = .44 mm

The wavelength of the 3.5 MHz transducer is much less than the wavelength of the 1.0 MHz transducer, so the axial resolutionof the 3.5 MHz transducer is superior. Axial resolution can also be calculated if the spatial pulse length is known. The axial resolution in mm is equal to half the spatial pulse length in mm. The use of short ultrasonic bursts then will improve the axial resolution of an ultrasound system. Lateral resolution is defined as the minimum distance between two structures lying perpendicular to the direction of sound propagation which will produce two distinct reflections. Lateral resolution is equal to the beam diameter, which varies with distance from the transducer face. Lateral resolution is therefore poorer in the far field due to the larger beam dimensions in the far field.

By choosing a higher transducer frequency, the axial resolution is improved but the rate of attenuation increases. Attenuation is the loss of acoustic energy by scattering or absorption of sound. The deeper the interrogation depth, the greater the loss of energy will be due to attenuation. A general guideline for estimating the degree of energy loss is 1.0 dB/MHz/cm. In other words, biological tissue casuses an energy loss of 1.0 dB/cm for each megahertz of ultrasonic frequency. A 1.0 MHz transducer will attenuate 10 dB at an imaging depth of 10 cm, while a 3.5 MHz transducer will attenuate 35 dB of sound energy at the same imaging depth.

Based upon the preceeding discussion, one can conclude that a compromise is needed when choosing an operating frequency. Higher frequency transducers have superior axial resolution, longer near fields, and reduced beam divergence in the far field. At the same time however, the penetration is poor due to the increased rate of attenuation. With imaging modalities then, it is clear that a compromise must be made when choosing the tranducer frequency. One must select the highest transducer frequency possible which will provide adequate tissue prenetration. The goal of the imaging examination is to obtain accurate structural information.

The Doppler Effect

When a sound source and receiver are moving relative to each other, there is a shift in the apparent frequency of the sound. This phenomenon is called the Doppler effect, in honor of the Austrian physicist who first described this frequency shift. When an ultrasonic signal is directed towards blood, the same effect is noted. If the red cells are approaching the transducer, the received ultrasonic signal will have a higher frequency than the transmitted signal. Conversely, if the red cells are moving away from the transducer, the received ultrasonic signal will have a lower frequency than the transmitted signal. The frequency shift can be calculated using the following equation:

$$Fd = [2F'v\ cos\beta]/c$$
$$(1-3)$$

where Fd is the frequency shift, F' is the transducer frequency, v is the red cell velocity, c is the acoustic velocity(1540 m/s), and ß is the angle between the beam and the blood flow. The equation may be rewritten to solve for the red cell velocity:

$$v = [cFd]/[2F'cos\beta]$$
$$(1-4)$$

When the angle between the ultrasonic beam and the blood flow under investigation is zero or close to zero degrees, the cosine term may be neglected. At larger beam-to-flow angles, the cosine term must be include in the equation otehrwise the velocity of the red cellls will be underestimated. The component of the red cell velocity along the beam path, vcosß, is called the radial velocity.

Spectral Analysis

A method of rapidly analyzing the complex frequency-shifted waveform is needed in Doppler echocardiography. The Discrete Fourier Transform or DFT is the most common method of waveform analysis, yielding information pertaining to the various frequency components and their relative intensity within the ultrasonic signal. Either the Fast Fourier Transform (FFT) or the Chirp-Z transform may be used to electronically compute the discrete Fourier transform. The FFT is a digital approach to the problem of computing the DFT, while the Chirp-Z algorithm represents an analog approach.

Whichever approach is implemented, the purpose is the same: to break down the complex Doppler waveform into its frequency components. One may regard the DFT as an electronic prism which separates the individual frequencies contained in the Doppler signal, just as the conventional prism separates white light into its various components. This process of component frequency analysis is known as spectral analysis, and the graphic display produced is called the spectrum or spectral trace.

The spectrum is displayed as an x-y plot on the viewing monitor. Time is represented on the x-axis, frequency or velocity is represented on the y-axis, and the signal intensity is indicated in shades of grey. If a black background is selected, an intense signal will be displayed in shades of grey which are close to white, as in conventional tissue imaging. A weak signal will be displayed in darker shades of grey. If a white background is selected, an intense signal will be displayed in shades of grey close to black.

The y-axis is usually divided into 64 or 128 points, each possessing a defined velocity or frequency value. The range of frequencies above and below the baseline is called the frequency window. If a low velocity flow is being analyzed, it is helpful to choose a low frequency window so that the 64 or 128 points are used to optimally display the low velocity information. Conversely, if a high velocity flow is being interrogated, a higher frequency window is needed in order to display the data correctly. The frequency or velocity resolution of these measurements is inversely related to the computation time of the spectral analyzer.

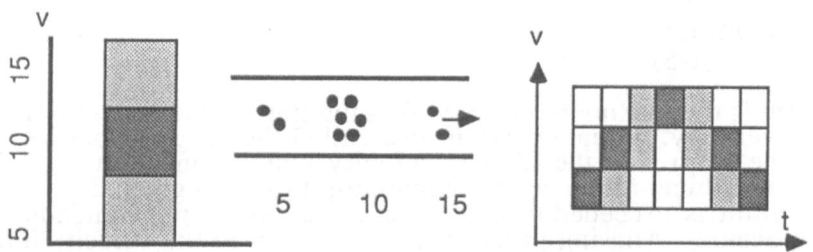

Fig 1-7. A simplified schematic which illustrates the concept of the display method. The blood flow in this vessel contains red cells which move at velocities in the 5, 10, and 15 cm/s range, respectively. Right. Most of the red cell scatterers are moving at 10 cm/s towards the transducer. This means that there will be more reflected ultrasonic energy in this frequency range than in the 5 or 15 cm/s range. Left. The spectral display. Time is displayed on the x-axis, and velocity in cm/s is displayed on the y-axis. Because a greater amount of ultrasound is reflected from red cells moving at 10 cm/s, a darker shade of grey is assigned to this range. Shades of grey are used to indicate signal amplitude in the spectral trace.

Pulsed Doppler Ultrasound

There are two basic ways of transmitting the Doppler signal. The signal is either continuously transmitted and received, or it is transmitted and received at discrete intervals. The pulsed mode will be discussed first. In pulsed Doppler ultrasound, the ultrasonic signal is transmitted for a specific length of time which is called the burst duration at constantly spaced intervals. The signal is reflected by all scatterers along the beam path, but may be selectively sampled by opening the receive gate at a certain time interval following signal transmission. This interval takes into account the amount of time needed for the pulse to travel to and from a selected depth. The volume of flow sampled at that selected depth is called the sample volume, range gate, or sample cell.

The axial dimension of the sample volume is determined by the burst duration and the period of time in which the receive gate remains open. The number of pulses emitted per second is termed the pulse repetition frequency. Since the ultrasonic pulse must travel to a certain depth and return before the next pulse is transmitted, the pulse repetition frequency is determined by the interrogation depth. To sample flow in a shallow interrogation site, a high pulse repetition frequency may be used because the roundtrip travel time of the pulse will be brief. To sample a deeper interrogation site, the pulse repetition frequency must be decreased to allow for the longer travel time. The value of the pulse repetition frequency is therefore limited by the interrogation depth. Range or depth resolution is provided with pulsed mode, since the interrogation depth is known. Transmission of an ultrasonic pulse occurs following the reception of the previous burst.

The maximum frequency which may be measured at a given depth is half the pulse repetition frequency; this value is known as the Nyquist frequency. Converted to velocity, the maximum measureable velocity is termed the Nyquist limit or Nyquist value. The Nyquist limit can be calculated at a certain interrogation depth (R) using the following equation:

$$Vm = c^2/[8F'R]$$
$$(1-5)$$

where Vm is the maximum velocity, F' is the transducer frequency and c is the acoustic velocity. Equation 1-5 is also called the range velocity product. It allows one to predict the highest velocity which can be measured using a specific transducer frequency for examining flow at a given depth. When the Nyquist limit is exceeded during the examination, a phenomenon known as aliasing occurs. Aliasing produces an ambiguity in the velocity information obtained (Figure 1-12)

In order to resolve velocities greater than the Nyquist value, one may consider only one sign of the Doppler shift. In other words, by examining flow in only one direction (either towards or away from the transducer), velocities up to twice the Nyquist value may be measured. This technique is called spectral unwrapping. A spectral unwrapping algorithm is available in most Doppler instruments to allow for an asymmetric Nyquist display of the spectrum. However, the audio signal will remain aliased unless an audio unwrapping option is employed. When the audio signal is aliased, one can no longer rely upon the audio signal for information regarding the beam-to-flow alignment. This is an important point which will be discussed further in the next chapter.

Pulsed mode then has the advantage or being capable of flow localization, but it is limited in that the maximum measureable velocity is determined by the pulse repetition frequency.

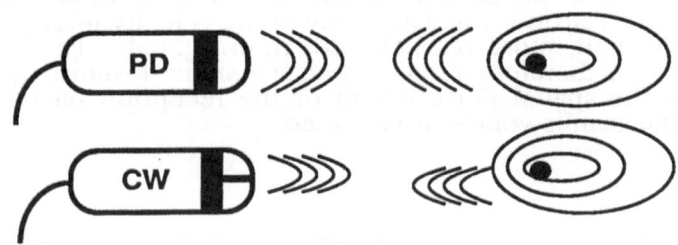

Fig 1- 8. Conventional Doppler modes. Pulsed Doppler ultrasound is transmitted and received through the same piezoelectric element. Pulsed mode has the advantage of range resolution, and the disadvantage of a relatively low limit on the the peak velocity which may be measured. Continuous mode is transmitted and received with different elements; there is no practical limit to the maximum velocity which can be measured. However, spatial resolution is not provided with continuous mode; the two techniques are complimentary.

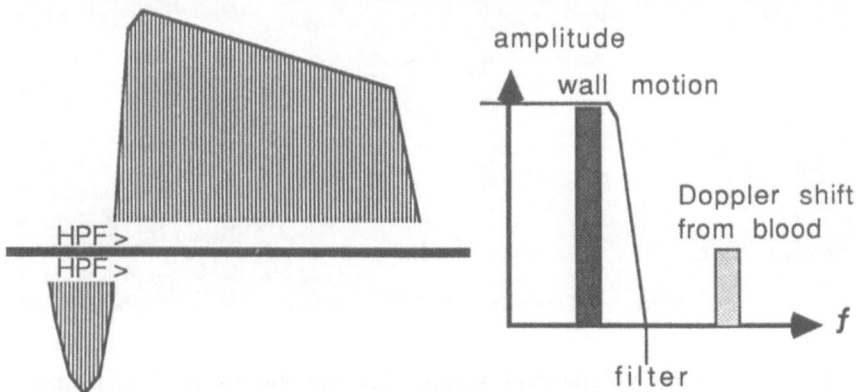

Fig 1- 9. When working with Doppler techniques a general problem is the seperation of backscattered signals from the blood , and specular reflections from tissue. High pass filtering (HPF) is used to remove low velocity high amplitude wall motion signals from the analyzed signal . The HPF should be set high (1 KHz to 1.5 KHz) when measuring high velocity flows to prevent saturation by the low velocity high amplitude signals.

9

The Sample Volume

As stated earlier, the axial dimension of the sample volume is determined by the length of the transmitted burst and the period of time in which the receive gate remains open. The ultrasonic burst length will be somewhat longer than the sinusoidal input to the transducer due to the ringing of the piezoelectric crystal. To change the axial dimension of the sample cell, the pulse burst duration or the reception time may be altered. The lateral dimensions of the sample volume are defined by the physical characteristics of the ultrasonic beam. Due to beam divergence, the width of the sample volume will be greater in the far field and the acoustic intensity will be less concentrated than in the near field. The lateral resolution will be poorer in the far field because of the increase in sample volume dimension.

The axial length of the sample volume is clinically important because it directly affects the sensitivity and accuracy of the velocity measurement. With a larger sample cell, more red cells are interrogated. The backscattered ultrasonic signal is therefore stronger, and the signal-to-noise ratio is higher. By increasing the spatial pulse length or the reception interval, the axial dimension of the sample volume is increased.

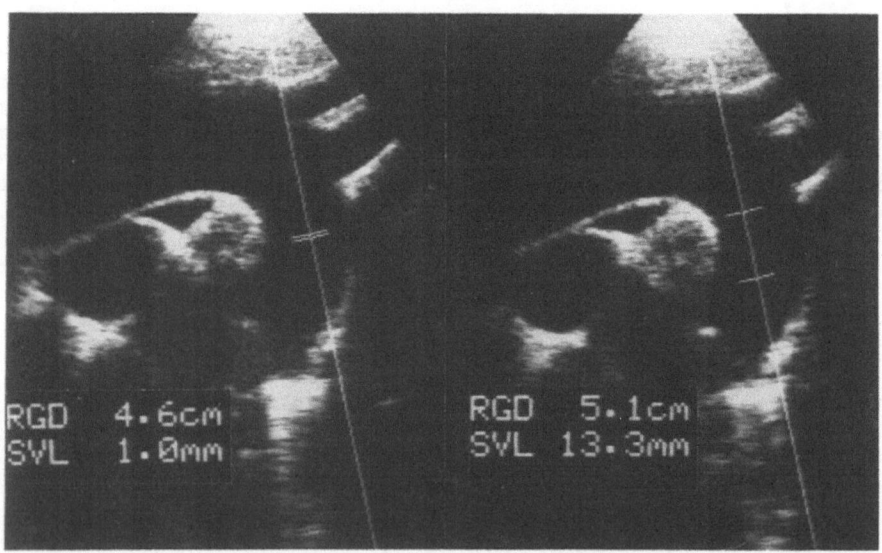

Fig. 1-10 . The sample volume dimensions. The volume of blood interrogated during pulsed mode transmission is known as the sample volume, range gate, or sample cell. The lateral and elevational dimensions of the sample cell are defined by the ultrasonic beam width. The axial dimension of the sample volume is defined by the pulse burst duration and the length of time in which the receiver gate remains open. It is possible to change the axial dimension or length of the range gate, as illustrated. (RGD = range gate depth, SVL = sample volume length).

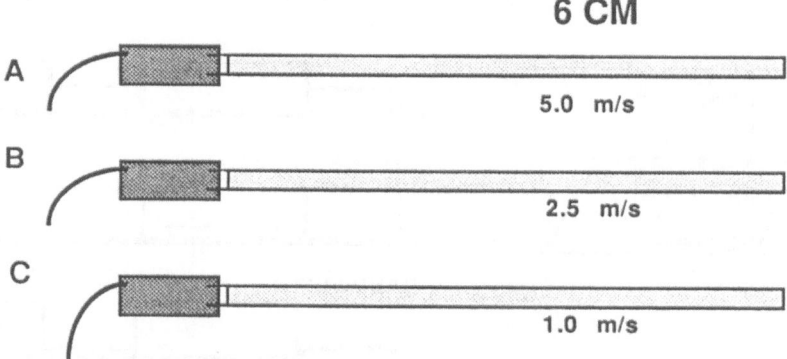

6 CM

A   5.0 m/s

B   2.5 m/s

C   1.0 m/s

Fig 1- 11 . The Range Velocity Product. The maximum velocity(Vm) which may be measured with pulsed mode is limited by the range velocity product:

$$(Vm)(R) = c^2/(8Fo)$$

where R is the depth of interrogation, c is the acoustic velocity, and Fo is the carrier frequency. By decreasing the carrier frequency, a higher velocity may be measured at the same given depth. The figure above shows the peak velcoity whigh may be measured at a 6 cm depth using a 1.0 MHz (A), 2.0 MHz (B), and 5MHz (C) carrier frequency.

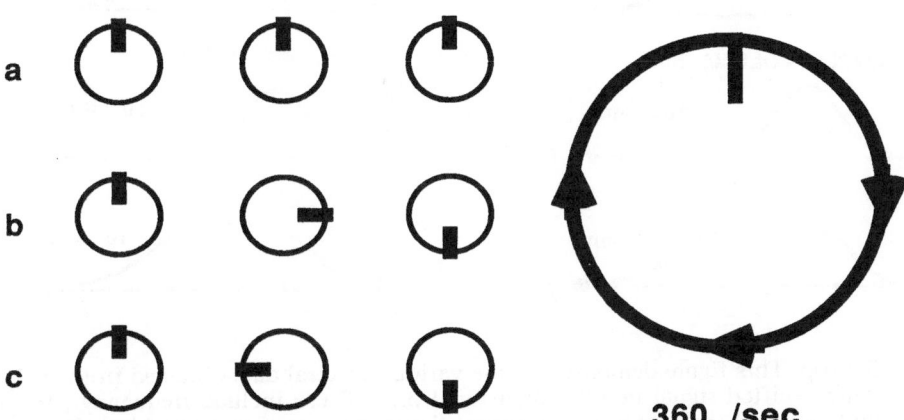

a

b

c

360 /sec

Fig. 1-12 . Aliasing. If a wheel rotates clockwise with a frequency of 360 degrees per second and is observed only at set time intervals, the sampling frequency (observation interval) can affect the information obtained (the direction of the wheel's rotation). A. The observation period is set at one second intervals. At each sampling period, the marker appears in the same position, hence the wheel appears to be stationery. B. The observation period occurs every 250 ms (the sampling frequency is 4 per second). The first three samples indicate that the wheel is moving in a clockwise manner, and the information obtained regarding the wheel's rotation is correct. C. The observation period occurs every 750 ms. The first three samples obtained indicate that the wheel is moving in a counter-clockwise direction, which is incorrect.

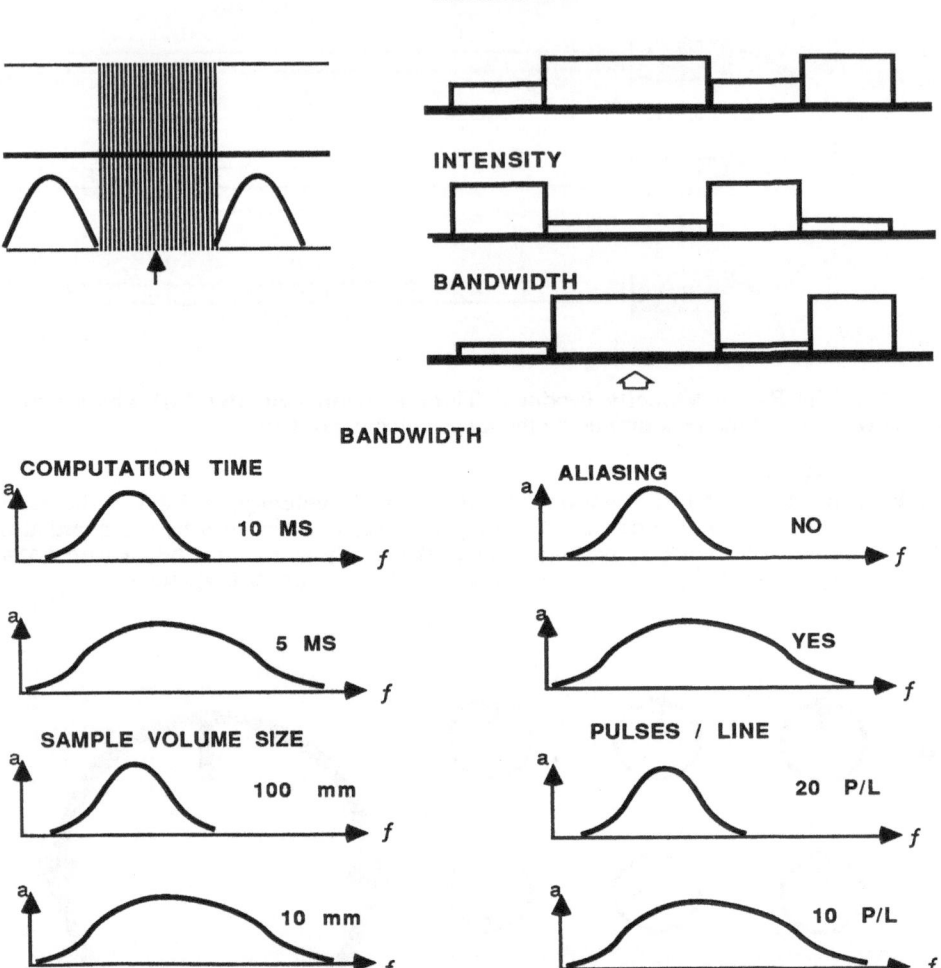

Fig. 1-13. Top. This figure demonstrates the various spectral data obtained from analysis of the frequency shifted signal in a 3 dimensional plot. These include frequency , frequency bandwidth (variance) , and amplitude. Bottom. There are several factors which effect spectral bandwidth such as frequency analysis time , sample volume dimension , and the presence of aliasing. These factors should be considered when interpreting the Doppler echocardiographic recordings.

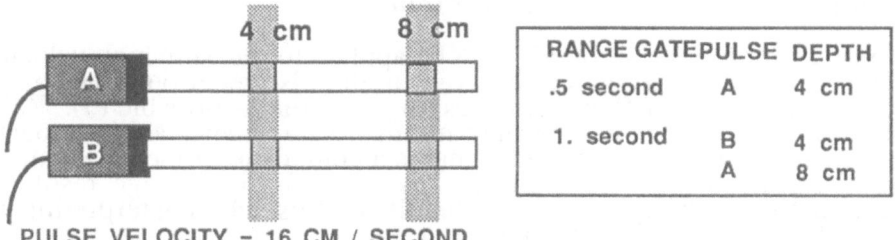

RANGE GATE	PULSE	DEPTH
.5 second	A	4 cm
1. second	B	4 cm
	A	8 cm

PULSE VELOCITY = 16 CM / SECOND

Fig. 1- 14. Range ambiguity.

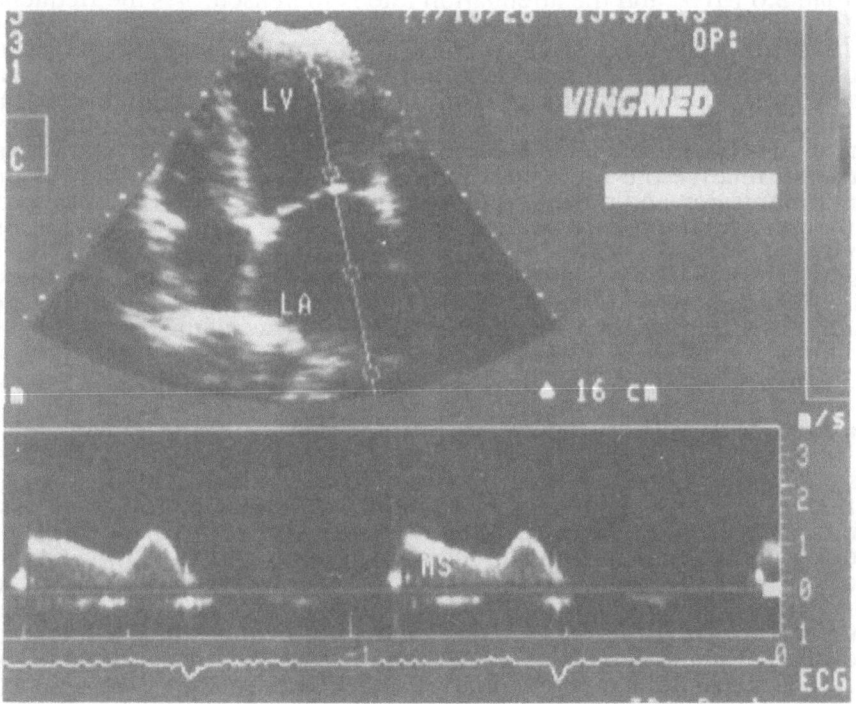

Fig. 1-15 . High pulse repetition frequency mode may be used to measure moderately high flow velocities, as in this case of mitral stenosis. The apical four chamber view is used and the positions of the range gates are indicated in the sector image. High pulse repetititon frequency mode has the advantage of a limited degree of spatial resolution when measuring increased flow velocities unlike continuous mode, where no spatial resolution is provided.

High Pulse Repetition Frequency Mode

The principle of range ambiguity can be applied to measure high velocities with pulsed Doppler ultrasound. If a very high pulse repetition frequency is utilized, measurement of flow velocities up to 5.0 m/s is possible (3). Range resolution is limited however, because multiple sample sites are interrogated along the beam path. The returned signal is a composite of the backscattered signals from these different sample sites. The limited range resolution inherent in this technique may create difficulties when interpreting the velocity information displayed in the spectrum.

High pulse repetition frequency mode has been shown by several investigators to consistently underestimate the peak flow velocities in adults with aortic stenosis (7,8). There are some features of this technique which are probably responsible for its inability to accurately record high flow velocities. The transducer frequency used with high pulse repetition mode is usually higher than 3.0 MHz, and the attenuation rate is increased. As the frequency of pulsing the piezoelectric crystal increases, the amount of energy present in each ultrasonic pulse decreases, thereby lowering the signal-to-noise ratio. The audio signal of high pulse repetition frequency systems still aliases at the Nyquist frequency. Unless an audio unwrapping option is available, the audio signal therefore is no longer useful in guiding the beam into a parallel alignment with the interrogated flow. A single piezoelectric crystal is used to transmit and receive the ultrasonic pulses at rapid rates, and there is nearly constant tranmission and reception of ultrasound. The crystal can not perform both functions simultaneously and saturation may occur, producing a loss of sensitivity.

High pulse repetition frequency mode can be successfully applied in the study of congenital lesions (3). The effects of ultrasonic attenuation are not as pronounced in this application due to the shallower interrogation depths encountered.

Continuous Wave Doppler Ultrasound

Pulsed Doppler instruments utilize a single piezoelectric element or group of elements working as a single element to function as the ultrasonic transmitter and receiver. In a continuous wave Doppler instrument, sound is continuously being transmitted and received so the pulse repetition frequency may be considered infinite. A dual or split piezoelectric element is neede in order to carry out simultaneous ultrasonic signal transmission and reception. Since the pulse repetition frequency is such a high value, there is no practical limit to the maximum flow velocity which may be measured. Pulsing of the transmitted continuous wave signal actually does occur, but the pulse repetition frequency is so high that the transmission is essentially continuous. If a single piezoelectric crystal is employed to transmit and receive ultrasound at these high pulse repetition frequencies, receiver saturation will result and the system sensitivity is compromised.

The prime advantage of continuous mode is its ability to measure high flow velocities which are necessary to measure gradients . Because the signal is constantly transmitted and received, range or spatial resolution is not possible. It is easier to assess beam-to-flow alignment with continuous mode than with pulsed mode since the entire length of the emitted beam may be considered the "sample volume" in continuous mode. The limitation of continuous wave Doppler is its lack of spatial resolution. In general the signal strength , or amplitude , from the peak blood flow velocity range is quite weak. Due to this the measurment of the peak blood flow velocity can be difficult in some situations , and may result in under estimation of the pressue gradient . High

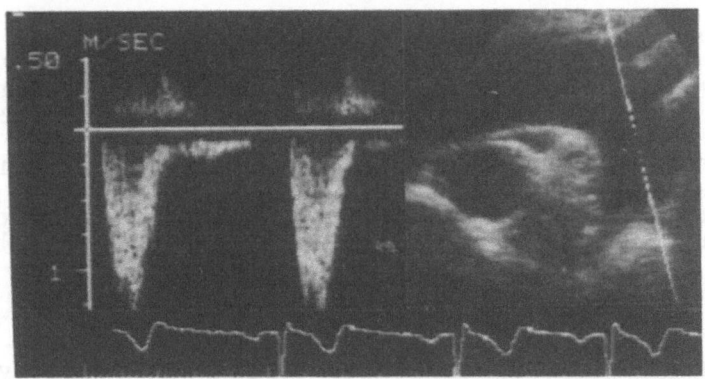

Fig. 1-16. Using continuous wave Doppler ultrasound, a split element is used to constantly transmit and receive the ultrasonic signal. There is no practical limit to the maximum velocity which may be measured. In this example, the continuous wave beam is positioned in the descending aorta, and the resulting spectral trace is displayed beneath the sector image. Compare the envelope of this trace to the pulsed mode trace in the same patient (Fig 1-). The positive flow in systole represents the flow into the neck vessels.

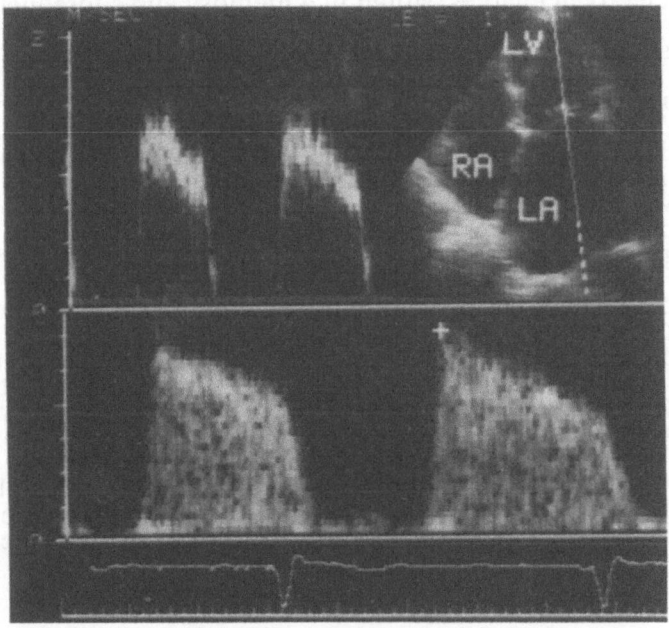

Fig. 1-17. Pulsed mode (top) and continuous mode (bottom) recordings of mitral flow in a patient with mitral stenosis. The pulsed mode recording of a given flow generally has a narrower spectral benadwidth than the corresponding continuous wave recording. The pulsed mode trace has been recorded with an expanded time base.

flow velocities can be reliably measured, they can not be localized. The wider beamwidths used in continuous mode facilitate detection of narrow jets which may be missed with pulsed mode. However, due to the wide beamwidths of continuous mode, two jets in close proximity to each other may be interrogated simultaneously.

Based upon this introductory discussion, it is clear that the optimal Doppler instrument for cardiovascular applications should combine both pulsed and continuous modes. Continuous mode may be employed to measure high flow velocities and to localize flows. Pulsed mode can be utilized to obtain range resolution.

IMAGING AND DOPPLER SYSTEMS: THE BASIC PRINCIPLES

An imaging system can basically be described as a pulsed-echo device; that is, it functions by generating and transmitting an ultrasonic pulse at specific time intervals. The rate at which these pulses are produced in one second is termed the pulse repetition frequency. The maximum pulse repetition frequency is determined by the acoustic velocity in tissue and the desired imaging depth. Following ultrasonic transmission, the returning echoes are received by the transducer for a certain period of time. The amplitude, direction, and arrival time of these reflected signals are used to construct an A-mode (amplitude mode) or M-mode (motion mode) display. In real-time imaging systems, this process is repeated by electronically or mechanically sweeping the ultrasonic beam through a fixed arc. Returning echoes from all interrogation depths are converted to electrical charges, stored in a memory and subsequently taken out of the memory to produce a visual display.

Imaging systems use the acoustic reflections from tissue to generate a display from which structural information is obtained. The Doppler shift of the received ultrasonic pulses is not used for extracting information. As discussed earlier, the Doppler shift occurs when a sound source and reflector are in motion relative to each other. The Doppler instrument processes these frequency-shifted ultrasonic pulses to determine the velocity and the direction of blood flow. Because of the beam-to-flow angle involved, the Doppler instrument actually measures the radial flow velocity. There are two methods of obtaining this information: by pulsing the ultrasonic signal or by continuously transmitting the signal.

In continuous wave transmission, ultrasonic signals are continuously being produced, transmitted and received. A voltage generator applies a continuous voltage to the piezoelectric crystal to produce the ultrasonic signal; a separate piezoelectric crystal is employed for signal reception. After the backscattered signal is converted to a voltage and amplified, it is passed to the receiver. The receiver compares the frequency-shifted signal to the reference signal produced by the voltage generator. The difference between the received signal and the reference signal is the frequency shift or Doppler shift. As stated in the Doppler equation (1-2), the frequency shift is proportional to the radial velocity of the scatterer and the ultrasonic carrier frequency.

The frequency-shifted signal is then sent to a phase detector, where it is compared to the reference signal in the direct channel and the reference signal in the quadrature channel. The reference signal in the quadrature channel has the same amplitude and frequency as the signal in the direct channel but is shifted 90 degrees in phase. The direct channel obtains its reference signal from the master oscillator, while the quadrature channel obtains its reference signal after the signal has passed through a $\pi/2$ phase shifter. This type of demodulation which employs two reference signals separated in phase by 90 degrees is called quadrature demodulation. By comparing the incoming signal with the two reference signals in the phase detector, the direction of blood flow can be determined. The signal is then passed to the spectral analyzer for analysis of its frequency components.

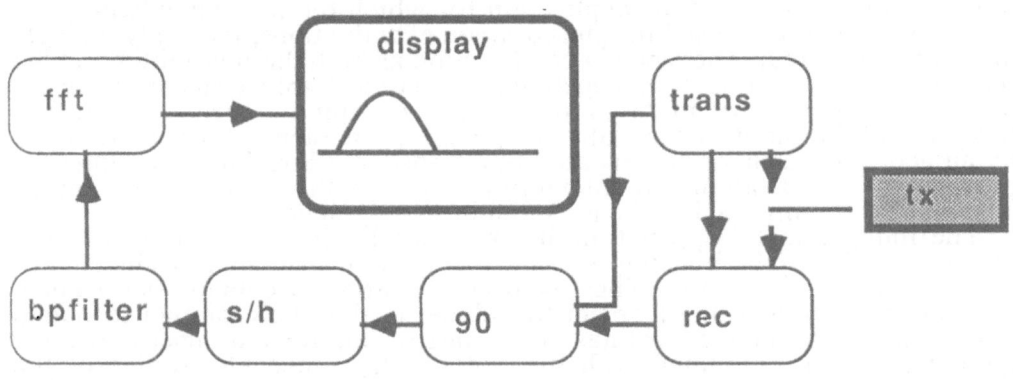

Fig. 1- 18. Simplified drawing of a Doppler ultrasound instrument

In pulsed mode transmission, ultrasonic signals are produced and transmitted at specific time intervals in the same manner as a pulsed echo imaging system. A single piezoelectric element or group of elements functioning as one element is employed for both signal transmission and reception. The voltage generator in a pulsed Doppler instrument contains a generator gate allowing the passage of voltage at certain time intervals. The voltage pulse then excites the piezoelectric crystal, resulting in the production of an ultrasonic pulse. The receiver also contains a gate which opens at selected intervals to allow for reception of the backscattered signals. Due to the presence of the receive gate, the flow velocity as well as the depth of the interrogated flow can be determined. The range gate depth or sample volume depth is operator-selected in pulsed Doppler systems. The pulse repetition frequency is limited by the acoustic velocity in tissue and the desired interrogation depth.

The optimal Doppler instrument uses low carrier frequencies with relatively long ultrasonic bursts for pulsed mode transmission and narrow bandwidth receivers.

The lower transducer frequencies allow a higher velocity to be measured at a given depth in pulsed mode, as shown in the range velocity equation (1-5). The spatial pulse length determines the axial dimension of the sample volume; a longer ultrasonic burst results in a larger sample volume, thereby improving the signal-to-noise ratio. At the same time, the use of longer ultasonic bursts degrades the axial resolution. This degradation in resolution is not a major concern in the design of a Doppler system because the blood flow velocity does not change appreciably with small variations in position.

These are opposing requirements to that of an optimal imaging system. The ideal imaging system utilizes the highest transducer frequencies possible which will result in adequate tissue penetration. Short spatial pulse lengths and wide bandwidth receivers are design requirements of the ideal imaging systems. The use of short burst lengths and high frequency transducers will improve the axial and lateral resolution. The ability to obtain accurate anatomical information is dependent upon a high degree of image resolution. The wide bandwidth receivers are needed for processing the broad range of ultrasonic signals produced by the various cardiac structures.

The choice of a piezoelectric element used in constructing the Doppler transducer depends upon the application for which the probe is intended. If the transducer will be used for pulsed mode examinations, then only a single element is required. The element can function as both the transmitter and the receiver. If continuous wave capability is desired, a split element or pair of elements is necessary in order to provide continuous transmission and reception of the ultrasonic signal. The piezoelectric elements are surrounded by an acoustic insulator and encased in a transducer housing. The potential problem of cross-talking or interaction between the transmit and recive elements is circumvented by the use of an insulating material.

The independent Doppler transducer is smaller in size than an imaging transducer; the probe housing is usually angled so that the transducer face remains in contact with the chest wall as the probe orientation is changed. These two features of the Doppler transducer enable the examiner to obtain high quality Doppler recordings from narrow intercostal spaces in most patients. When combined with the specifically tuned electronics of the Doppler instrument, it is easy to understand why the independent Doppler system generates superior Doppler recordings.

The ideal Doppler transducer and imaging transducer utilize different types of backing material behind the piezoelectric elements. In an imaging probe, the element is usually backed with a damping material to remove the lower amplitude portion of the signal thereby reducing the spatial pulse length. This results in an improvement in the axial resolution. At the same time, this causes a reduction in signal amplitude and sensitivity. In Doppler applications, the backscattered signal from blood has a much weaker intensity than the reflected signals from tissue interfaces. Use of a damping material will further decrease the amplitude of the Doppler signal, and this decrease in amplitude may be significant.

In a combined Doppler and imaging system, compromises must be made in the design specifications. Either a phased array or mechanical scanning format can be selected when designing such a system. Generally it is less difficult to acheive adequate image and Doppler resolution when mechanical sector technology is chosen. The piezoelectric elements used in a constructing a mechanical transducer are larger than those used in a phased array transducer. The choice of transducer frequencies is broader with mechanical sector systems so the optimal frequency for a given application can be selected. The Doppler cursor can be steered through the sector arc in a mechanical system, while it may be fixed in a phased array system. If an annular array transducer is used in conjunction with mechanical sector technology, a high degree of simultaneity between the different modalities is possible.

Color Flow Analysis

In a pulsed Doppler examination, flow is interrogated within a specific region known as the sample volume. The velocity, direction, and flow characteristics of the blood within this particular region can be determined. Continuous wave Doppler ultrasound enables one to measure high flow velocities, but no range resolution is obtained. Both conventional Doppler techniques utilize spectral analysis to extract information regarding the flow velocity, component signal intensity, and flow direction. Spatial orientation of the interrogated flow, however, is not provided. Pulsed Doppler ultrasound provides a small degree of spatial orientation, but the information is limited to a single intracardiac site without reference to concurrent hemodyanmic events.

Color flow analysis uses the Doppler-shifted signals from red cell scatterers to determine the direction, velocity and relative density of the red cells. In this respect, it is similar to conventional Doppler techniques.The color flow information is obtained by a multi-gated pulsed Doppler methods which will be described in this chapter. The major difference between color flow imaging and conventional pulsed mode lies its ability to provide spatial orientation of flow. The spatial relationships between the interrogated flow and the adjacent anatomical structures can be examined in real-time. In color flow analysis, flow is sampled at many sites which differ in their axial and lateral position within the sector image. The flow signal is analyzed by an autocorrelator technique which in effect yields a coarse form of spectral analysis. The processed flow signal is then input to the two-dimensional image memory, and the resultant sector image displays the flow information superimposed upon the tissue image.

MULTI-GATED PULSED DOPPLER TECHNIQUE

In conventional pulsed mode, an ultrasonic signal is transmitted along a single line of propagation. The sample site is localized by opening the receive gate at a specific point in time, taking into account the roundtrip travel time. In color flow analysis, several lines of transmission are utilized, with multiple sample sites along each line.

Ideally the pulsing and flow sampling process should be repeated as often as possible along each transmission line. As the number of pulses per line is increased, the accuracy of the velocity estimated is improved. Random noise is also reduced by an increase in the number of pulses. This results in an increase in system sensitivity. The color flow methods of pulsing and sampling is demonstrated schematically in Fig 1-8 .

It is important to keep in mind that the number of pulses transmitted per line and the number of acoustic lines are parameters which ultimately limit the sector frame rate. Another limiting factor is the desired interrogation depth. To avoid range ambiguity, the pulse repetition frequency must

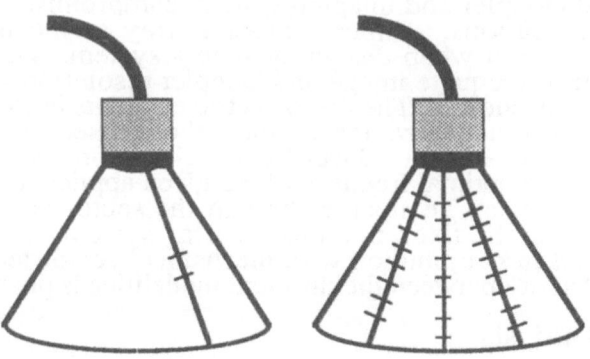

Fig. 1- 19 . In conventional pulsed Doppler a single range gate is sampled on a single line of interogation. For color flow mapping several range gates along several scan lines.

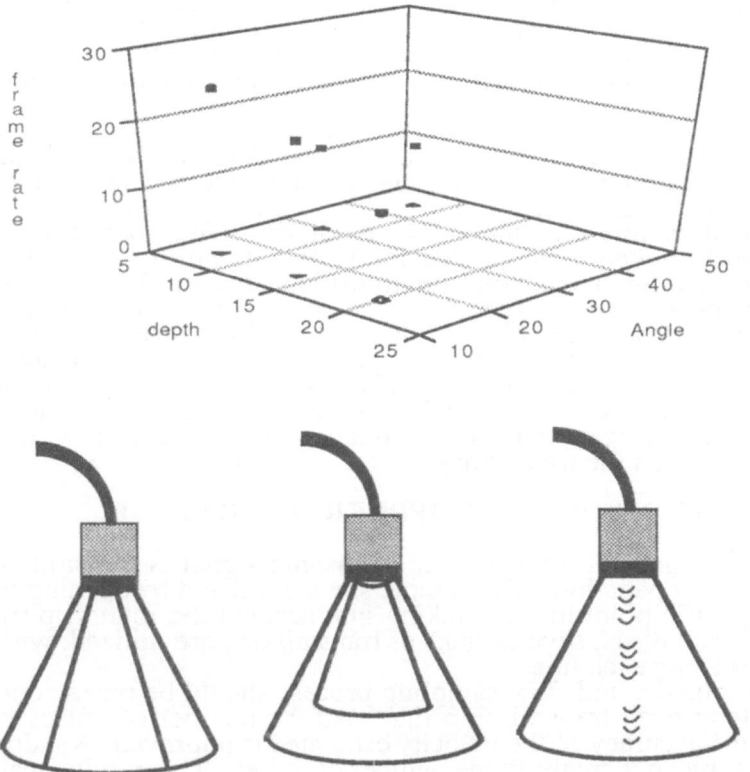

Fig. 1- 20 . Effects of scan depth , tissue and blood flow imaging sectors angles , and number of pulses per line. The graph demonstrates the relationship between these variables .

be reduced with increasing depth, as with conventional pulsed mode. As the pulse repetition frequency decreases, the maximum measureable velocity decreases. The frame rate may be maintained at greater imaging depths by reducing the number of acoustic lines, thereby reducing the sector angle. Figure 1-20 demonstrates the relationship between frame rate, acoustic line density, and depth. One will note a decrease in frame rate as the angle is increased , the depth is increased , the number of pulses per line increased , or the low velocity reject threshhold decreased .

The backscattered signal from blood has a weaker intensity than the signals reflected from tissue interfaces. These strong tissue signals must be removed from the received Doppler signal, otherwise receiver saturation may occur. High pass filters are used in color flow analysis to remove these low frequency but high intensity signals originating from the motion of the cardiac and vessel walls.

Autocorrelation

In conventional pulsed mode, the complex backscattered signal from blood is analyzed by either the Fast Fourier transform or Chirp-Z method. While these techniques are accurate and relatively easy to implement, they are essentially too slow for color flow applications. Rapid analysis of the incoming signal is essential in color flow imaging and may be acheived at the expense of frequency resolution. Autocorrelation is the technique used for color flow signal processing. The autocorrelator extracts the mean frequency shift from the backscattered signal. After the incoming signal is filtered, it passes to the quadrature detector for phase detection so that the directional information may be extrapolated. The outputs from the direct channel and the quadrature channel are then sent to the autocorrelator, where they are passed through delay lines and multiplied together with the two outputs from the phase detector. Integration of the two outputs from the multiplier circuit results in the extraction of the mean Doppler frequency. The mean flow velocity can therefore be estimated.

It is possible to obtain information relating to the freqency bandwidth (variance) and the signal amplitude (back scattered signal strength) as well as the mean frequency . The optimal way to analyze the signal is to consider all these parameters together , as the signal to noise ratio is improved and the seperation of mild aliasing and low velocity turbulent flows is possible.

The extracted velocity and directional information is overlaid upon the tissue image by means of a color scale. In the most commonly used color assignment, shades of red indicate flow towards the transducer while shades of blue indicate reversed flow or flow away from the transducer.(Figure 1-23) Each individual shade represents a specific range of velocity. An area shaded in light blue for example has a higher flow velocity than an area shaded in dark blue. When the blood flow velocity exceeds the Nyquist value, color aliasing occurs. A forward flow may then be depicted in shades of blue, with the lower velocity regions of forward flow depicted in shades of red.

The color assignment of the flow imaging instrument used by the author is modulated in up to 128 steps. In some applications, a broader range of color shades may facilitate the extraction of flow information. Areas where there is no flow are depicted in black, therefore black may be considered the baseline or "no flow" color. When searching for a low velocity flow, it may be helpful to assign only unmodulated red and blue to the flow image. It is the authors opinion that one of the most important factors in selecting a color map for clinical applications is that it offers a perceptual clarity of the data which permits the operator to analyze the flow structure under investigation.Using this color scheme, even very low velocities will be detected against the black background.

Variance

In conventional pulsed mode, disturbed flow is indicated by the presence of a wide bandwidth audio signal or a wide bandwidth spectrum. One must be careful however, to distinguish the effects of frequency aliasing from the wide bandwidth signal of turbulent flow. Color flow analysis uses a variance scale to indicate the presence of disturbed flow. Degrees of variance are indicated in shades of green. Turbulent forward flow is then coded yellow (red + green) while turbulent reverse flow is coded in shades of turquoise (blue + green). As the flow becomes more disturbed, a brighter shade of green is assigned to the display. When high velocities occur in conjunction with turbulence, color aliasing will be observed, thus creating a mosaic pattern in the flow display. There are some inaccuracies in the estimation of variance due to the short sampling times and the small sample volumes used in color flow analysis. Transit time effects and color aliasing must also be considered in the interpretation of the variance display. On a perceptual level, the variance display is helpful in the localization of jets.

The presence of color aliasing must be considered when interpreting the flow display. Using the conventional color assignment (where red indicates flow towards the transducer), forward flow velocity exceeding the Nyquist limit will be depicted in blue. If the flow velocity is much greater than the Nyquist limit, color aliasing or wraparound may occur more than once. The value of the velocity can not therefore be accurately estimated.

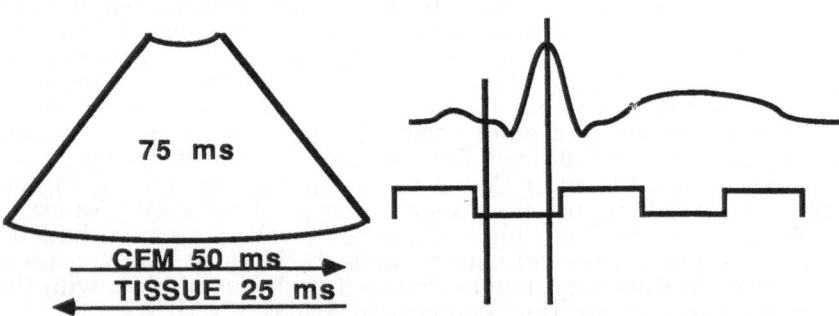

Fig. 1-21. it takes a certain period of time to collect the ultrasonic information necessary to construct both the tissue and flow image. In this figure we see the time/image histogram from an image that took 75 ms to build. If an indication of the collection time is not displayed some temporal mismatch between the ECG gate and the displayed frame can ocurr.

The Color Flow Imaging System

Either mechanical sector technology or phased array technology may be utilized in the construction of a color flow imaging system. In the past, phased array transducers were thought to be the only type of transducer which could be applied in flow imaging. Mechanical sector technology was regarded as unsuitable for flow imaging applications, but the feasibility of such technology has been established. The color flow system used by the author features a mechanically scanned annular array transducer. There are some advantages to the use of an annular or ring array transducer which will be discussed.

The annular array transducer contains a variable number of concentric piezoelectric elements which are acoustically shielded from each other. The number and size of the rings may vary. The concentric configuration of the elements enhances the potential for beam focusing.

The ultrasonic beam decays as it travels through the body due to attenuation of acoustic energy. The beam profile becomes less well delineated due to divergence and the presence of side lobes. These effects may be controlled to some extent by focusing the beam with an acoustic lens. It is also possible to perform electronic focusing by phasing the transmission sequence of the phased array or annular array elements. By the same technique, one can also dynamically focus the received signal. The beam is electronically steered

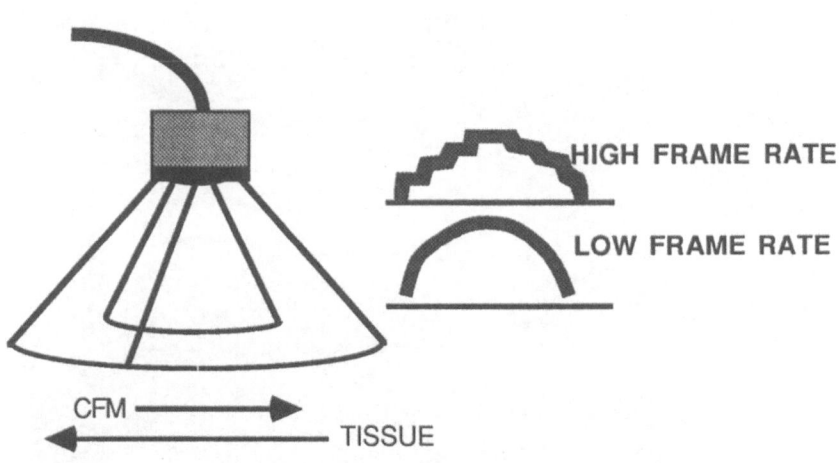

Fig.1-22 . Anytime more than one ultrasound modality is used certain trade offs in the quality of one mode or the other (or both) must be made. For instance , if a triplex mode is used it takes a certain period of time to collect data to build the tissue image , a certain period of time for the color flow image , and a period of time for the conventional Doppler. Different situations require optimization of one mode or the other , and the echocardiographer must decide which is more important for a given patient . Generally the more time one spends on a given mode the better the quality of that mode will be .

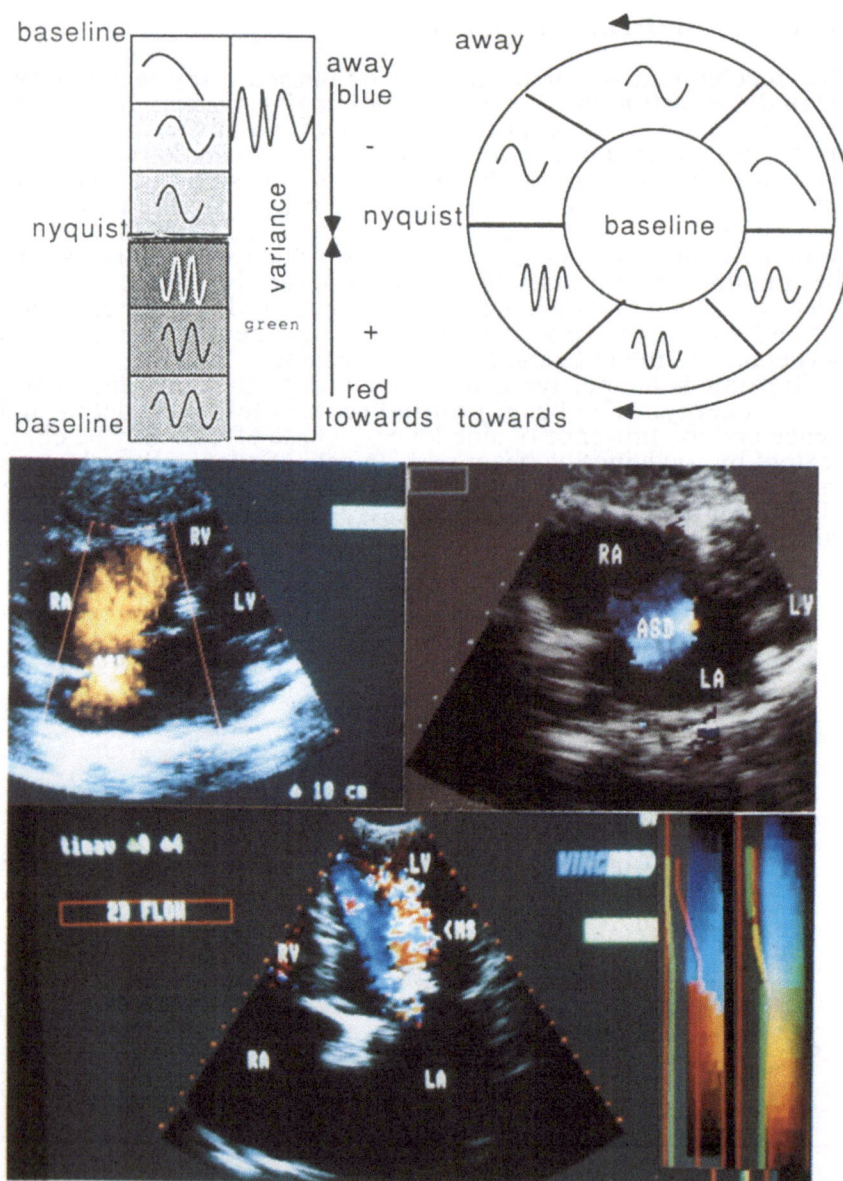

Fig. 1- 23. The flow map most frequently used is the red / blue with variance (green) , and rainbow , in which the various colors are assigned to a specific velocity range . If a turbulent or severely aliased signal is present the red for forward flow , and blue for away flow will mix with green for variance resulting in a mosaic pattern

in a phased array system, while it is mechanically steered in an annular array system. An advantage of mechanically steering the beam is that the effective aperture is not reduced as with electronic beam steering. This reduction occurs when the ultrasonic beam is steered off the central vector. The result is a decrease in the lateral resolution of the phased array system.

Conventional phased array transducers can not focus in the elevational plane while annular array transducers have that capability due to the concentric element configuration. The clinical significance of this may be illustrated with the following example. If two flows are proximal to one another, but one is out of the imaging plane, flow may still be sampled from that out-of-plane flow in a phased array system. This may result in contamination or mixing of the target flow signal with the out-of-plane flow signal. The elevational focusing of the annular array transducer prevents this from occurring.

Each ring or element of the annular array transducer may be assigned a different focal point, and the rings contribute to form a highly collimated beam. The resultant ultrasonic beam has a very long focal zone, and there is less attenuation of acoustic energy. Penetration is thereby improved. A higher frequency annular array transducer can thus be used at greater imaging depths than the conventional type of transducer. Due to the concentric configuration of the elements, the beam can also be focused in the axial, lateral, and elevational planes.

The ultrasonic signal travels as a series of positive and negative pressure states in a wave with convex wavefronts. This wavefront reaches the transducer face out of phase due to this wave geometry. In a phased array transducer, the piezoelectric elements are relatively small in size. The signal must be averaged at a delay line to account for the out-of-phase returned signal. Because of the small element configuration, some of the elements sample positive pressure components while others sample negative components. The dynamic range of the system or the ratio of the largest signal amplitude to the smallest signal amplitude is reduced. Some of the system's dynamic range must be used at the delay line to average the returned signal. Annular array transducer, in contrast, use larger piezoelectric elements. The phase difference of the wavefront is averaged at the transducer face. This means that the entire dynamic range is available for image and flow processing.

In color flow systems, it is necessary to pulse the ultrasonic signal for both tissue imaging and flow imaging. Timing of the ultrasonic pulses is therefore a critical design consideration, and there is a time lag between the display of sector information and flow information. Usually this time lag is negligeable from a clinical standpoint.

Sample Volume Dimensions in Color Flow Analysis

Color flow analysis is a multi-gated pulsed Doppler technique. Therefore, it is subject to the same considerations and limitations of conventional pulsed mode. The size of the sample volume used in color flow analysis affects the sensitivity of the flow measurement.

By increasing the size of the sample volume, a greater number of red cells are interrogated. The intensity of the backscatttered Doppler signal is augmented, improving the signal-to-noise ratio. The estimation of variance is also improved with the use of larger sample volumes. As in conventional pulsed mode, transit time effects may become significant when small sample cells are employed. The transit time effect is caused by red cell motion across the ultrasonic beam, resulting in spectral broadening. This makes spectral broadening a less reliable indicator of turbulence in conventional pulsed mode. In a similar manner, transit time effects make the estimation of variance less reliable in color flow imaging.

Color M-mode

It is possible to superimpose flow information on the M-mode display rather than the two-dimensional display. The overall sensitivity of the color M-mode is superior to color flow imaging because only one line of interrogation is used to perform the examination. Consequently, more pulses per line may be used in the former method, resulting in an improved signal-to-noise ratio. The accuracy of the velocity and variance estimation is also improved. The time delay between the tissue display and the flow display is decreased in the color M-mode format. Although the temporal resolution is superior to the two-dimensional flow format, the disadvantage is the limited spatial resolution. Only one line of tissue and flow information is provided.

An application problem arises when performing the color M-mode examination. The optimal M-mode requires that the transducer should be perpendicular to the tissues being imaged, while the transducer should be parallel to the flow being interrogated for the optimal Doppler study. Flow is not necessarily parallel to the vessel walls, and it is difficult to predict its orientation relative to the anatomic structures. A compromise in the quality of the M-mode and the Doppler information is necessary. By using an "off-axis" transducer position, it is generally possible to obtain an adequate color M-mode recording. If no cine-loop feature is available on the color flow system, the color M-mode capability is useful as a temporal reference.

Data Storage and Documentation

Conventional Doppler recordings may be made by means of a hardcopy device such as a strip chart recorder, Polaroid camera, or thermal printer. Dynamic recordings can be stored on a videotape recorder. Color flow information on a frozen sector image can also be saved for later interpretation by taking pictures. Although the size of the photograph is small and the relative cost per photograph high, the quality of reproduction is acceptable.

A means of reviewing color flow images in real-time is necessary as well, and a videotape recorder can be used for this purpose. However, there is noticeable tissue and flow image degradation with videotape recorders.

The system used by the author (Vingmed CFM 700, Vingmed AS, Norway) allows the last 64 frames of flow information to be stored in a digital memory. Upon playback, the information may be reviewed in forward or reverse order. The playback speed may be selected as frame-by-frame, normal speed or greater than normal speed. This stored information may also be placed in a cine-loop format for detailed observation. There is no noticeable tissue or flow image degradation in the cine-loop format. Electrocardiographic gating of the cine-loop function is also possible for detailed temporal information.

Because hemodynamic events occur so rapidly, a means of reviewing flow information in a frame-by-frame or cine-loop format is needed for accurate interpretation. The digital archiving and retreival system used by the author offers the best solution at this time to the problem of color flow storage and analysis.

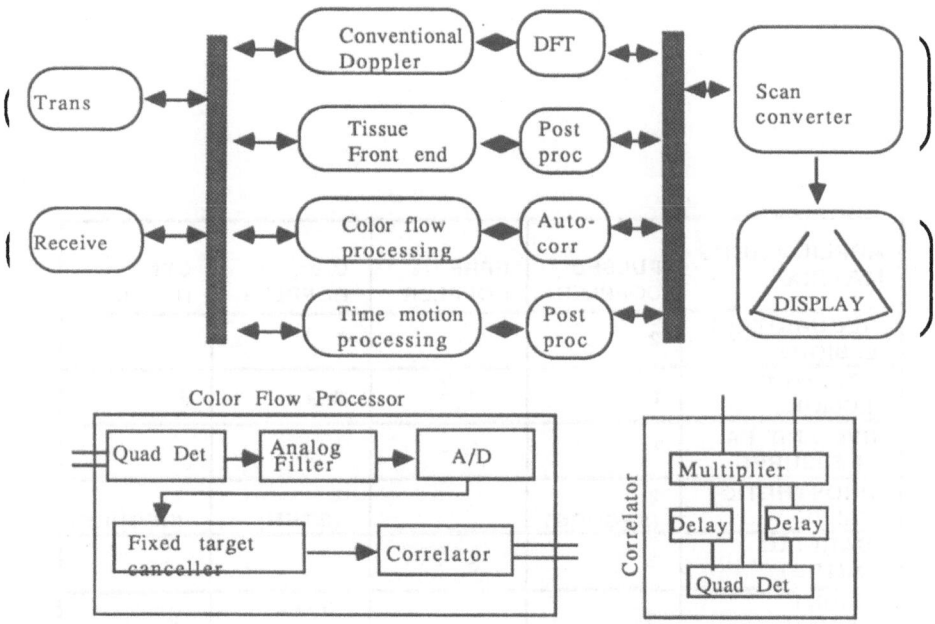

Fig.1-24 A simplified schematic of a Phased Annular Array color flow mapping device. This system configuration permits rapid time sharing and a wide range of signal processing capabilities. Coupled with the annular array tranducer technology , signifigant increases in Doppler sensitivity may be realized

LIMITATIONS OF COLOR FLOW ANALYSIS

In order to use any diagnostic modality well, one must be aware of the potential drawbacks and limitations of that modality. Color flow analysis is a pulsed Doppler technique and is therefore subject to the limitations of aliasing, range ambiguity, and transit time error. The flow signal display is influenced by the system sensitivity, gain settings, and the high pass filter settings. The time-sharing scheme employed to generate the tissue image and the flow image influences the resulting display. Beam characteristics such as the focal zone or the side lobe intensity may also affect the accuracy of the flow information. The use of different color assignments by different flow imaging systems makes image comparison difficult. These points are related to technical considerations alone. The hemodynamic status and size of the patient will also influence the quality of the flow and tissue images. The left ventricular outflow of an obese patient will obviously be more difficult to image than that of a healthy adolescent. Nevertheless, color flow analysis is a valuable addition to conventional Doppler techniques in the investigation of cardiovascular flow. The spatial orientation provided by color flow mapping can be a valuable source of information on hemodynamic events. Color flow analysis allows one to obtain a global assessment of intracardiac flow dynamics. The objective of the flow imaging examination is flow localization, not flow velocity measurement.

APPLICATIONS MATRIX	PULSED DOPPLER	HPRF DOPPLER	C.W. DOPPLER	CFM DOPPLER
REGURGITANT LESIONS	2	1	1	2
STENOTIC LESIONS	1	3 -	3 +	1
RVs AND PA PRESSURES	1	3 -	3 +	
PROSTHETIC VALVE	2 - (REGURG)		3 + (STEN)	2 (REGURG)
CARDIAC OUTPUT	3	3 -	3 -	
SHUNT LESIONS	3		3 + (PRESS)	2
QUALITATIVE 1 SEMI-QUANTITATIVE 2 QUANTITATIVE 3				

Table 1-1. This table represents a brief overview of useful techniques in the setting of various pathologic settings. The main point to consider is that no one technique is useful in all situations.

References

1. Angelsen BA. Analog estimation of the maximum frequency of Doppler spectra in ultrasonic velocity measurements. Report 76-21W, Div. of Engineering Cybernetics, Norwegian Inst of Technology, Univ of Trondheim, Norway (1976).

2. Baker DW. Two-dimensional echo imaging and pulsed Doppler blood flow detection: A comprehensive approach to cardiovascular diagnosis. In Cardiovascular Diagnosis by Ultrasound, edited by Hanrath P, Bleifeld W, Souquet J, Martinus Nijhoff, 1982.

3. Snider AR, Stevenson JG, French JW, et al. Comparison of high pulse repetition frequency and continuous wave Doppler echocardiography for velocity measurements and gradient prediction in children with valvular and congenital heart disease. J Am Coll Cardiol 1986

4. Stewart WJ, Galvin KA, Gillam LD, et al. Comparison of high pulse repetition frequency and continuous wave Doppler in the assessment of high flow velocity in patients with valvular stenosis and regurgitation. J Am Coll Cardiol 1985;6:565.

5. Chapman JV. Clinacal Evaluation of the Doppler Power Spectrum. Eur Rev of Biomed Tech 8,3 ; 168, 1986

6. Chapman JV, Brun P, Meguira A. Initial Clinical Evaluation of a Phased Annular Array Color Flow Mapping System. Int Cong on Card Doppler, Kyoto ; 161, 1986

7. Hatle L, Angelsen B. Doppler Ultrasound In Cardiology. Lea & Febiger, 1982

CHAPTER 2

On the Design of 2D Flow Imaging Systems.
Bjorn A.J. Angelsen Dr. Tech.

1. Introduction.

To generate a 2D velocity image takes inherently longer time than to generate a 2D structural image. One way to describe the reason for this, is that we have to observe a scatterer for a periode of time to be able to determine its velocity, and the accuracy of the velocity estimate increases as the time we observe the scatterer increases. We can draw an analogy to how the motion of an aeroplane or a star,far away in the sky, is observed. They appear to stand still, except if you observe them over a periode of time so you can see that they have moved. The same is true if we want to determine a Doppler shift in frequency of an ultrasonic echo: The accuracy of the frequency estimate, Df, is inversely proportional to the time we observe the signal, T.

$$Df= 1/T \quad (1)$$

Thus, while we for a structural image fire a single pulse in each direction, and does a single sample of the received amplitude for each pixel (short for picture element), we have to fire several pulses in each direction and observe the motion over a periode of time, $\approx$ msec, for flow imaging.

2.Technical Problems.

Apart from this difference, there are three major technical problems in 2D imaging of blood velocity:

i) The signal from blood is much weaker than the signal from tissue. In order to do a practical analysis of the signal, we have to remove the signal components from the tissue. This can be done since the tissue is moving much slower than the blood, and thus produces a lower Doppler shift. Therefore a high-pass filter that removes the low Doppler frequencies, will remove the tissue components from the signal.
One could argue: By pulsing and range gating one gets a temporal or spatial separation of the signal from the tissue and blood so that high-pass filtering is not nessecary. However, there are always multipath echos, or reverberations, which adds a tissue component to the signal from the blood-filled cavities and contaminates the signal from blood.
In the signal analysis we could use a separate high-pass filter for the signal from each pixel. This is called parallel processing because several processing units (high-pass filters) are working parallel in time. The concept is simple, but the size and the cost of the instrument then becomes proportional to the spatial resolution of the instrument.

The complexity of the instrument can be reduced if we use a single unit to process the signal from each pixel and chew on the data as the echos are arriving. This is called serial processing and has been used in similar situations in radar to remove echos from targets that does not move (Fixed Target Canceller, FTC).

The essence of the FTC is that the received signal from one pulse is stored and subtracted from the signal from the next pulse, so that if the targets have not moved, the signal is cancelled. In our case we do not only want to cancel the signal from fixed targets, but also from slowly moving targets i.e. the muscular tissue which moves slower than the blood. In conjunction with the discussion above, we must observe the signal from the tissue over a periode of time to determine its velocity, and therefrom decide whether it is so low that the signal should be rejected. This requires that we must store the signal from several pulses if we want a slowly moving target canceller.

A typical Doppler frequency from the tissue is 600 Hz, and if we want a frequency accuracy of 300 Hz, we need according to Eq. (1) to observe and store the signal for a periode of

$$T = 1/Df \approx 3 \text{ msec} \quad (2)$$

At present, digital storage is the only practical method to store a signal for such a period of time, but present technology limits the dynamic range of digital techniques by the limited resolution (number of bits) that can be obtained in fast A/D converters. To get a compact high-pass filter with a large dynamic range, the present instrument uses a combination of analog and digital techniques.

ii) The second problem is to determine the Doppler shift for all pixels in the image in a compact way, so that the size and cost of the instrument can be attractive. As with high-pass filtering, a single processor for each pixel gives a conceptually simple, but voluminous solution. The ideal solution is here as well to use serial processing, by which one unit processes the signal from all pixels in series as the echos arrive.

The present instrument estimates the mean Doppler shift, the rms bandwidth of the Doppler shift, and the intensity of the Doppler signal. The above parameters are estimated because they are simple to estimate with a serial processor, and what we really want to know is the maximum blood velocity in each pixel, unobscured by frequency aliasing due to the pulsing of the beam. At the University of Trondheim, there is a heavy effort going into research for velocity estimation. The color flow mapping instrument therefore has a modular structure so that new developments in velocity estimation will fit into the structure.

iii) We have above touch onto the third problem: The ability to quantify large velocities without entering into aliasing problems. To obtain range resolution in flow imaging, the ultrasonic beam must be pulsed. This introduces the well known phenomenon of frequency aliasing as in regular pulsed Doppler, where Doppler shifts above the Nyquist limit is mapped onto Doppler shifts of the opposite sign. The only known method to avoid this phenomenon is either to use **high pulse repetition frequency Doppler** by which we get the range uncertainty of multiple sample volumes, or use **CW Doppler,** by which the range resolution is completely lost.

The present instrument uses a time sharing method by which regular Doppler measurements and imaging is done intermittently at such a rate that they appear simultaneous to the user. Due to a proprietary and patented **MSE technique** (Missing Signal Estimator) invented at the University of Trondheim, the timesharing is masked from the user. By this method it is possible to do flow imaging to obtain a geometrical visualisation of the flow, while the operator with the track ball can select an area in the image where either LPRF, HPRF, or CW Doppler can be done to quantify the velocity to do gardient measurements and so forth, together with the moving image.

3. Scan Methods.

To obtain an image of blood velocities in a plane, one must obviously be able to insonify all points of the plane. This can in principle be done by flooding the field with ultrasound, i.e. transmitting such a **spread beam** that it covers the whole field, as illustrated in Fig. 1. We could then use an array of multiple elements as receiver and process the signal from the array elements in such a way that we obtain the velocity from the whole field, as illustrated in the figure.

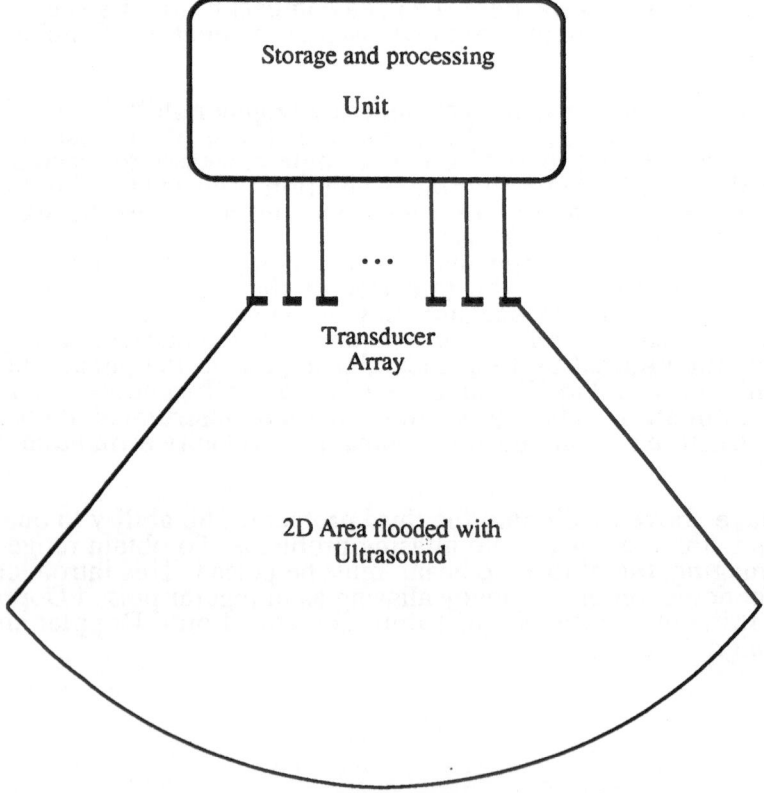

Fig. 2-1. 2D flow imaging using a broad beam to flood the area.

There is a severe practical limitation to this approach in that the transmitted intensity drops heavily with depth because the beam is spreading. In order to obtain sufficient intensity in the far-field, the intensity in the near-field becomes prohibitively large. To avoid this we have to transmit a **concentrated beam**, and in order to probe the whole field, we have to sweep or step the beam in some fashion over the whole image field.

With a **mechanical scanner** the beam can not be stepped, but must be swept continuously. With a **phased array** on the other hand, the beam direction can only be stepped. It has been argued that flow imaging can not be done with a mechanical scanner since the Doppler shifts generated by the transducer motion would cause problems, and that one has to step the beam direction so that the beam stands still during the measurement. However, this is a false argument, and in fact the limitations are the same for the continuous mechanical and the stepped phased array scanner.

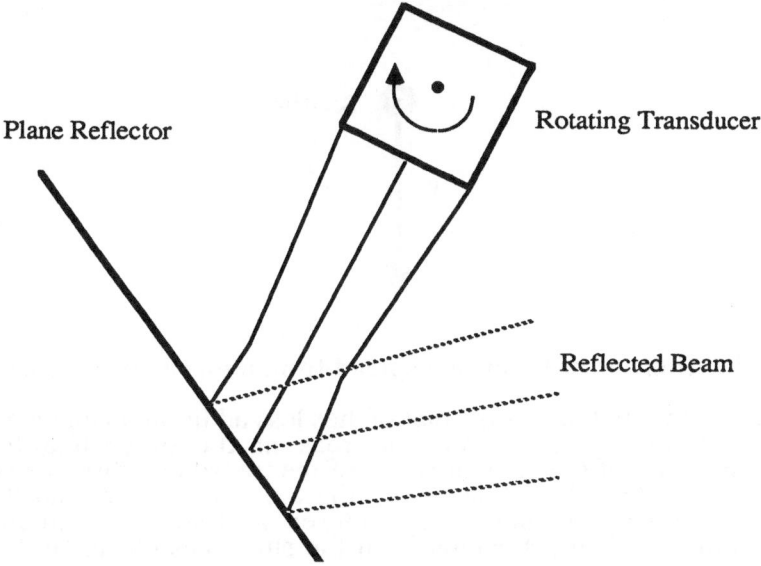

Fig. 2-2. Rotating transducer with a skewed reflector.

One illustration that has been used for this argument is shown in Fig. 2. It illustrates a plane reflector that is skewed with respect to the beam so that the cross section between the beam and the reflector gets closer as the beam sweeps, and the plane would be observed as a moving reflector generating a Doppler shift. However, there is an error in the argument because with such a plane reflector, the reflected beam will be at an angle, as illustrated, and will not be picked up by the transducer.

A better way to analyse the situation with a continuously moving mechanical scanner, is to decompose the transducer face into so small sub-areas that the velocity due to transducer rotation is essentially constant over these areas. This is illustrated in Fig. 3. The signal from the transducer can then be seperated into components from these sub-areas. The Doppler shift in frequency for each sub-area is caused by the relative velocity between the scatterer and the sub-area.

The total signal is the sum of the components from the different sub-areas, and since the velocity varies over the transducer face, we will get a distribution of Doppler shifted frequency components from a scatterer, as illustrated in Fig. 4, instead of the single Doppler shift for the stationary transducer.

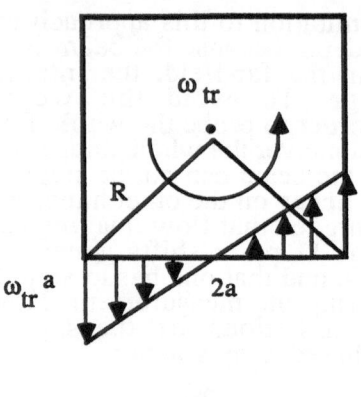

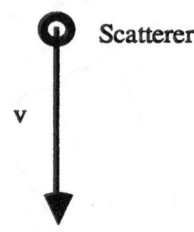

Fig. 2-3. Analysis of frequency spread from a mechanical transducer.

The sub-areas close to the axis of rotation has less additional Doppler shifts due to transducer rotation than the sub-areas at the outer boarder of the transducer. Because of the circular shape of the transducer disc, the size of the sub-areas decreases with distance from the axis of rotation, and the largest intensity in the Doppler signal is centered around the frequency for a stationary transducer, which stems from the sub-areas closest to the axis of rotation.

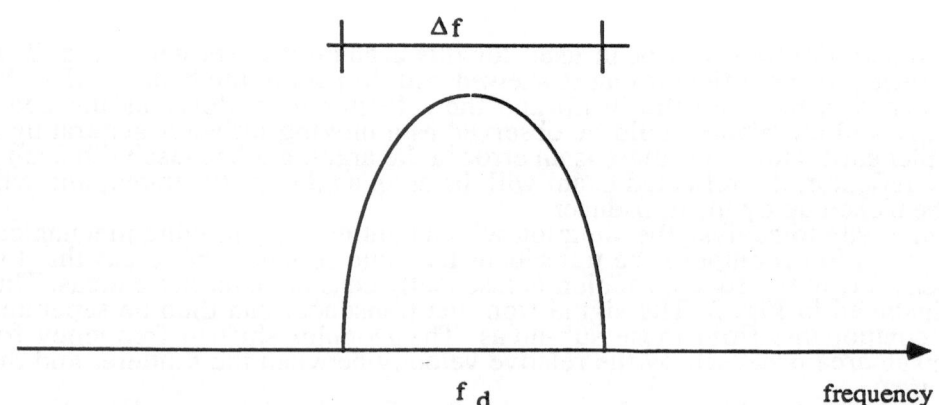

Fig. 2-4. Frequency spread due to transducer rotation.

34

For Nyquist sampling, the angular width of the transducer, Df, is

$$Df = l/4a \quad (3)$$

where l is the wave length, and a is the radius of the transducer face. We use a rotary velocity of the transducer of w_{tr}. The time, T_b, it then takes to collect the data with a continuous sweep for a beam width, is

$$T_b = Df/w_{tr} \quad (4)$$
or
$$w_{tr} = Df/T_b = l/4aT_b \quad (5)$$

The maximum additive velocity of a sub-area due to the transducer motion is then

$$Dv = w_{tr}a = l/4T_b \quad (6)$$

This gives an additional Doppler shift according to the Doppler formula of

$$Df = 2f_0 2Dv/c = 1/T_b \quad (7)$$

where f_0, is the transmitted frequency, c is the ultrasonic velocity, and $l = c/f_0$. For the phased array, we step the beam direction in descrete steps so that the beam stands still for a periode T_b during the measurement. Since we have a limited record of data, the accuracy in the frequency estimate is

$$Df = 1/T_b \quad (8)$$

Thus we get the same frequency spread for a phased array scanner with a stepped sweep, as for a mechanical scanner with a continuous sweep of the beam, and there is no theoretical basis for choosing one method above the other in this respect. However, with a continuous mechanical sweep one can use a causal high-passfilter, while one with a phased array scanner must use a noncausal filter to achieve the resolution in Eq. (8). This simplifies the implementation of the high-pass filter for a mechanical scanner . The choice is therefore mainly a practical one of cost and other performances.
It is easier to get a good beam definition with a mechanical than with a phased array scanner, and with a mechanically scanned ring array it is possible to get dynamic focussing transverse to the scanning plane in contrast to the phased array where we can only do dynamic focussing in the scan plane. Phased array transducers have traditionally bean smaller with easier access than the mechanical transducer, but this is merely a practical problem which has been largely overcome in later designs.

References

1. Angelsen BAJ , Kristoffersen K , Torp H . 2 D-flow Imaging with an Annular Array Scanner. 2 nd Int. Congress on Cardiac Doppler , (Abstract)Kyoto 1986

2. Linker D.T., Skjerpe T , Samstad S , Rossvoll O , Chapman J.V., Kristoffersen K, Angelsen B.A.J . Color Flow Mapping with an Annular Array Transducer : An Approach Integrated with CW and Pulsed Doppler in Adult and Pediatric Patients . 2nd International Congress on Cardiac Doppler (Abstract), Kyoto 1986

3. Angelsen B.A.J., Torp H, Kristoffersen . Technical Principles and Approaches to Color Doppler Flow Imaging . 7th Symposium on Echocardiography (Abstract) , Rotterdam 1987

4. Linker D.T., Rossvoll O , Chapman J.V. , Angelsen B.A.J. Sensitivity and Speed of CFM verses CW Doppler in the Detection of VSD . 7th Symposium on Echocardiography (Abstract) , Rotterdam 1987

5. Linker D , Angelsen B.A.J.,Johansen H.C., Lønstad H., Torp H. Computer Analysis of 2D Tissue and Flow Images.(Abstract) Heart and Vessels Supplement 3: 1-52 1987

6. Angelsen B.A.J., Kristoffersen k, Torp H. Diagnostic Information in the Color Flow Images .(Abstract) Heart and Vessels Supplement 3: 1-52 1987

7. Chapman J.V., Brun P. , Meguira A ,Torp H , Angelsen B.A.J. A new method of Indicating Disturbed Flow in a Color Flow Mapping System . (Abstract)Heart and Vessels Supplement3: 1-52 1987

CHAPTER 3

INTRACARDIAC FLOW DYNAMICS

Phillip Brun M.D.
Albert Meguira
Andreas Strauss M.D.

The principles that govern fluid motion in normal blood vessels can still be best approached by using the classic Poiseuille model. This law states that the ratio of the pressure gradient (P1 - P2) to flow (Q) is a function of the tube dimensions and the viscosity (μ) of the moving fluid:

$$\frac{P1 - P2}{Q} = \frac{8\mu L}{\pi(r^4)}$$

where r is the radius of the tube and L is the length of the tube. The ratio of pressure gradient (P1 - P2) to flow (Q) is also defined as the vascular resistance (R).

$$R = \frac{8\mu L}{\pi(r^4)}$$

The most important factor affecting vascular resistance is the vessel caliber since changes is resistance are inversely proportional to the fourth power of the vessel radius. The other two factors, viscosity and tube length, have a much lesser impact upon the vessel resistance. Viscosity can be thought of as the internal friction between adjacent blood layers, and remains essentially constant under physiological conditions. The vessel or tube length is also constant in blood vessels. Although Poiseuille's law strictly refers to a steady laminar flow in a rigid cylindrical tube, it can be regarded as a simplified model in the study of pulsatile blood flow in an elastic system.

There are several reasons why Poiseuille's model is applicable in the study of hemodynamics. First, the pulsatile flow in the cardiovascular system can be understood by extension of the principles of steady flow. Secondly, the pressure and flow pulse waves can be dealt with as steady flow upon which pulsations are superimposed.

At the velocities existing in the normal vascular tree, the blood flow is almost always laminar. This means that the flowing blood column streams in a series of concentric cylindrical layers strictly parallel to the tube walls (Fig 1). Each layer has its own velocity; the highest velocity is found in the core layer and the velocity diminishes with distance from the core layer. At the vascular wall, a stationery fluid layer is encountered. This symmetrical distribution of velocities around the central tube axis gives the well-known parabolic flow profile. The decrease in velocity from the vessel core to the wall is referred to as the velocity gradient (dv/dx, v and x being the velocity and radius of any specified cylindrical lamina of fluid, respectively). Each cylindrical layer exerts a forward force or stress on the immediately adjacent layer flowing at a slower velocity.

This stress is called shear stress (G) and can be referred to as the moving force (F) per unit surface of contact between adjacent lamina (S):

$$G = F/S$$

The slower moving lamina exerts a drag or backward force on the faster moving inner lamina; this backward force is the viscous retarding force. In order to maintain a steady flow, the shear force must overcome the viscous resistive force. The shear stress and the velocity gradient are greatest at the vessel wall and zero in the central axis of the vessel. The greater the velocity gradient, the greater is the shear stress. This can be expressed formally as:

$$G = \mu \ (dv/dx)$$

The proportionality term μ is defined as the coefficient of viscosity. In many cases, there is a linear relationship between the velocity gradient (shear rate) and the applied shear stress. This is true of water and other fluids. The existence of a linear relationship implies that viscosity is a constant value, being an inherent physical property of the liquid and independent of the shear rate. These fluids are referred to as Newtonian or ideal fluids.

In non-Newtonian fluids, viscosity is not constant but depends upon the shear rate. Blood is not a Newtonian fluid, for at low shear rates the viscosity rises exponentially with a further fall in shear rate (Fig 2). Furthermore, in very small tubes like the vessels of the microcirculation with a diameter less than 0.5 mm, the viscosity diminishes with decreasing tube diameter. This phenomenon is termed the Fahreus-Linquist effect. Nevertheless, under physiological shear rates encountered in arteries and arterioles (80-100/s), the hemodynamic behavior of blood resembles that of a Newtonian fluid. The CGS (centimeter-gram-second) unit of viscosity is the poise (P);, in honor of the work of Poiseuille. The SI (International System) unit of viscosity is the Pascal-second (Pa.s) which is equivalent to the newton per square meter (N/sq-m). The viscosity of water at 20 degrees Centigrade is close to 0.01 P and the value for blood with a hematocrit of 45% at 37 degrees Centigrade is 0.04 P (0.004 Pa.s).

Entrance Flow

In a straight circular tube, the time-steady laminar flow of a Newtonian fluid produces a parabolic velocity profile. But even in a steady laminar flow, the parabolic distribution of velocitites is not invariably present. At the entrance to the tube from a reservoir, the velocity profile of a steady flow is blunt or flat. All the concentric layers or fluid elements move at the same velocity comparable to a coherent plug (Fig. 3-2). The boundary layer of this blunt profile is extremely thin and there is markedly increased shear stress at the vessel wall.

This situation is present in the aorta and in the initial part of small arteries branching off from larger ones. As the fluid

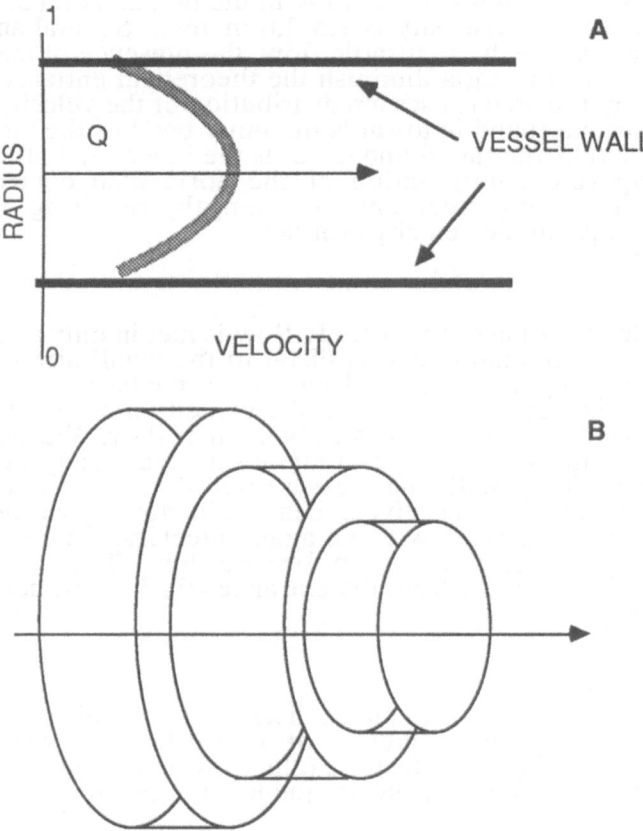

Fig. 3-1 . A Parabolic velocity profile in steady laminar flow. B. Three dimensional representation of laminar flow.

moves along the tube, the velocity of the fluid near the wall slows down and the blunt portion of the profile in the center diminishes. This causes the development of a parabolic velocity profile remote from the entrance. The distance from the entrance required for the development of a parabolic velocity distribution is termed the entrance or inlet length, and this phenomenon is termed the entrance or inlet effect. The theoretically calculated entrance length for steady flow in the human aorta at physiological mean flow velocity and viscosity is 1.5-2.0 meters. Several anatomical and physiological factors such as pulsatile flow, the presence of major branches, and the curvature of the aorta diminish the theoretical entrance length. The curvature of the aortic arch causes a redistribution of the velocity profile. The highest velocities are found in towards the inner bend of the ascending aorta, while the lowest velocities are found towards the inner bend of the descending aorta. The tapering configuration of the aorta also contributes to the shortening of the theoretical entrance length, resulting in an earlier development of a parabolic velocity profile.

Pulsatile flow

In practice, the condition of time-steady flow is met in only a relatively small part of the arterial circulation that is distal to the small arterioles. In large arteries, the flow is highly pulsatile. Thus, one of the basic assumptions of the Poiseuille model is violated. Therefore, the velocity profile will not be of the same parabolic form that is found in steady laminar flow. We can consider the pulsatile flow as the result of the summation of a steady and oscillatory pressure gradient. The oscillating pressure will cause the flow to accelerate until a maximum velocity is acheived, then it will slow down, stop, accelerate in a reverse direction, then slow down again, etcetera. In contrast, a steady pressure gradient will result in a mean forward flow. The velocity profile of such a pulsatile flow remote from the entrance (fig.2) will depend upon the angular frequency w:

$$w = 2\pi f$$

where f is the frequency of oscillations. The velocity profile therefore is also dependent upon f. This phenomenon of pulsatile flow was analysed by Womersley who introduced the factor a (alpha) which summarizes the various physical factors involved; i.e. the frequency f, the tube radius r, and the viscosity μ:

$$a = r[(2\pi f)/\mu]^{1/2}$$

This parameter a is in fact the ratio between the inertial and viscous forces. Thus, if a is small, the flow is dominated by viscous forces such as the flow in the peripheral circulation. If a is large, then the flow is dominated by inertial forces such as the slow in large arteries where a is greater than 10.

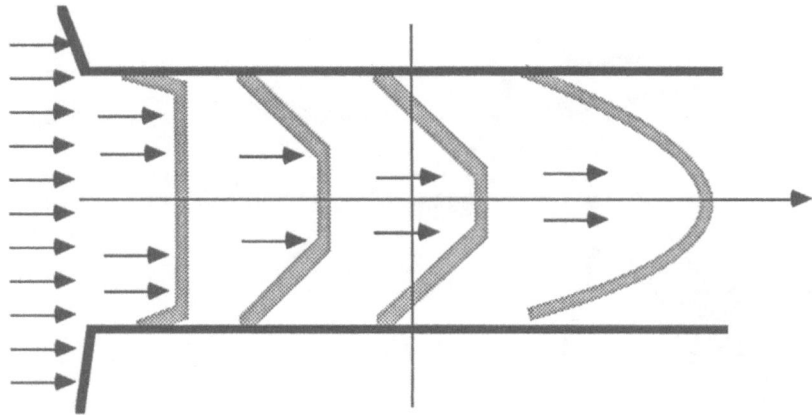

Fig. 3-2 . The influence of the entrance region of the flow velocity profile which develops.

Furthermore, the velocity profile will vary instantaneously. However, in a somewhat simplified manner, the time-mean velocity profile built up by a pulsatile flow will consist of a relatively blunt nonsheared central core with high inertia and a peripheral layer of low velocity laminae near the wall. This peripheral layer exhibits low momentum and high viscous drag. Thus, the fluid in pulsatile flow behaves like a solid mass sliding inside an outer layer of sheared viscous liquid which surrounds it (fig.1). Its velocity profile, remote from the inlet can be compared to the profile of a steady flow within the entrance length, that is, a fluid which has not had time to become completely established.

Turbulent Flow

If the flow rate in a steady or pulsatile flow increases beyond a certain critical threshold, the orderly layered pattern of laminar flow is disrupted and replaced by an irregular random motion of the fluid elements called turbulence. In turbulent flow, fluid particles move radially as well as axially and form rapidly changing eddies and vortices. The factors determining the attainment of the critical threshold between laminar and turbulent flow are the tube diameter (D), the mean velocity (V), the density of the fluid, and the fluid viscosity. These variables are expressed as a dimensionless quantity called the Reynold's number (Re):

$$Re = (VD)/v$$

where v is the kinematic viscosity or the ratio of the fluid density to the viscosity. The higher the Reynold's number, the greater the probability of turbulence. The critical value of Reynold's number referred to as causing turbulent flow to develop is usually in the neighborhood of 2300. This is an experimentally determined value and is dependent to a large degree upon the experimental conditions. The Reynolds number represents in fact the ratio between the inertial

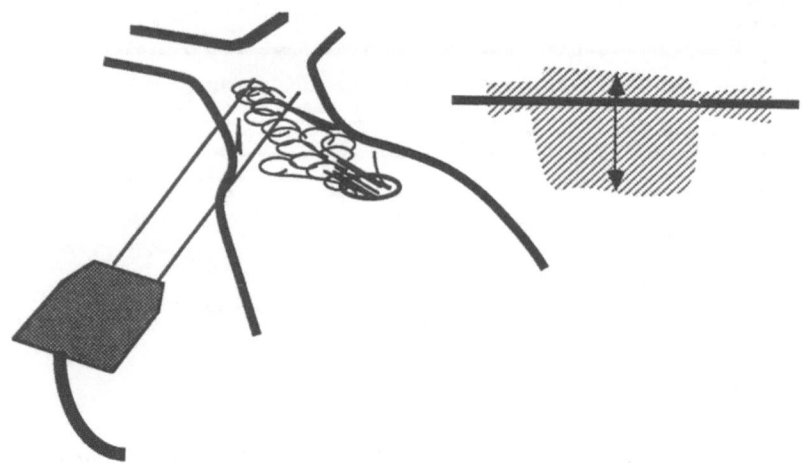

Fig. 3-3 . The term " series effect " has been used by Goldberg and coworkers to describe the occurence of turbulent flow at a site distal to the origin of the turbulence . In the clinical setting one might find turbulent flow in the pulmonary artery which results from a ventricular septal defect in the right venticular outflow tract.

forces (the numerator) and viscous forces (the denominator), emphasizing that the maintenance of steady laminar flow depends on the balance between both forces. When inertial forces increase unduly compared to viscous forces, turbulence develops.

The type of velocity profile that may be seen in turbulent flow is represented in Fig 5. The velcoity profile is much flatter than the corresponding profile in laminar flow but there is still a region of shear near the wall. The proportion of the flat front varies with the degree of turbulence. Although the distinction between laminar and turbulent flow is clear-cut, many transitional stages can occur. A turbulent flow is strictly referred to as a condition where disturbance involves all the flowing liquid and, in cases of pulsatile flow, exists throughout the cycle.

For all the intermediate stages where the flow is neither clearly laminar nor clearly turbulent, the term disturbed flow is used. From a practical point of view, the knowledge of the presence of turbulent flow is important for several reasons. First, it broadens the instantaneous velocity distribution in the vessel because negative, positive, and zero velocities are present. Secondly, the pressure-flow relationship is no longer linear in turbulent flow; turbulent flow requires the application of a larger pressure drop per unit length than in laminar flow. Finally, a part of the energy dissipated in turbulent flow appears as acoustic energy, causing the development of cardiovascular murmurs.

Propagation of the Pressure Pulse and the Windkessel Model

The propelling force that determines blood flow through the vessels is the pressure difference between the root of the aorta and the right atrium. As the right atrial pressure is close to zero, this pressure difference can be approximated by the mean aortic pressure. The latter can be referred to as a steady or diastolic pressure upon which an oscillatory component or pressure pulse is superimposed. The pressure generated by the heart during systole decays in a nearly exponential manner in diastole. This slow diastolic pressure fall in the aorta is easy to understand if we remember that the large arteries have elastic walls. A portion of the blood ejected in systole is stored in the arteries as in a reservoir, and is then forced into the periphery during diastole. The theoretical model for this event is called the Windkessel model. This model compares the large arteries to a compliant chamber whose volume (V) is proportional to the instantaneous pressure P. In the aorta itself, the instantaneous pressure is the instantaneous aortic blood pressure:

$$V = CP$$

where C is a constant of compliance or capacitance. Furthermore, in this model, the peripheral circulation can be represented by the constant resistance R. The total flow volume ejected by the heart with each stroke (Qt) is the sum of the compliant flow stored by the distending aorta (dV/dt) during systole and the systolic flow rate through the periphery (Qp):

$$Qt = Qp + dV/dt = P/R + (C)(dP/dt)$$

During diastole, the stroke volume Qt is zero so the equation may be re-written:

$$P/R + (C)(dP/dt) = 0$$

The solution of this differential equation for the diastolic instantaneous blood pressure yields the following proportionality:

$$P \cdot e^{-t/RC}$$

This proportionality states that the diastolic pressure in the arteries falls off exponentially with time; such a decay is closely realized in practice.
As the pressure wave travels down the aorta, it changes in shape and becomes progressively delayed. This delay is mainly due to the elasticity of the walls of the large compliant arteries. The delay decreases with diminishing arterial wall elasticity and the the velocity of the pressure wave propagation increases. On the other hand, the amplitude of this pressure wave increases giving rise to the apparent paradox that systolic pressure rises with distance from the heart. This process of pressure pulse amplification down to

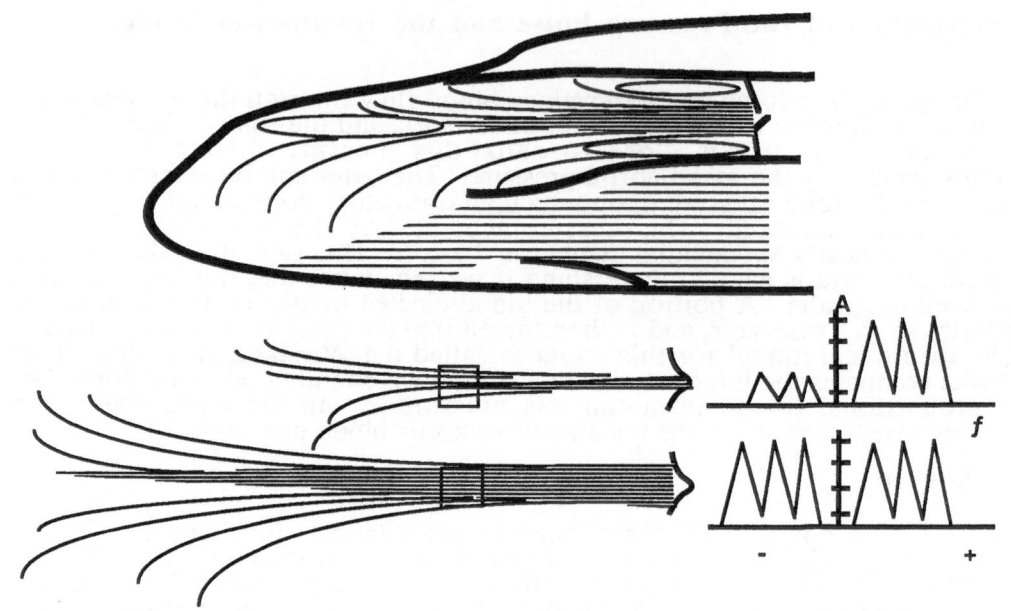

Fig.3-4. Generally , the regurgitant flow will extend further into the retrograde chamber and the power / velocity distribution is more even in a large regurgitation .

third branch generation from the aorta is due partially to wave reflections at different bifurcation sites and partially to gradual tapering and stiffening of the arterial tree.

In contrast to the peaking of the pressure pulse, the flow or velocity waveform decreases and becomes progressively attenuated as it travels through the arterial system. In summary, wave reflection causes enhancement of the transmitted pressure amplitude but is the source of reversal of flow velocity. This flow reversal can be easily recorded in the femoral artery with Doppler ultrasound methods.Such a velocity pattern is typical for arteries supplying territories of high vascular resistance. In contrary, the velocity (or flow) waveform in arteries with low peripheral resistance contains a significant diastolic flow component . This waveform can be encountered in the internal carotid and renal artery as well as in arteries with pronounced vasodilatation. In these arteries, the shape of the flow wave is very similar to that of the pressure wave, presenting the same exponential decay pattern.

Clinical Applications Using Doppler Ultrasound

The basic concepts of fluid dynamics discussed in this section can be applied in the study of the cardiovascular system with Doppler ultrasound. Two major applications of Doppler ultrasound are the assessment of the pressure gradient across an obstruction and the measurement of cardiac output. The pressure gradient can be assessed by using the modified Bernoulli equation, and its derivation is fully explained in Chapter 5. In order to estimate the cardiac output, the velocity profile existing at the sampling site must be considered.

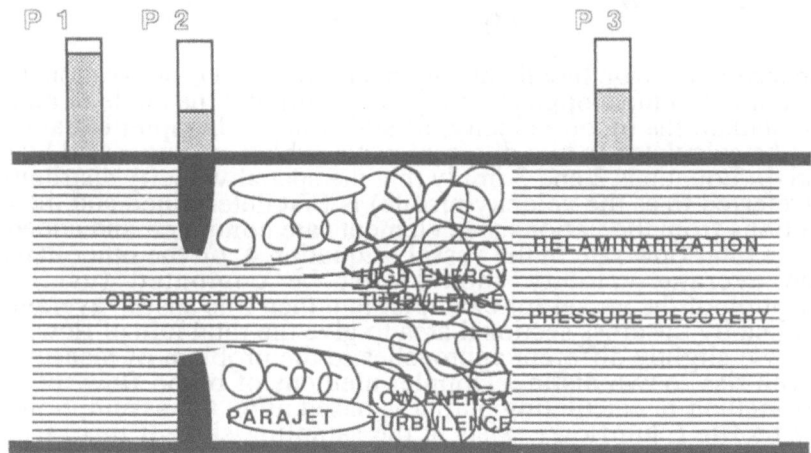

Fig.3-5 . Flow through an obstruction.

Cardiac Output

Our purpose is not to describe the most accurate method of measuring cardiac output or the potential sources of error involved in output estimation. Instead, we will discuss the basic equations used in measuring flow output by Doppler techniques, taking into account the essential factor which is the velocity profile.

Consider blood flowing through a vessel with a cross sectional area A, as shown in Figure 6 . The rate of blood flow (Q) through an element of the cross-section ΔAi is simply:

$$Q = (Vi)(\Delta Ai)$$
$$(1)$$

where Vi is the blood velocity at that given cross section. The total rate of flow is then calculated as the sum of all the contributions across the vessel cross section:

$$Q = \Sigma[(Vi)(\Delta Ai)]$$

$$(2)$$

If the area cross sectional elements become very small, we can replace ΔA_i with dA, and rewrite the equation as follows:

$$Q = \int_A V dA \qquad (3)$$

This equation can also be written in a slightly different form:

$$Q = [(\int_A V dA)/(\int_A dA)] \times [\int_A dA] = (V)(A) \qquad (4)$$

∇ is the spatial average blood velocity over the vessel cross sectional area A.

Measurement of the Doppler or frequency shift and the angle of attack allows one to calculate the blood velocity, as stated in the Doppler equation. Blood flow can be calculated in two different ways, which are suggested by equations 2, 3, and 4. Equations 2 and 3 imply that the spatial velocity distribution in the vessel (referred to as the velocity profile) is first determined and then the flow contributions from the various area elements are computed and added together to give the total flow rate in the vessel. Equation 4, on the other hand, implies that the average velocity should first be computed (using uniform insonification of the vessel for example) and then this spatial average velocity is multiplied by the cross sectional area to give the total rate of flow.

These two slightly different approaches to the problem of measuring output have given rise to two distinct Doppler methods of blood flow measurement. Another method of calculating output is based upon the assumption that a flat velocity profile (plug flow) exists at the sampling site. If this assumption is valid, then the Doppler measurement becomes relatively easy. The Doppler shift can be measured by a variety of methods, but typically the maximum frequency envelope is obtained using real-time spectral analysis. If a flat velocity profile is assumed, then the mean and maximum frequency (or velocity) are theoretically the same.

Flow Through An Obstruction

Normally in a steady flow, the presssure drop through a vessel segment is proportional to the flow rate and to the resistive forces encountered in this segment. As the fluid is forced through a convergent stenotic region, the pressure drop increases. This latter effect is due to the fact that the same flow volume must traverse a diminished cross sectional area. This is only possible if the spatial mean velcity increases. The increase in velocity results in a rise of the kinetic energy of the fluid elements. The amount of kinetic energy dissipated through an obstruction corresponds to the presssssure drop at the site of the obstruction. Considering the pressure and velocity to be constant over the cross-section, the pressure drop (P1 - P2) can be written as:

$$P1 - P2 = 1/2(p)(V2^2 - V1^2)$$

where p is the density of blood, and V2 and V1 represent the blood velocity distal and proximal to the obstruction, respectively. As discussed in Chapter 3, this equation may be simplified to yield the modified Bernoulli equation:

$$P1 - P2 = 4 \, V2^2$$

The blood flow through an obstuction is laminar, presenting a blunt velocity profile (Fig. 3-5). This flatness is due partially to the convergence of the streamlines and partially to the pulsatility of the flow. Immediately downstream from the obstuction, three flow zones may be distinguished: the jet, the prajet, and the zone of developed turbulence. In the jet itself, the flow is laminar. The width of the jet is smaller than the stenotic orifice diameter. Immediately distal to the stenosis, between the jet and the vessel wall, lies a zone called the parajet area. The parajet consists of stagnant fluid areas and vortices passing retrograde towards the obstruction. The post-jet flow disturbance is a zone of developed turbulence where vortices and eddies form, and the fluid elements are engaged in an irregular random motion.

II. THE CLINICAL MEASUREMENT OF FLOW VOLUME

The flow volume (Q) at a given vessel cross section is defined as the product of the spatial mean blood flow velocity (v) and the inner cross sectional area of the vessel (A):

$$Q = vA$$

In order to calculate the volume of blood flow by Doppler techniques, the angle between the Doppler beam and the blood flow under investigation must be considered if a parallel alignment between the beam and the flow path is not possible:

$$Q = (vA)/cos\text{ß}$$

where ß is the beam-to-flow angle. Generally however, it is possible to acheive a nearly parallel beam-to-flow alignment when sampling flow in the ascending aorta from the suprasternal window. This reduces the potential for error in the flow volume calculation because there is no reliable way to estimate ß during the Doppler echocardiographic examination. Blood flow is not necesarily parallel to the vessel walls, and the beam-to-flow angle varies in three dimensions.

An accurate estimation of the mean blood velocity requires that the aortic lumen be uniformly insonified by the Doppler beam. This is not possible in the adult ascending aorta; the aortic diameter is much greater than the ultrasonic beam width. Estimation of the flow volume by Dopppler techniques therefore requires that a flat velocity profile exists in the ascending aorta distal to the aortic annulus. This is a reasonable assumption because the Doppler sampling site is located in a flow inlet, where a blunt profile is likely to exist.

When this assumption of a flat velocity profile no longer is valid, then cardiac output measurements based upon the recorded flow velocity are not possible.

The assumption of a flat velocity in the ascending aorta implies that the spatial mean velocity will be nearly the same value as the maximum velocity recorded in the center of the aortic lumen. The maximum flow velocity (Vm) may then be substituted for the spatial mean velocity in the flow volume equation:

$$Q = Vm \times A$$

To calculate the cardiac output (CO) at the aortic valve level, the following equation is used:

$$CO = FVI \times A \times HR$$

where FVI is the flow velocity integral, or area under the aortic flow curve and HR is the heart rate. The cross sectional area of the aorta used in the output equation may be obtained from the appropriate M-mode or two-dimensional recordings, and several methods of estimating the area have been suggested. Calculation of the area from the M-mode diameter of the aortic root is simple, but a circular cross sectional area is assumed. The value of the obtained diameter changes appreciably with a change in placement of the M-mode cursor. Any error made in the diameter measurement will be squared in the area calculation. A direct measurement of the aortic valve orifice from the two-dimensional image is difficult in most patients

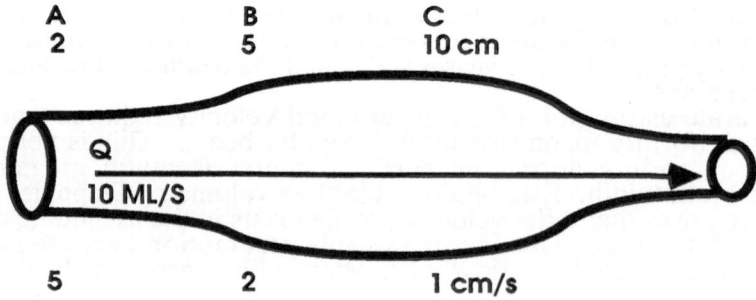

Fig.3-6. In a closed flow circuit, the flow velocity , cross sectional area , and flow volume are interdependent. This figure demonstrates this relationship.

due to limitations in image resolution. There is also an inherent problem in orifice planimetry, since the angle between the sector plane and the orifice is unknown. Probably the best approach is a combination of two-dimensional and M-mode recordings of the aorta. The M-mode cursor may then be positioned at the level of the aortic orifice, and the aortic diameter measured from the M-mode recording made at this level. Ihlen and coworkers (6) obtained good correlations with invasive measurements of cardiac output when the M-mode diameter at the aortic orifice was used in the area calculation. Overestimation of cardiac output occurred when the M-mode diameters measured in the proximal and distal aortic root were used to estimate the aortic area. Stewart et al obtained better correlations with roller pump outputs in open chested dogs when the annulus diameter rather than the sinotubular diameter was used in the Doppler calculation of aortic area (7). Since the estimation of the orifice area represents the largest source of error in the calculation of the cardiac output, care should be taken in obtaining an accurate M-mode recording. The cardiac output at the aortic valve level can not be estimated by this method in patients with aortic valve abnormalities.

In the ideal situation, the aortic cross sectional area and the flow velocity integral should be measured simultaneously in order to minimize error in the output calculation. However, this is not practical since different transducer positions are used to obtain the optimal M-mode recording and the optimal Doppler recording. The M-mode recording is most often obtained from the third or fourth left intercostal space, while the Doppler recording is obtained from the suprasternal transducer position. Pulsed mode should be used to record the aortic flow velocity curve rather than continuous mode so that range resolution is preserved and a narrow bandwidth signal obtained.

Doppler Summary	meas1	meas2	meas3	avg/c
VTI ao cm	13.21			13.21
VTI pa cm	13.64			13.64
Hrt rate ao	70.00			70.00
Hrt rate pa	69.00	71.00		70.00
FCsa ao cm2	3.14			3.14
FCsa pa cm2	3.14			3.14
CO VTI ao lm				2.90
CO VTI pa lm				2.99
SV VTI ao l				.04
SV VTI pa l				.04
Q pa/ao VTI				1.03

Fig.3-7 The volumetric flow perameters may be calculated online in many ultrasonic instruments. This Qp-Qs ratio was obtained in a normal adult.

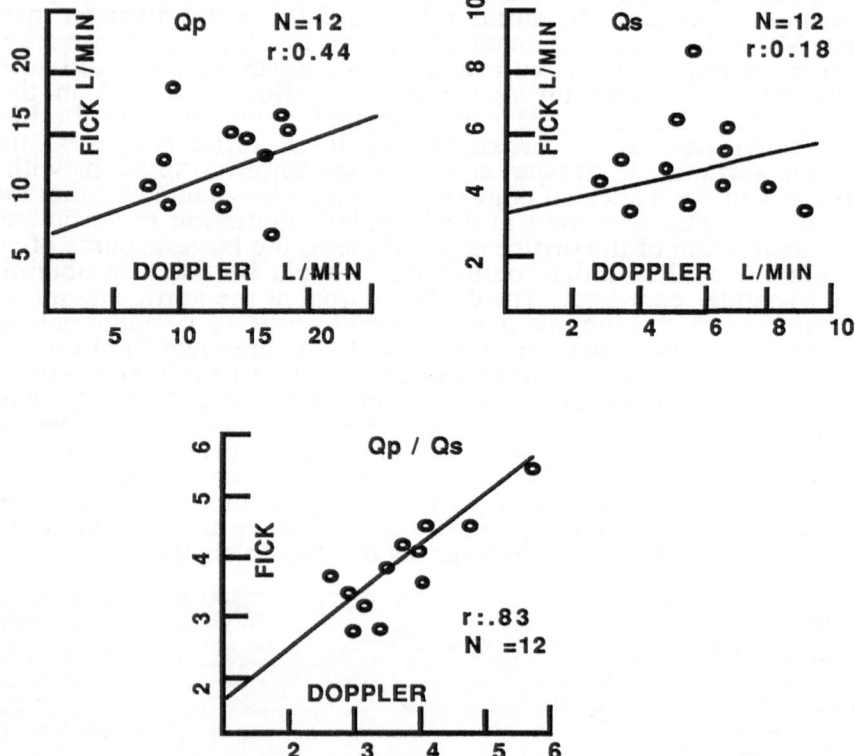

Fig.3-8. In this study the cardiac output across the pulmonic valve and the aortic valve measured by Doppler ultrasound techniques and by the Fick method were compared. A disappointing correlation was obtained , though a slightly better comparison was obtained at the pulmonic site. The Qp / Qs ratio however , correlated quite well .

The appearance of the opening and closing movements of the aortic valve on the amplitude display facilitate the positioning of the sample volume. When the sample volume is placed at the orifice level, the opening and closing spikes will have approximately the same amplitude. The audio signal should contain mainly high frequencies, and the recorded spectral pattern should have a narrow bandwidth. A slight degree of spectral broadening may be demonstrated during flow deceleration; this is caused by inherent flow instability. The flow velocity integral should be calculated for five to ten beats, and the average value used when estimating the cardiac output.

The Pulmonary Output

The pulmonary output is calculated in the same way as the aortic output; the pulmonary cross sectional area and the pulmonary flow velocity integral must be determined in order to estimate the Doppler-derived output. The pulmonary diameter is best estimated from the two-dimensional image when the patient is rolled into an extreme left lateral position. By placing the transducer in the third or fourth left intercostal space, one may usually obtain an adequate Doppler recording of pulmonary flow. Pulmonary flow varies with respiration, and slight changes in the peak flow velocity will normally be recorded. As with the aortic method of estimating output, five to ten flow velocity integral should be measured and the average value used when determining the pulmonary output.

The Mitral Valve Method

Cardiac output may also be estimated by determining the pulmonary venous return at the mitral orifice level. The Doppler recording of mitral flow is obtained from the apical window, and the sample volume is placed slightly downstream from the mitral annulus. The flow velocity integral is calculated for five to ten beats, and the mean value obtained. Because the size of the mitral orifice changes throughout diastole, a corrected orifice area (Ac) is used in the output equation:

$$CO = FVI \times Ac \times HR$$

The corrected mitral valve area is computed using Fisher's method (8). The maximal mitral orifice (A) is determined by planimetry of the appropriate short-axis still frame of the mitral valve. A standard M-mode recording of the mitral valve is then obtained in which the anterior and posterior leaflets are clearly visualized. The ratio of the mean leaflet separation (Ln) to the maximal leaflet separation (Lm) is then derived. The corrected mitral orifice area is calculated as:

$$Ac = (Ln/Lm) \times A$$

The cardiac output at the mitral level may then be determined once the mean flow velocity integral and the orifice area are known.

Zhang et al (9) reported good correlations with invasive estimates of cardiac output using this technique. However, this method is not applicable in patients with mitral valve disease.

It is also possible to estimate the cardiac output at the tricuspid valve level, but in practice it is difficult to implement. The major problem with this approach is the lack of a clearly defined way to measure the size of the tricuspid orifice. Nevertheless, Gillam et al (10) have suggested that the Doppler-derived outputs measured at the tricuspid and mitral orifices can correlate equally well with simultaneous thermodilution measurements of cardiac output. De Boo and coworkers have also been successful in measuring flow at the tricuspid orifice with Doppler techniques in normal adults (11). However, two orthogonal views of the tricuspid orifice were needed in order to estimate the orifice area with an ellipsoid formula.

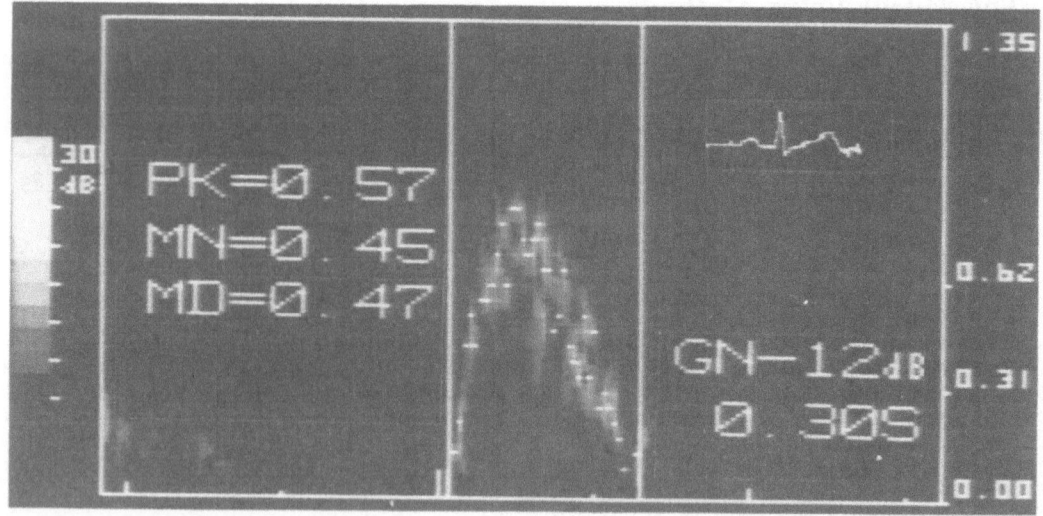

Fig. 3-9. The mean velocity, or average velocity of flow over a specific time interval is used to obtain the flow volume. In a symmetric flow curve this is approximately the ejection time multiplied by the peak velocity divided by two.

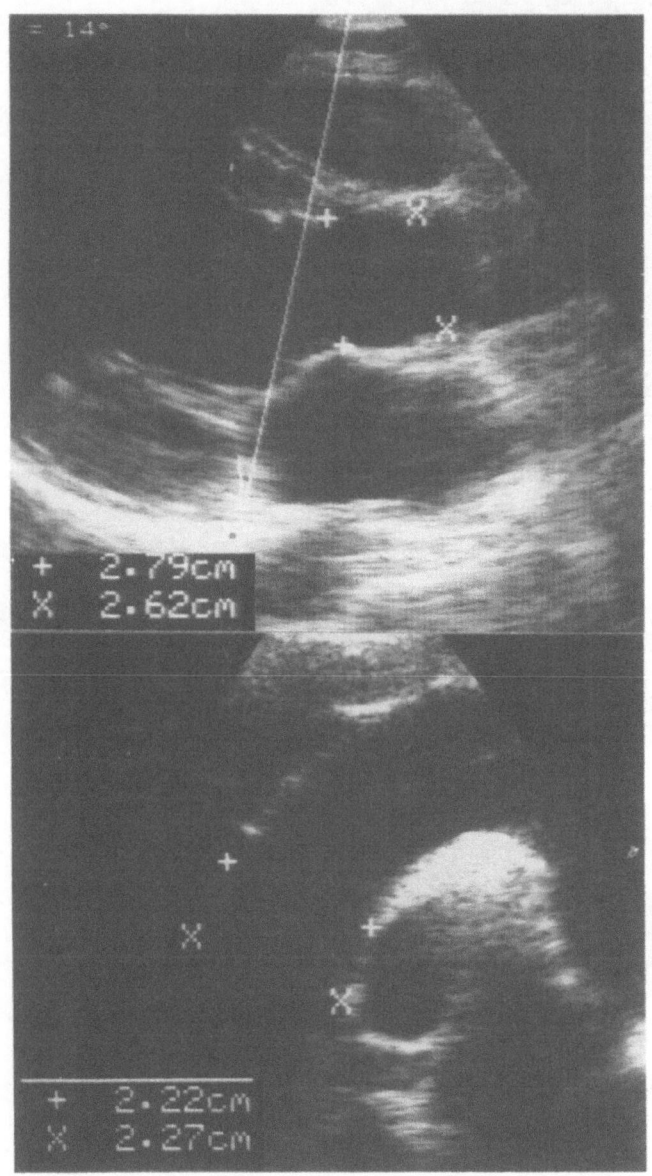

Fig. 3-10. The flow cross sectional area may be measured from either the parasternal long axis or from the suprasternal notch. While the suprasternal notch permits the flow and the aortic diameter to be measured from the same transducer position, it is generally easier to measure the aortic diameter from the parasternal position.

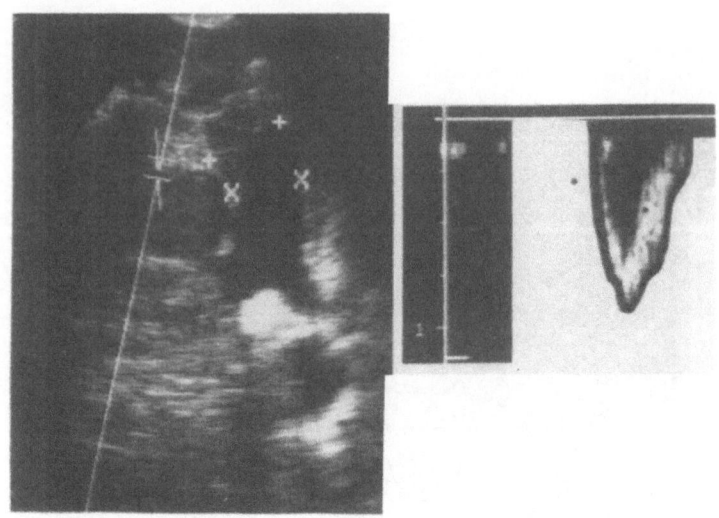

Fig.3-11. The examination technique for measuring the pulmonary flow volume.

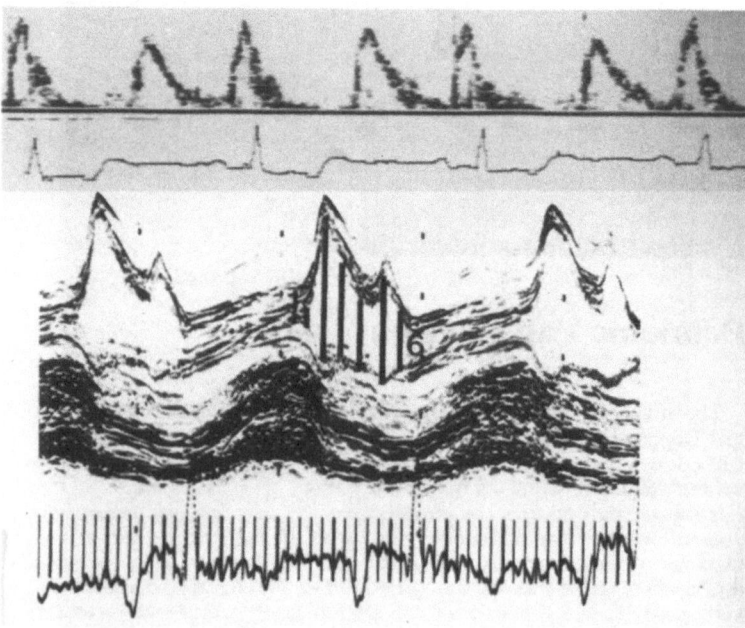

Fig. 3-12 The mitral valve examination technique requires measurements from the M-mode , the two dimensional image , and the flow velocity curve . While in theory , open-chested dogs , and in certain pediatric applications this method works well, in the normal adult patient too many measurements (read as possible sources of error) are encountered.

References

1. Caro CG, Pedley TJ, Schroter RC, Seed WA. The Mechanics of the Circulation. Oxford University Press, London, 1978.
2. Gill, Robert W. Measurement of blood flow by ultrasound: Accuracy and sources of error. Ultrasound Med & Biol 11;4:625-41, 1985.
3. Hatle L, Angelsen BAJ. Doppler Ultrasound in Cardiology: Physical Principles and Clinical Applications (2nd ed), Lea & Febiger, Philadelphia, 1985.
4. McDonald DA. Blood Flow in Arteries(2nd ed). Edward Arnold, London, 1974.
5. Milnor WR. Hemodynamics. Williams & Wilkins, Baltimore/London, 1982.
6. Ihlen H, Amlie JP, Dale J, et al. Determination of cardiac output by Doppler echocardiography. Br Heart J 52:54-60, 1984.
7. Stewart WJ, Jiang L, Mich R, et al. Variable effects of changes in flow rate through the aortic pulmonary and mitral valves on valve area and flow velocity: Impact on quantitative Doppler flow calculations. J Am Coll Cardiol 6;3:653-62, 1985.
8. Fisher DC, Sahn DJ, Friedman MJ, et al. The mitral valve orifice method for noninvasive two-dimensional echo Doppler determinations of cardiac output. Circulation 67:872-7, 1983.
9. Zhang Y, Nitter-Hauge S, Ihlen H, Myhre E. Doppler echocardiographic measurement of cardiac output using the mitral orifice method. Br Heart J 53:130-6, 1985.
10. Gillam LD, Ascah KJ, Wilkins GT, et al. Which cardiac valve provides the best Doppler estimate of cardiac output in humans (abstr)? Int Symp on Doppler Echocardiography: 25, July 1986.
11. De Boo, Van Mill GJ, Van der Werf T. An improved noninvasive method to assess the ratio of pulmonary to systemic flow in adults using pulsed Doppler echocardiography (abstr). Fourth Int Cong on Echocardiology: 88, April 1984.

CHAPTER 4

THE NORMAL EXAMINATION
James V. Chapman

The Imaging Windows

In order to interrogate blood flow across the cardiac valves in an organized manner, a standard protocol for the routine Doppler ultrasound examination should be established. The imaging windows utilized in the course of a Doppler examination will first be described. Since blood flow is not parallel to the anatomic structures, it is often necessary to interrogate flow from several transducer positions in order to record the true peak flow velocity. When obstruction is present, the value of the peak flow velocity may differ markedly from one imaging window to another.

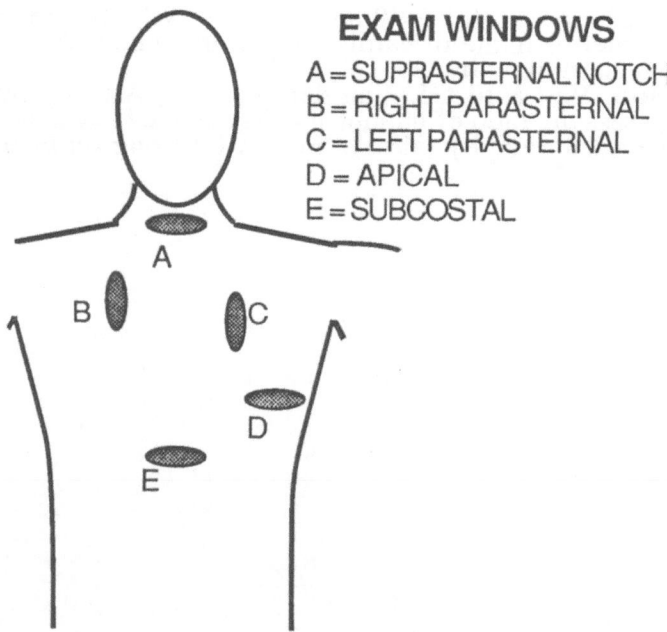

EXAM WINDOWS
A = SUPRASTERNAL NOTCH
B = RIGHT PARASTERNAL
C = LEFT PARASTERNAL
D = APICAL
E = SUBCOSTAL

Fig. 4-1. The most commonly used examination windows are illustrated above. The patient is normally rolled into a left lateral decubitus position when imaging from the left parasternal (C) or apical windows (D). The subcostal (E) and suprasternal (A) views are most easily obtained when the patient is supine. The patient should be rolled into a right lateral position when imaging from the right parasternal window (B).

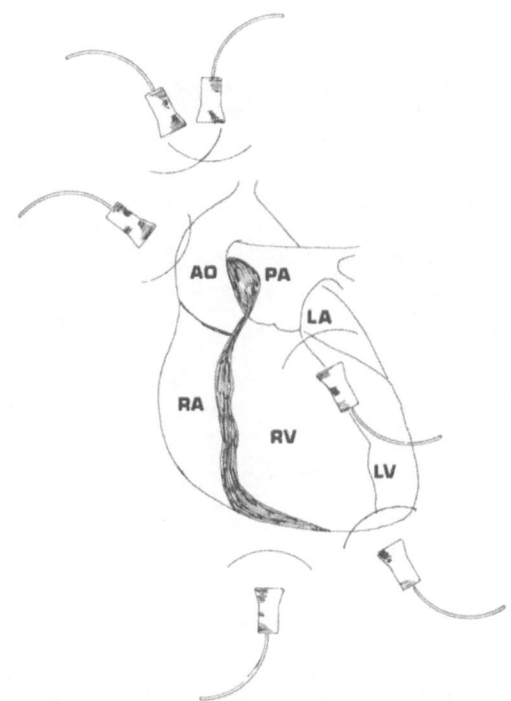

Fig. 4-2. The transducer orientation relative to the cardiac structures for the examination windows in figure 4-1 are illustrated above.

The Left Parasternal Window

The patient is rolled into the left lateral decubitus position with a pillow behind his back for support. The transducer is placed in the third or fourth intercostal space and angle superiorly. With medial angulation, the tricuspid flow may be examined from this position. With lateral angulation, the right ventricular outflow and the pulmonary flow may be interrogated. In young patients, these flows can be obtained with relative ease from either the supine or left lateral position.

The Apical Window

The patient is placed in either the supine or left lateral position. The point of maximal impulse is palpated, and the transducer is placed over this point or slightly beneath it. The mitral flow, left ventricular outflow and aortic flow can be selectively examined depending upon the angulation and sample volume position. With inferomedial angulation, the tricuspid flow can be examined. It is sometimes possible to record flow in the inferior vena cava and pulmonary veins from the apical window.

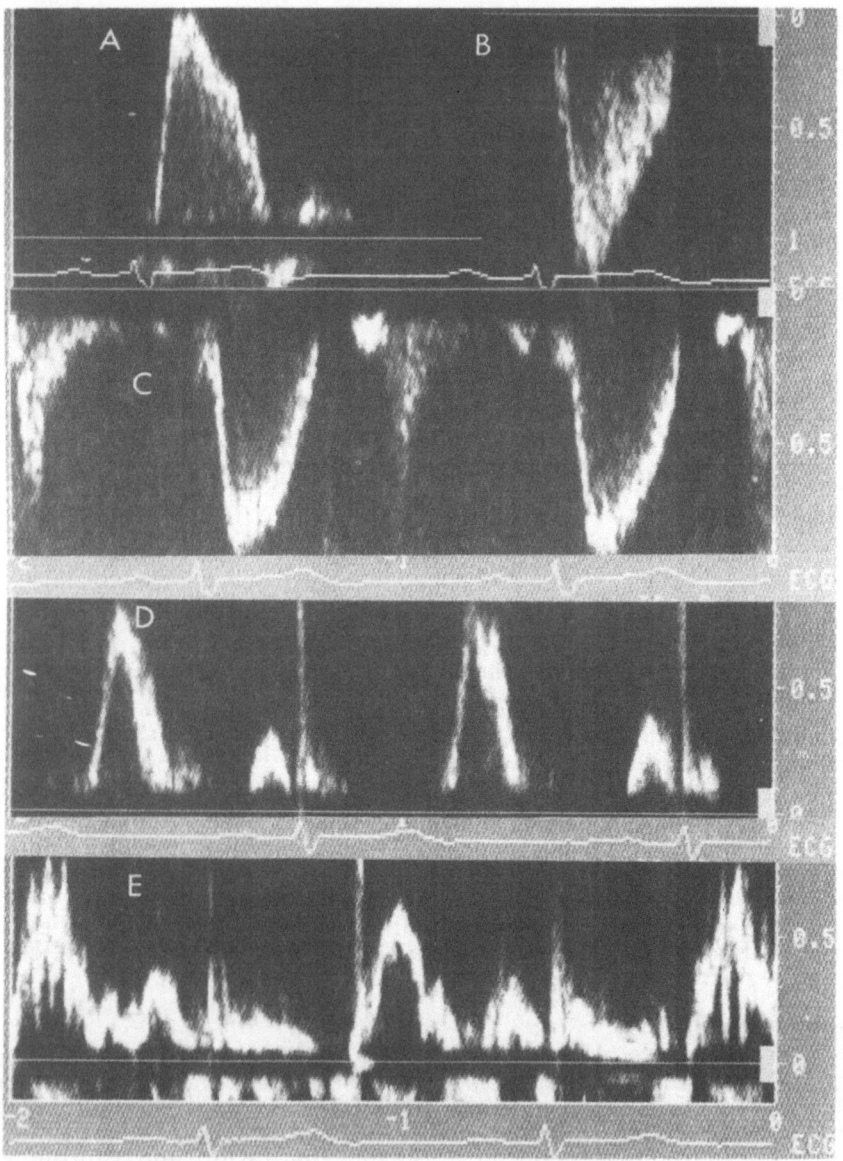

Fig. 4-3. In this series of spectral analysis tracings the normal flow across the A) Ascending aorta , B) the descending aorta , C) the left ventricular outflow tract , D) the mitral valve , E) and the tricuspid valve are demonstrated.

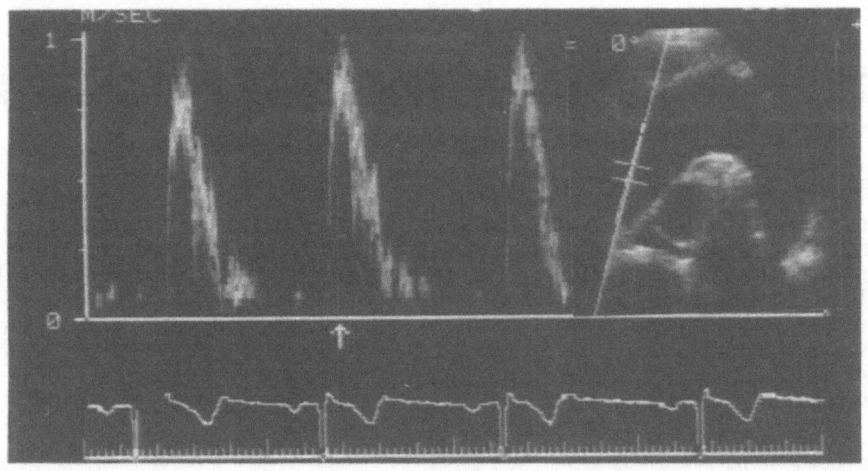

Fig. 4-4. Pulsed mode recording of normal flow in the ascending aorta obtained from the suprasternal window. Note the narrow bandwidth of the flow velocity curve, with a slight degree of spectral broadening during flow deceleration.

The Subcostal Window

The patient is placed in a supine position with his knees elevated. The transducer is placed just below the xiphoid process, and angled towards the left shoulder. Flow in the pulmonary artery, right ventricular outflow tract and caval veins may be selectively examined from this position. Infrequently, an adequate recording of aortic flow may be obtained from this position.

The Suprasternal Window

The patient is placed in a supine position with the neck slightly extended if possible. The probe is placed in the suprasternal notch. Flow in the ascending aorta, descending aorta, and superior vena cava may be examined from this imaging window. In older patients, it is sometimes helpful to turn them slightly laterally or to have them sit up and lean forward slightly.

The Right Parasternal Window

The parient is rolled into a right lateral position with a pillow behind his back for support. The probe is positioned in the second or third intercostal space and angled inferomedially. Flow in the ascending aorta can be interrogated from this position.

The Right Supraclavicular Window

The patient is placed in the supine position, and the transducer is placed next to the right sternocleidomastoid muscle. Flow in th superior vena cava can be examined from this position.

Characteristics of Normal Blood Flow

Normal blood flow across the valves of the heart, through the cardiac chambers, and into the the great vessels is laminar. In laminar flow, the flow cross-section may be represented as a large number of concentric layers. These layers do not travel at precisely the same velocity, and red cells do not cross from one fluid layer to another. Because of the effects of viscous friction, the fluid layer adjacent to the vessel or chamber wall moves at a reduced velocity. In this simplified model of cardiac flow, we consider the velocity of the fluid layer nearest to the wall to be zero. The core layer moves at the highest velocity, and the velocity of each layer decreases as a function of distance from the center of the lumen.(See fig.3-1).The resultant profile which develops is parabolic in configuration. If most of the fluid layers are traveling at the same velocity (except for the layer nearest to the wall), a blunt or flat velocity profile develops.

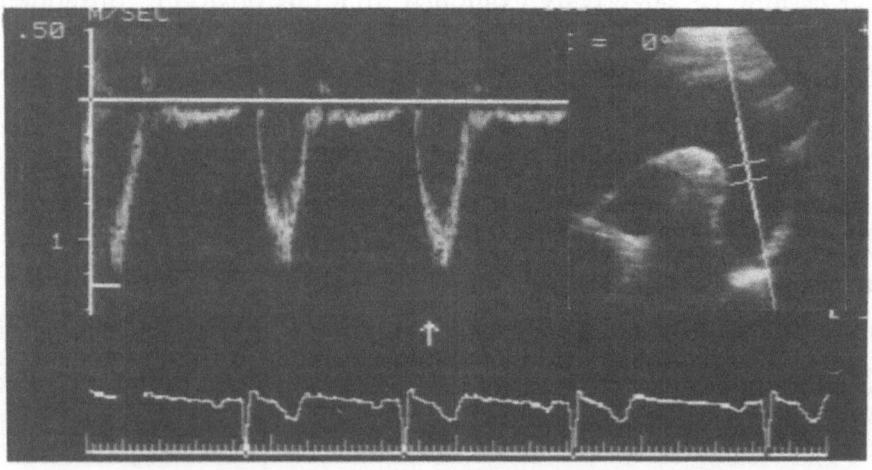

Fig. 4-5. Pulsed mode recording of normal flow in the descending aorta recorded from the suprasternal tranducer position. A low amplitude diastolic flow is also recorded. Usually, diastolic flow towards the transducer is recorded in early diastole.

When a blunt velocity profile exists, the maximum flow velocity may be assumed to approximate the spatial mean velocity. If a parabolic flow profile actually exists, this assumption is no longer valid. The maximum flow velocity measured in the center of the lumen is appreciably greater than the spatial mean velocity in such a case. The value of the core flow velocity is higher than the velocity of the neighboring layers. A parabolic or a flat profile may be found in laminar flows.

As the flow velocity increases due to the presence of an obstruction, the laminar flow configuration becomes unstable. Mixing of the fluid layers begins to take place. There is motion now of the red cells in a direction transverse to the flow plane. Consequently, there are two components needed to describe the flow pattern. The first is a slowly varying term for the forward flow; the second component is a rapidly changing term for the transverse displacement of red cells. The flow itself is described as turbulent. Because there is random motion transverse to the flow plane, considerable energy losses occur. Turbulent flow may therefore be considered to be an inefficient flow regime.

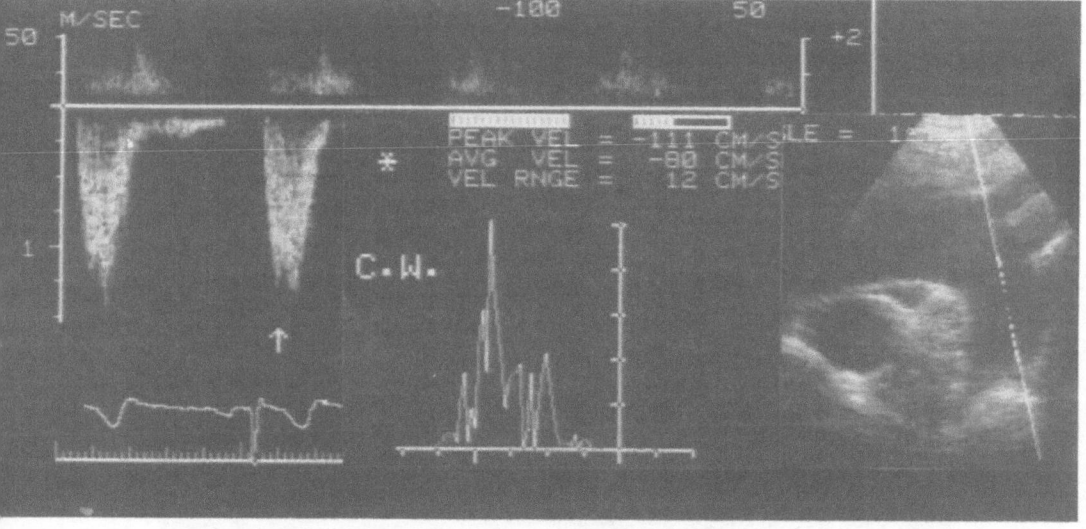

Fig. 4-6. Recording of normal flow in the descending aorta with continuous wave Doppler. The peak flow velocity is 1.35 m/s, and a relatively wide spectral bandwidth is noted. This is due to the larger area of flow sampled . In early diastole, low amplitude reverse flow (flow towards the transducer) is recorded. The diastolic flow away from the tranducer throughout the rest of diastole is also a normal finding.

Aortic Flow

Flow in the ascending aorta may be sampled from the suprasternal, apical or right parasternal windows. Occasionally, a good quality Doppler recording may be obtained from the subcostal window, despite the fact that the aortic lumen appears perpendicular to the transducer. In the normal patient, the best recording is usually obtained from the suprasternal long-axis plane. In this view, the ascending aorta is located on the left side of the sector, the transverse aorta is located at the top of the sector, and the descending aorta is located on the right side of the sector. Often the aortic valve is clearly visualized from the suprasternal window.

To obtain a pulsed mode recording of aortic flow, the sample volume is placed in the ascending aorta just distal to the valve. The transducer angulation is changed slightly until a narrow bandwidth audio signal is heard. A flow velocity recording should be made when the flow boundary or flow envelope is well-defined and consistent from beat to beat. The clarity of the audio signal is the best guide for assessing a parallel alignment to flow. If an optimal beam-to-flow angle can not be acheived from this position, the right parasternal window should be used. The transducer is placed in the second or third right intercostal space and angled so that the ascending limb of the aorta is visualized. The peak aortic flow velocity ranges from 0.7 to 1.6 m/s in normal adults; the normal range is slightly higher in children.

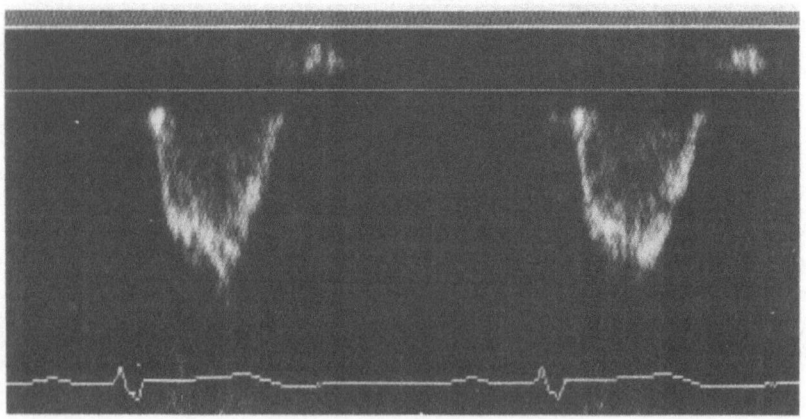

Fig. 4-7. Pulsed mode recording of normal flow in the descending aorta. The peak flow velocity is 1.25 m/s, and a fairly narrow spectral bandwidth is noted. In early diastole, low amplitude reverse flow (flow towards the transducer) is recorded, and in systole a small degree of spectral broadening is noted . This is due to a deceleration instability and is a normal finding.

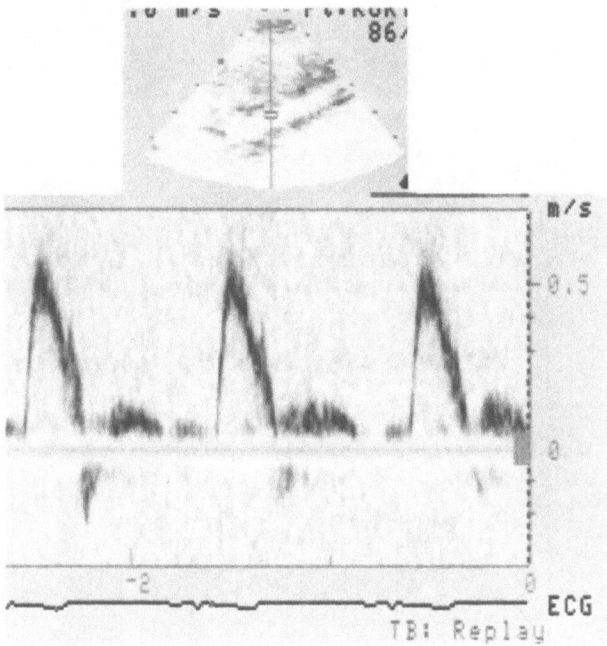

Fig.4-8. This normal abdominal aortic flow study was obtained from the subcostal transduer position. The flow velocity is underestimated due to the beam to angle to flow. This is one of the few instances where the angle correction may be used on the assumption that flow will follow the structure used for the angle estimation.

With color flow imaging, a red flow bolus may be seen in the ascending aorta moving towards the suprasternal notch in systole. The flow profile appears flat as the flow crosses the valve, but gradually assumes a parabolic configuration with increasing distance from the valve. A skewing of the flow profile towards the inner bend of the ascending aorta may sometimes be noted. No flow is detected in the transverse aorta due to the perpendicular beam/flow alignment.

The pulsed mode recording of flow in the descending aorta is shown in Fig. 5. The sample volume is placed in the lumen of the descending aorta distal to the subclavian artery. By relying upon the audio signal and the spectral bandwidth for flow orientation, an optimal narrow bandwidth spectrum can be recorded. The peak flow velocity in the descending aorta is usually slightly less than that in the ascending aorta.

In the color flow investigation, the systolic flow in the descending aorta is seen as a blue flow bolus moving away from the transducer. The flow profile may appear to be skewed towards the outer bend of the descending aorta.

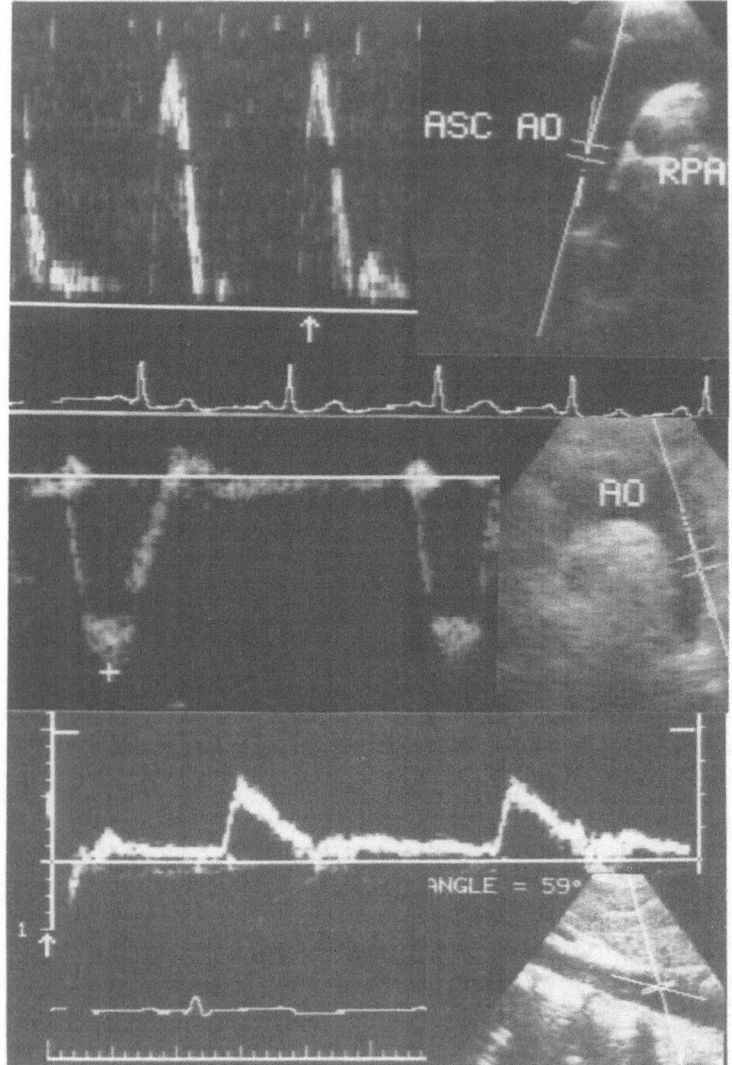

Fig.4-9. Pulsed mode recordings of aortic flow obtained from three locations. Top. Pulsed mode recording of flow in the ascending aorta recorded from a modified suprasternal long axis view. Middle. Pulsed mode recording of flow in the descending aorta. Spectral unwrapping has been used to resolve the peak flow velocity. Bottom. Pulsed mode recording of flow in the abdominal aorta obtained from the subcostal window using high pulse repetition frequency mode.

Pulmonary Flow

Pulmonary flow is best examined from the left parasternal or subcostal imaging window. To obtain a pulsed mode recording, the sample volume is positioned slightly downstream from the pulmonary valve. From this sampling site, a negative flow velocity curve is recorded in systole. The peak flow velocity in adults lies in the 0.6 to 1.3 m/s range, as established by Hatle and coworkers. The maximal velocity may exceed this range in normal children. If the sample volume is situated too close to the valve cusps, the valve movements will interfere with the recording of the pulmonary flow signal.

The pulmonary flow velocity curve has a more rounded contour than the aortic flow trace, and the peak pulmonary velocity occurs later in systole. However, the shape of the pulmonary flow curve is affected by changes in sample volume placement within the arterial lumen. If the sample volume is too close to the vessel wall, a marked systolic flow reversal can be recorded. When the sample volume is positioned in the center of flow, the audio signal is clear and the contour of the flow pattern is consistent. In normal individuals, the contour does not change appreciably as the sample volume is moved away from the pulmonary valve cusps.

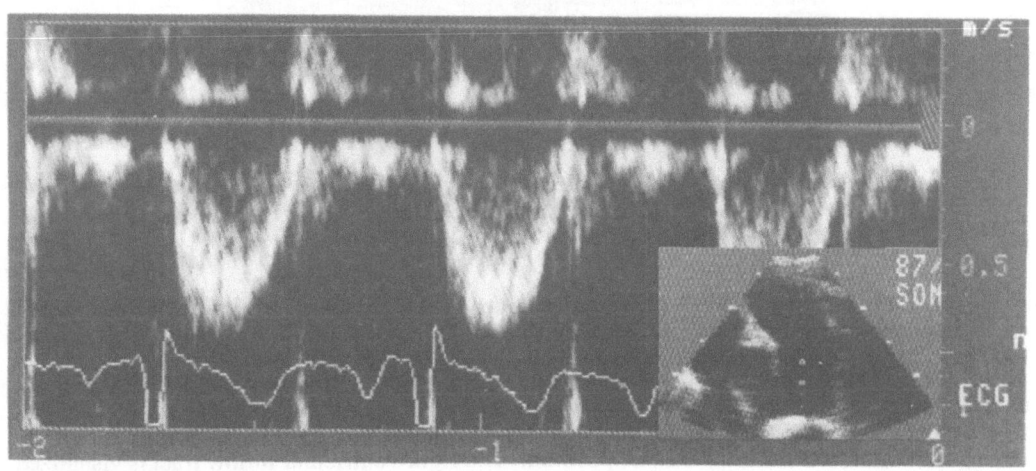

Fig. 4-10. Pulsed mode recording of normal pulmonary artery flow in a young adult. The peak velocity is approximately 0.7 m/s but increases slightly with inspiration. The opening and closing movements of the pulmonary valve are clearly recorded in the third beat.

After recording a well-defined pulmonary flow curve, the right ventricular ejection time and the pulmonary acceleration time can be measured. The right ventricular ejection time is defined as the period in which systolic pulmonary flow takes place; it is the interval from the beginning to the cessation of pulmonary flow. The pulmonary acceleration time is defined as the time interval required for the development of the peak flow velocity. It is measured as the period of time elapsed between the beginning of the flow trace and the peak of the flow trace. Generally the pulmonary artery acceleration time is greater than110 ms in normal subjects (1 ,8). In the presence of elevated pulmonary artery pressssure, the acceleration time is decreased. The ratio of the acceleration time to the right ventricular ejection time may also be calculated. The value of these time intervals may vary from beat to beat, and a mean value should be calculated to minimize error.

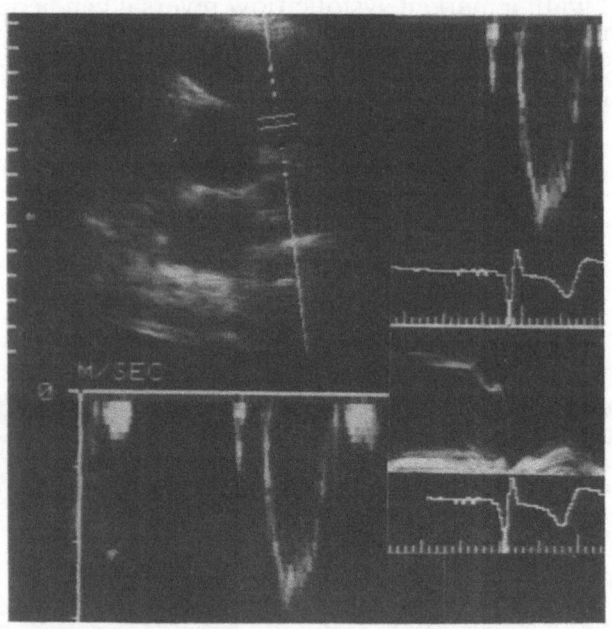

Fig. 4-11. Left. Normal pulmonary artery flow recorded from the third left intercostal space in an adult patient. The sample volume is placed slightly distal to the pulmonary valve, and a negative flow velocity trace is obtained. Note the pre-systolic low amplitude dip in the flow velocity curve. Bottom left. The M-mode recording of the pulmonary valve made from the same position. The pre-systolic flow in the Doppler recording and the A wave in the pulmonary valve echo occur at the same point in the cardiac cycle. Right. Normal biphasic tricuspid flow recorded from the same position. The right ventricular inflow tract is visualized, and the sample volume is placed downstream from the tricuspid valve. The passive filling component (first "v") is greater than the atrial filling component (second "v"). The M-mode recording of the tricuspid valve echo is also shown.

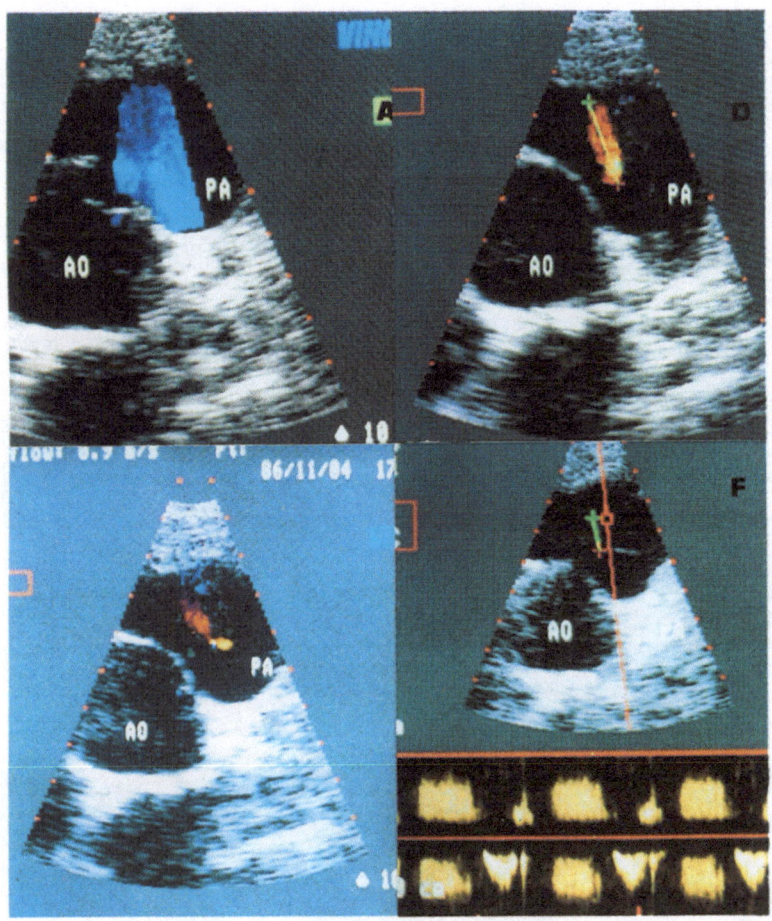

Fig. 4-12. Color flow analysis of normal pulmonary artery flow recorded from a parasternal short axis position. Shades of blue represent flow away from the transducer, while shades of red and gold represent flow towards the transducer. Top left. Normal systolic flow into the pulmonary artery is seen. Top right. In diastole, a small flamelike flow coded in shades of red and gold is recorded. This represents the presence of physiological pulmonary insufficiency.

Bottom left. The regurgitant flow recorded in late diastole. The flow extension is much less than in the preceeding diastolic frames, but the signal is still clearly recorded. Bottom right. Color flow mapping and conventional pulsed mode. The sample volume is positioned in the area where the regurgitant flow is detected with color flow analysis. The typical pulsed mode flow pattern in physiological pulmonary insufficiency is recorded. The regurgitant signal is well recorded in mid- to late-diastole, but is not recorded in early diastole.

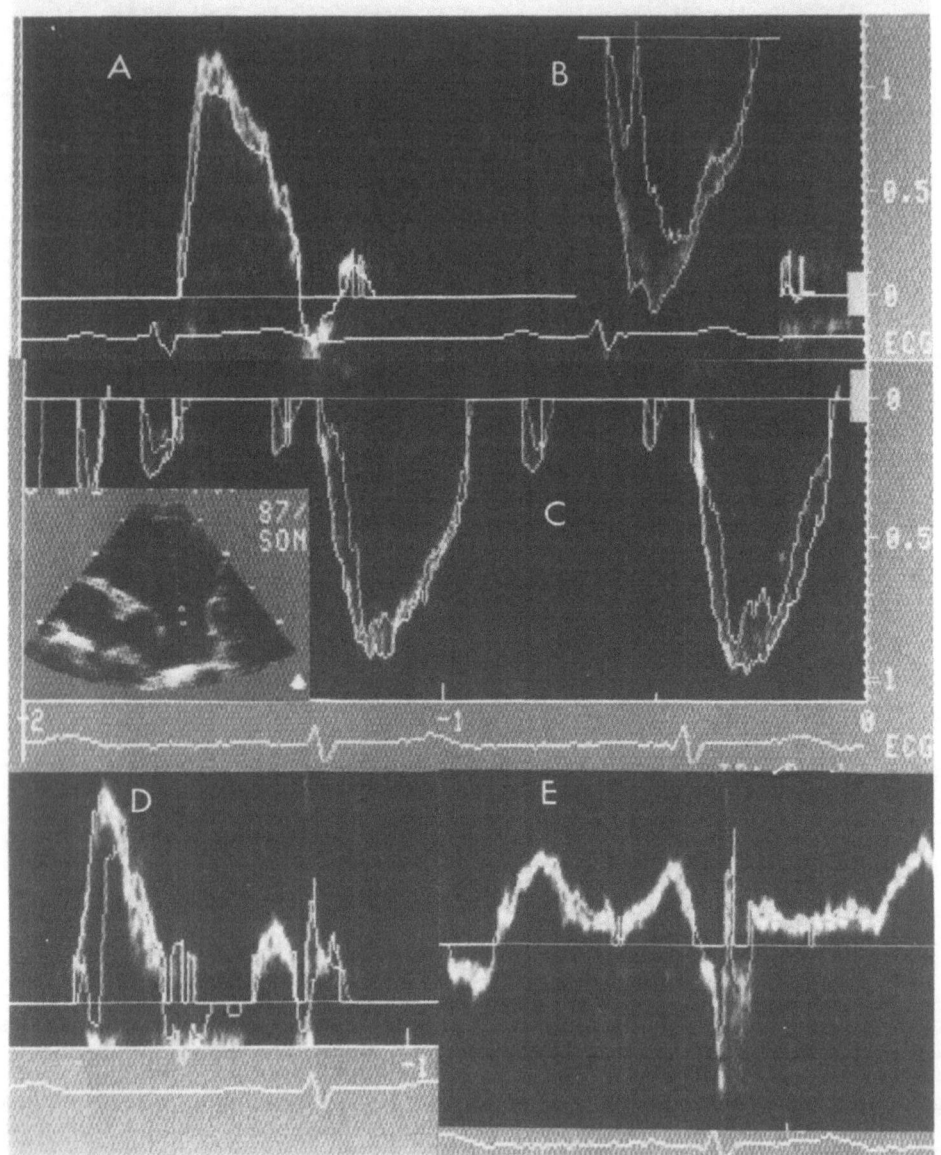

Fig. 4-13. In this series of figures the mean and maximum frequency estimators have been derived from the Doppler spectrum. A good alignment to flow is indicated when the two curves are are of an approximate velocity. (A) ascending aorta , (B) descending aorta , (C) pulmonary artery flow , (D) mitral flow , and (E) tricuspid flow.

Frequently in normal individuals, a weak positive diastolic flow signal can be detected when the sample volume is slightly proximal to the pulmonary valve (fig.12). This low velocity flow signal is best recorded in mid- to late-diastole, and has a pattern resembling pulmonary regurgitation. This signal indicates the presence of an insignificant pulmonary insufficiency which is described as physiological. The weak diastolic signal of physiological insufficiency is confined to a very small region behind the pulmonary valve.

The color flow mapping study of pulmonary flow is also performed from the parasternal or subcostal window. A systolic flow bolus in shades of blue is seen in the pulmonary artery. The flow profile in the right ventricular outflow tract may appear to be skewed, becoming flat as the flow crosses the pulmonary valve. Slightly distal to the valve, a parabolic flow profile may be visualized. The core flow velocity may exceed the Nyquist value, and color aliasing may be observed in the center of the flow bolus.

The physiological pulmonary insufficiency detected with conventional pulsed mode can also be demonstrated with color flow imaging. The regurgitant flow is represented as a small red flame originating from the valvular level. The flow is localized to a discrete area behind the pulmonary valve, extending for approximately 1.0 cm into the right ventricular outflow tract. The orientation of the jet changes throughout diastole, hence its flame-like appearance. This change in spatial orientation probably causes the early diastolic dropout of the regurgitant signal in conventional pulsed mode.

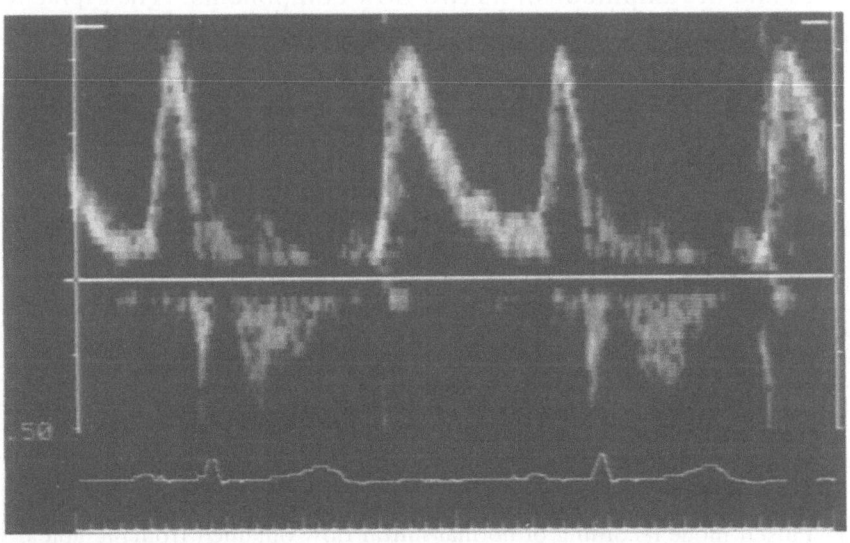

Fig. 4-14. Pulsed mode recording of normal mitral flow obtained from the apical window. The normal mitral flow pattern is biphasic in sinus rehythm, with a peak occurring furing rapid filling and a peak occurring after atrial contraction.

Mitral Flow

The pulsed mode recording of mitral flow is obtained from the apical window. The sample volume is placed slightly distal to the mitral annulus so that the valve movements will not interfere with the blood flow signal, and a diastolic flow velocity curve is recorded. The normal mitral flow is biphasic; there is a passive filling component and a component occurring after atrial contraction. The passive filling component has a higher peak velocity than the atrial flow component, lying in the range of 0.6 to 1.3 m/s in adults. The passive filling component is also known as the E wave, while the atrial component is known as the A wave.

Charbel et al (5) calculated the ratio of E wave peak velocity to the A wave peak velocity in normal subjects and in patients with compromised left ventricular function. In the normal control group, a mean E/A ratio of 1.1 was calculated. The mean E/A ratio in the group with reduced left ventriculat function was 0.7. Gardin and coworkers (6) demonstrated an increase in A wave velocity in severe hypertensives when compared to mild hypertensive and normotensive subjects. Visser et al (7) found an inverse relationship between the E/A ratio and the Killip class in the setting of acute myocardial infaction. The pulsed Doppler recording of mitral flow therefore appears to be a sensitive indicator of alterations in the left ventricular filling pattern. It is essential however, to be certain of correct beam-to-flow alignment and sample volume positioning when recording mitral flow. Movement of the heart during the cardiac cycle may cause a shift in the sample volume position. The sample volume may then be located on the atrial side of the orifice rather than the ventricular side. This positional change will alter the configuration of the mitral flow pattern and the amplitude of its two flow components. The biphasic nature of left ventricular inflow is dependent upon the cardiac rhythm. In the presence of atrial fibrillation, the A wave will be absent.

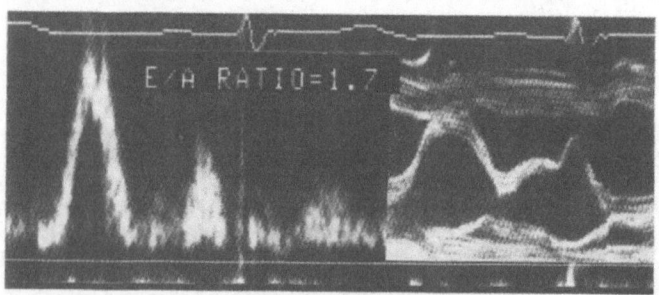

Fig. 4-15. Pulsed mode recording of normal mitral flow obtained from the apical window. The normal mitral flow pattern is biphasic in sinus rehythm, with a peak occurring furing rapid filling and a peak occurring after atrial contraction. The first peak is termed the E wave or E component, and the second is called the A wave or A component. When atrial fibrillation is present, the A wave will not be recorded.

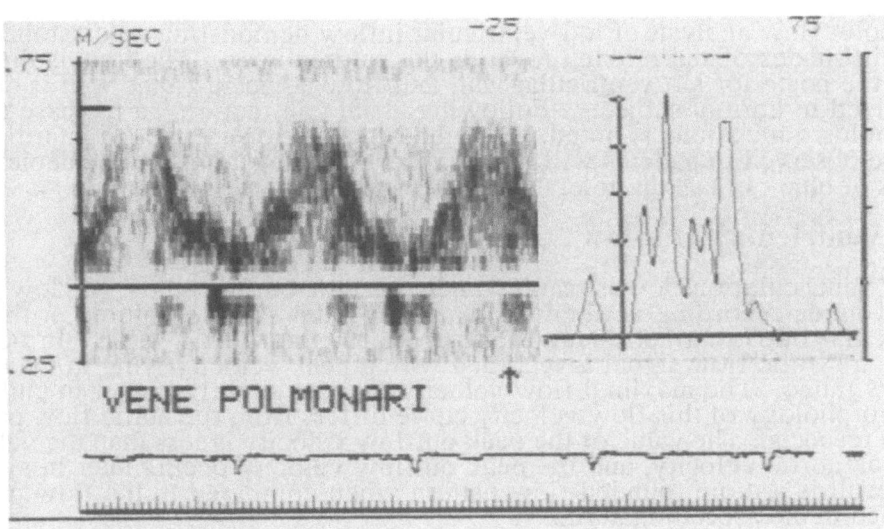

Fig.4-16 The flow in the pulmonary veins can often be sampled from the apical transducer position. The frequency bandwidth of this recording is quite wide as the power spectrum (inset) demonstrates. When flow mapping with conventional pulsed Doppler for a mitral regurgitation the pulmonary veinous flow may be confused with the low velocity wide bandwidth signal of the maximum regurgitant jets systolic extension into the lef atrium..

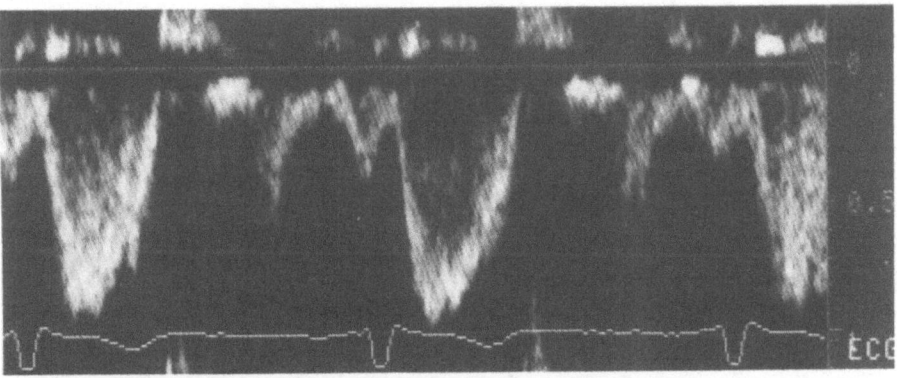

Fig. 4-17 . Pulsed mode recording of left ventricular outflow recorded from the apical window. The sample volume is placed approximately 1.0 cm behind the aortic valve, and a negative flow velocity curve is obtained. The peak velocity of left ventricular outflow in this example is 0.9 m/s. The negative biphasic flow pattern recorded in diastole represents the mitral flow signal.

71

The color flow analysis of left ventricular inflow demonstrates a diastolic flow bolus in shades of red moving towards the cardiac apex. The flow is directed along the posterior left ventricular wall and flow adjacent to the wall is clearly visualized in normal subjects. Following atrial contraction, an increase in the flow bolus dimensions is noted. Flow eddy formation in mid- to late-diastole may be observed in patients will low heart rates. The eddies will be depicted in shades of blue. In late diastole, the flow direction reverses.

Left Ventricular Outflow

Left ventricular outflow is usually interrogated from the apical window. The pulsed mode recording is obtained by placing the sample volume in the left ventricular outflow tract about 1.0 cm beneath the aortic valve. In normal adults, a sytolic flow signal is recorded with a peak velocity lying in the 0.7 to 1.1 m/s range. The maximal flow velocity may be slightly higher in children. The morphology of this flow velocity curve differs from the aortic flow pattern in two respects. The value of the peak outflow velocity is less than the value of the peak aortic velocity, and the peak outflow velocity occurs later in systole. The result is a more rounded flow pattern when compared to the flow pattern recorded in the ascending aorta.

As the sample volume is moved closer to the aortic valve, the closing valve spike and then the opening valve spike originating from cusp movement through the sample volume is detected. It is not uncommon to record mitral flow in diastole along with systolic left ventricular outflow. This flow contamination is due to the proximity of the inflow and outflow circuits. The mitral flow signal can be differentiated from the signal of aortic insufficiency on the basis of timing and peak velocity. The signal of aortic regurgitation begins immediately after aortic valve closure, but mitral flow does not begin until after isovolumic relaxation. The peak mitral velocity is significantly lower than the peak regurgitant flow velocity.

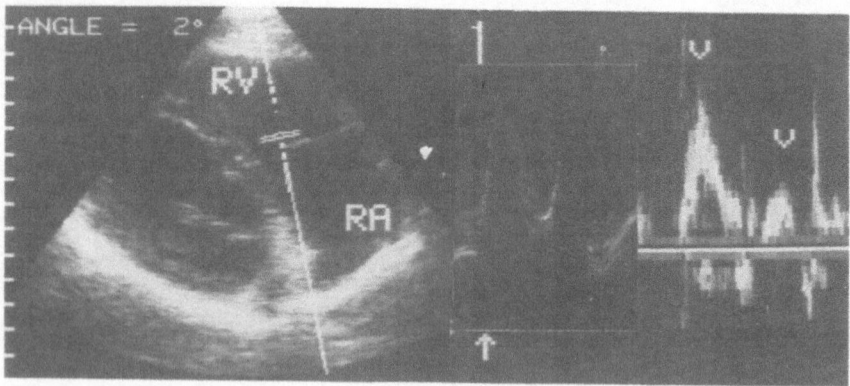

Fig. 4-18. Pulsed mode recording of normal tricuspid flow obtained from the apical window. The peak velocity is approximately 0.6 m/s, and the value of the peak flow velocity is seen to vary with respiration. (LA = left atrium, LV = left ventricle, RV = right ventricle, RA = right atrium).

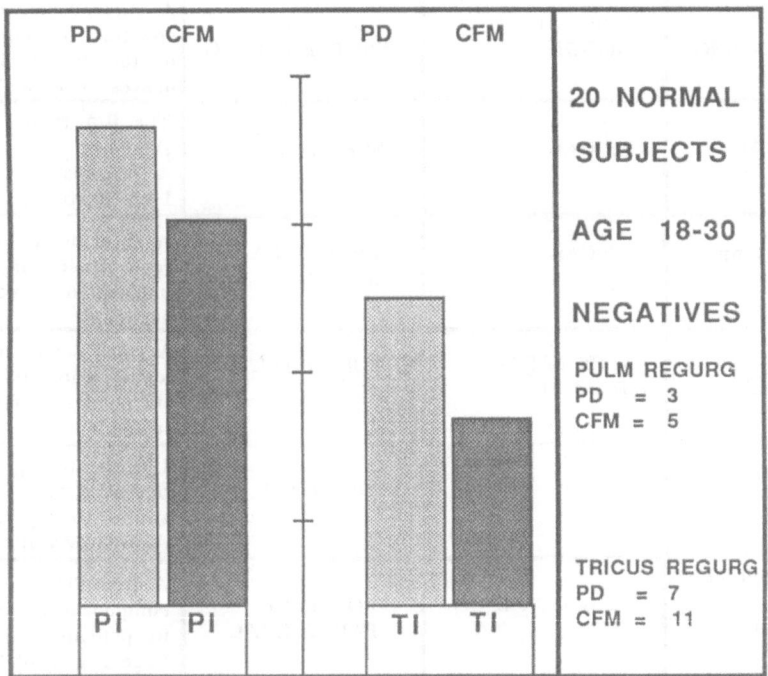

	PD	CFM		PD	CFM	
						20 NORMAL
						SUBJECTS
						AGE 18-30
						NEGATIVES
						PULM REGURG PD = 3 CFM = 5
	PI	PI		TI	TI	**TRICUS REGURG** PD = 7 CFM = 11

Table 3-1 .   The occurence of pulmonary and tricuspid regurgitation in normal subjects is frequently noted. In this series of healthy young subjects the frequency of both tricuspid and pulmonary regurgitation is demonstrated. The presence of a normal pulmonary regurgitation is more common than tricuspid , and the conventional pulsed Doppler appears slightly more sensitive than color flow mapping in detecting these small regurgitations   .

	FACTORS TO CONSIDER		
SITE	**TRANSDUCER POS.**	**ALTERNATIVE**	**NOTE**
ASCENDING & DESCENDING AORTA	SUPRASTERNAL NOTCH	RIGHT PS LAX FOR THE ASC. AO	A slight degree of spectral broadening in the deceleration phases is normal
MITRAL VALVE	APICAL	SUBCOSTAL	The E-A ratio should be > 1, < 1 indicates LVd dysfunction
TRICUSPID VALVE	APICAL	LEFT PARA-STERNAL	A small degree of regurgitation is not uncommon in normal subjects
PULMONIC VALVE	LEFT PARA-STERNAL	SUBCOSTAL	A small degree of regurgitation is not uncommon in normal subjects
LV OUTFLOW TRACT	APICAL	SUBCOSTAL	Use the timing of AoV & MV spikes to seperate AI from MV flow
INFERIOR VENA CAVA & HEPATIC VEINS	SUBCOSTAL	LOW LEFT PARSTERNAL	A diastolic flow component is seen in patients with large degree of TI

Table 3-2 . When screening intracardiac flows for abnormalities by Doppler ultrasound , there are common findings to be aware of , which indicate a pathological situation is present . These include high velocity flows , distirbed flows ,and regurgitant flow signals . A few specific details regarding the interrogation of flow at various localized sites are listed in this table. If one sets up a routine exam method , a relatively small amount of time is added to the echocardiographic study. The Doppler examination adds a great deal of information regarding the patients hemodynamic state , relative to the added exam time .

The color flow analysis of left ventricular outflow may be performed from the apical window or from an intermediate transducer position between the apex and the left sternal border. By late diastole, a flow bolus in shades of blue is visualized in the left ventricular cavity. When left ventricular ejection occurs, there is movement of this bolus into the outflow tract. The peak outflow velocity may exceed the Nyquist value, resulting in color aliasing.

Tricuspid flow

The pulsed Doppler recording of tricuspid flow or right ventricular inflow may be obtained from the apical or left parasternal imaging window. The sample volume is placed slightly downstream from the tricuspid valve, and a positive biphasic diastolic flow pattern is recorded. As with the mitral flow pattern, the passive filling component has a higher amplitude than the atrial flow component. The tricuspid peak velocity is less than the mitral peak velocity, lying in the 0.3 to 1.7 m/s range. Tricuspid flow varies with respiration; this characteristic helps distinguish tricuspid flow from mitral flow when using an independent Doppler transducer to perform the examination.

As with pulmonary flow, a high incidence of physiological tricuspid insufficiency has been noted. The holosystolic regurgitant flow signal is usually detected when the sample volume is positioned directly behind the tricuspid valve. The signal intensity is weak because of the small regurgitant flow volume, and the signal is localized to a discrete area in the right atrium. When the pulmonary artery pressure is within normal limits, the peak velocity of the regurgitant flow will be less than 2.5 m/s.

Continuous mode should be employed to record the maximal regurgitant velocity.

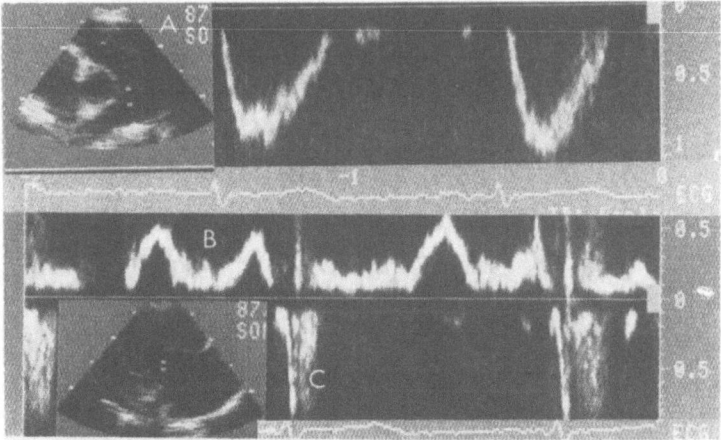

Fig.4-19 Top. Normal pulmonary artery flow examined from the left parasternal transducer position. From the same position the tricuspid flow can be interogated. (B) In diastole and,(C) systole. A small regurgitant flow is detected. This is not an uncommon finding in young healthy adults. The flow is of a very weak intensity and is localized in the area proximal to the valve.

Color flow analysis of tricuspid flow is also performed from the parasternal or apical windows. A diastolic flow bolus in shades of red will be seen in the right ventricular cavity. The flow is usually more clearly delineated from the parasternal window, probably because of the reduced interrogation depth. When physiological insufficiency is present, a small systolic jet in shades of blue appears at the level of the tricuspid annulus. The jet extension is about 1.0 cm in physiological insufficiency and the jet width is narrow (less than 1.0 cm).

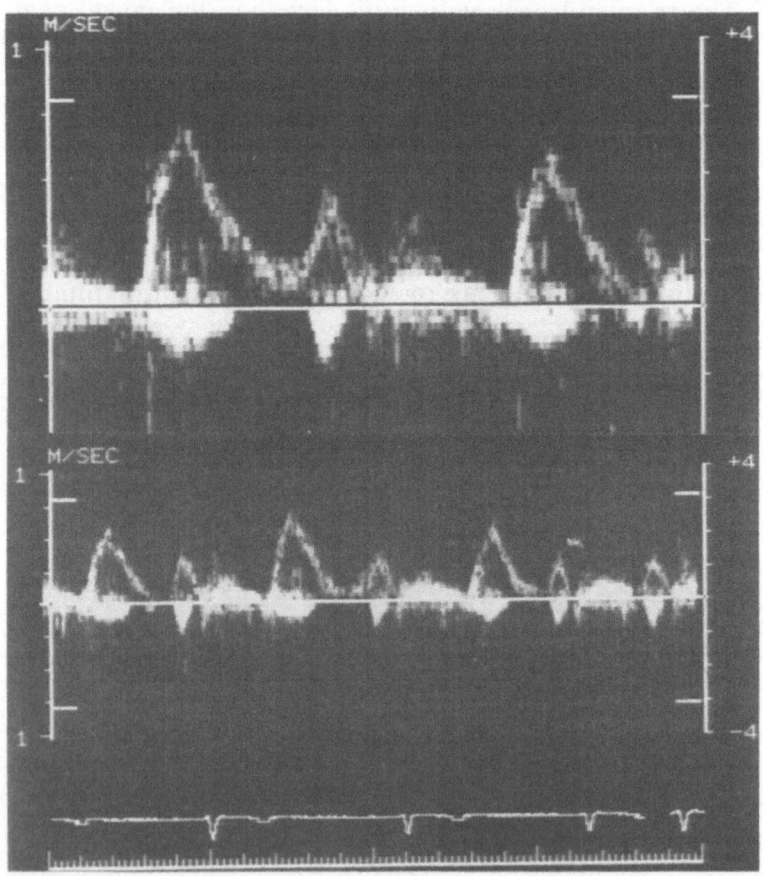

Fig. 4-20. Pulsed mode recording of normal tricuspid flow obtained from the apical window. The peak velocity is approximately 0.7 m/s, and in the bottom panel the value of the peak flow velocity is seen to vary with respiration.

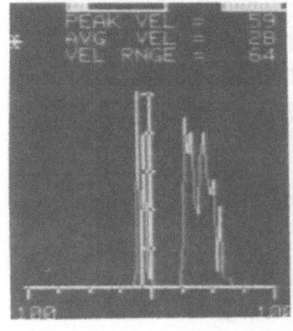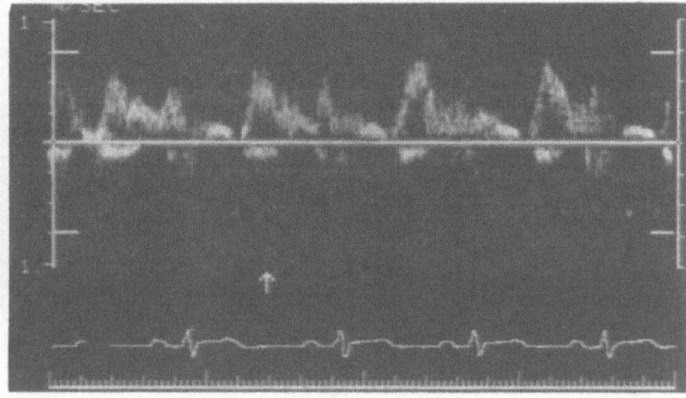

Fig. 4-21. Pulsed mode recording of normal tricuspid flow obtained from the apical window. The peak velocity is approximately 0.6 m/s, and the value of the peak flow velocity is seen to vary with respiration. (LA = left atrium, LV = left ventricle, RV = right ventricle, RA = right atrium). The power spectrum display demonstrates a narrow bandwidth signal (computed from spectral line indicated by the arrow).

The Caval Veins

The pulsed mode recording of flow in the superior vena cava may be obtained from the right supraclavicular, suprasternal, or subcostal windows. The supraclavicular window usually provides the best beam-to-flow orientation. The normal flow pattern in the superior vena cava and the hepatic veins consists of four components; there are two anterograde and two retrograde flows. The retrograde flow occurs following the P wave and the T wave of the electrocardiogram. These two components are termed the a wave and the v wave, respectively. The anterograde systolic flow is called the x wave, and usually has the highest velocity. The anterograde diastolic flow component is called the y wave. When recording at a small angle to flow, the peak velocity of the x wave ranges from 0.5 to 1.3 m/s in normal adults. This value may be higher in children and adolescents.

Flow in the inferior vena cava may be detected from the apical, parasternal, or subcostal window. The velocity pattern is similar to that of the superior vena cava, but the quality of the Doppler recording is suboptimal. The reason for this poor quality is the large beam-to-flow angle encountered. From the subcostal position, a positive or negative flow velocity curve can be generated with slight changes in transducer position. The transducer is nearly perpendicular to flow from this position, and the flow direction changes with minor alterations in position. Flow velocity in the caval veins increases with inspiration, although it is easier to demonstrate this when recording flow in the superior vena cava.

The color flow analysis of flow in the superior vena cava is performed from the right supraclavicular or suprasternal

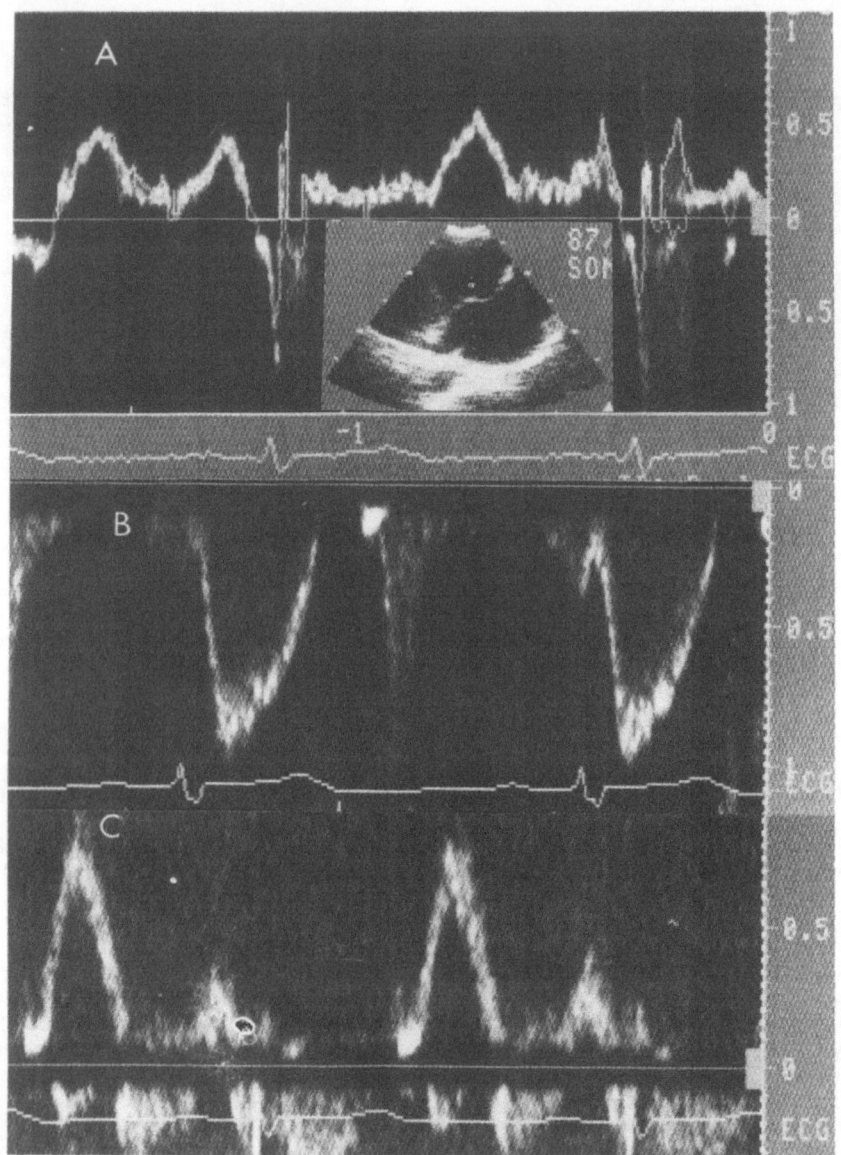

Fig.4-22. From the apical exam window one may interrogate the tricuspid valve (A) , the left ventricular outflow tract (B) , and the mitral valve.

window. A flow bolus in shades of blue is visualized in diastole, followed by a short period of flow reversal after atrial contraction. Systolic flow is depicted in shades of blue, and the flow reversal occurring after the T wave may not be visualized. Flow in the inferior vena cava is difficult to image with color analysis due to the near perpendicular beam-to-flow alignment.

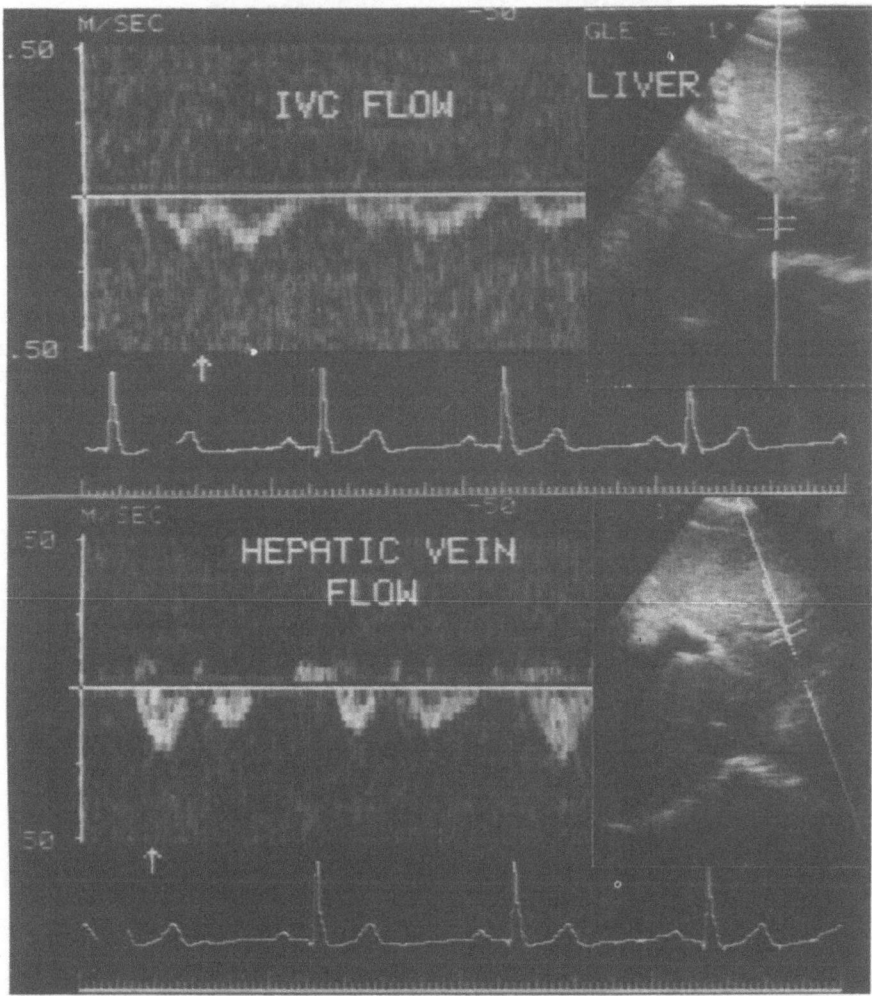

Fig. 4- 23. Top. Pulsed mode recording of normal flow in the inferior vena cava obtained from the subcostal window. A negative biphasic flow pattern is recorded, with one peak occuring in systole and the other in diastole. The flow velocity is relatively low, but this is probably due to the fact that a parallel alignment with vena caval flow is not possible from this position. (IVC = inferior vena cava). Bottom. Pulsed mode recording of normal flow in the hepatic veins recorded from the same position.

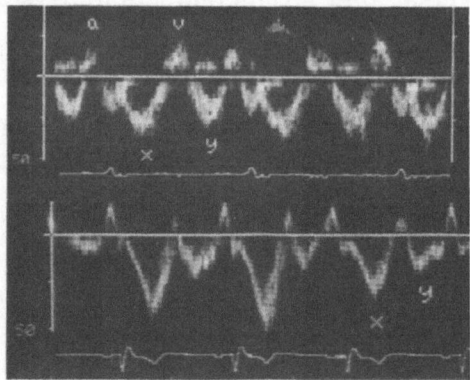

Fig.4-24 . Top. Pulsed mode recording of normal flow in the inferior vena cava obtained from the subcostal window. A negative biphasic flow pattern is recorded, with one peak occuring in systole and the other in diastole. Bottom. Pulsed mode recording of normal flow in the hepatic veins recorded from the same position.

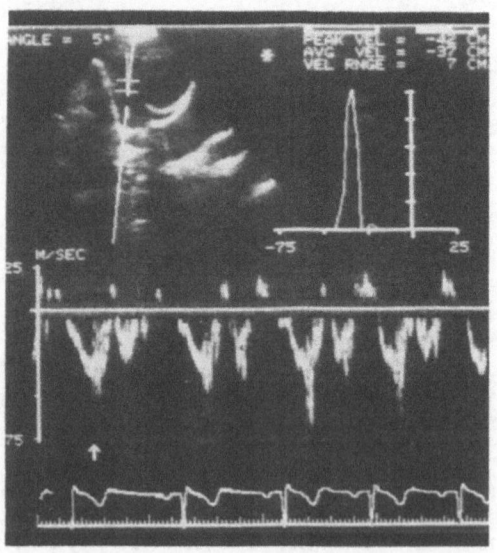

Fig. 4-25. Normal pulsed mode recording of flow in the superior vena cava obtained from the suprasternal window in a normal patient. A more optimal beam-to-flow alignment is possible when recording flow in the superior vena cava than in the inferior vena cava. Consequently, a relatively narrow bandwidth signal is detected and the peak flow velocity is higher in the superior vena cava. It is also easier to record the short period of flow reversal following the P and T wave of the electrocardiogram in the superior vena cava.

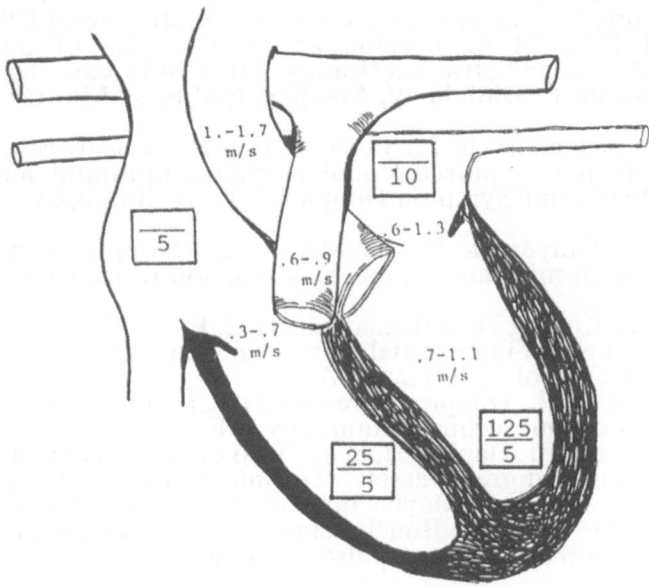

Fig. 4-2.6 The normal range of flow velocities recorded in adults with pulsed Doppler ultrasound, as reported by Hatle et al. The normal ventricular systolic and diastolic pressures (in mm Hg) are indicated within the square boxes. The normal mean pressure (in mm Hg) in the left and right atrium is also indicated.

References

1. Hatle L, Angelsen B, Tromsdal A. Noninvasive assessment of the pulmonary artery systolic pressure with Doppler ultrasound. Br Heart J 1981;45:157.
2. Pearlman AS. Evaluation of ventricular function using Doppler echocardiography. Am J Cardiol 1982;49:324.
3. Lynch J, Sagar K, Wann L. Tricuspid regurgitation in normal subjects: Prevalence and possible mechanism (abstr) J Am Coll Cardiol 1986;7,2:145A.
4. Redel DA. Clinical value and limitations of pulsed Doppler echocardiography in pediatric cardiology. In Cardiovascular Diagnosis by Ultrasound. Hanrath P, Blefeld W, Souquet J(editors) Martinus Nijhoff, The Hague, 1982.
5. Charbel G, Vandenbossche JL, Lenaers A, et al. Non-invasive assessment of left ventricular filling by pulsed Doppler echocardiography and radionuclide angiography (abstr), Intl Symp on Doppler Echocardiography, July 1986, 58 ; Munich.
6. Gardin JM, Drayer JI, Rohan MK, et al. Doppler evaluation of left ventricular filling in mild and severe hypertension (abstr) J Am Coll Cardiol 1986,7;2:185A.
7. Visser CA, de Koning H, Delemarre B, et al. Pulsed Doppler-derived mitral inflow velocity in acute myocardial infarction: An early prognostic indicator (abstr) J Am Coll Cardiol 1986,7;2:136A.
8. Hatle L, Angelsen B. Doppler Ultrasound in Cardiology: Physical Principles and Clinical Application, second edition, Lea & Febiger, Philadelphia 1985.
9. Tajik AJ, Seward JB, Hagler DJ, et al. Two dimensional real time ultrasonic imaging of the heart and great vessels: Technique, image orientation, structure identification and validation. Mayo Clin Proc 53;271-303, 1978.
10. Kalmanson D, Veyrat C, Bouchareine F, et al. Noninvasive recording of mitral flow velocity patterns using pulsed Doppler echocardiography. Br Heart J 39;517, 1977.
11. Baker DW, Rubenstein SA, Lorch GS. Pulsed Doppler echocardiography: Principles and applications. Am J Med 63;69, 1977.
12. Pickoff AS, Bennett V, Soler P, et al. Detection of pulmonary venous flow by pulsed Doppler echocardiography in children. Am Heart J 105;8226, 1983.

CHAPTER 5

APPLICATIONS IN ACQUIRED HEART DISEASE

James V. Chapman
Aurelio Sgalambro M.D.

Determination of the Pressure Gradient

There is a direct relationship between the frequency shift, Fd, and the maximum red cell velocity (Vm), as expressed in Equation 1-2:

$$Vm = [cFd]/[2F'\cos\beta]$$

where c is the acoustic velocity, F' is the transducer frequency, and ß is the angle of incidence between the ultrasonic beam and the blood flow. When obstruction to flow is present, an increase in red cell velocity will occur. By accurately recording the peak transvalvular flow velocity, the pressure gradient existing across the valve can be estimated noninvasively.

Hatle and coworkers have demonstrated that the modified Bernoulli equation can be used to determine the transvalvular pressure gradients. The modified Bernoulli equation is:

$$P1 - P2 = 4 \ (Vm)^2$$

(5-1)

where Vm is the maximum flow velocity recorded across the valve, P1 is the pressure proximal to the valve, and P2 is the presssure distal to the valve. Some confusion may arise regarding the derivation of this simplified equation. The Bernoulli equation is written as follows:

$$P1 - P2 = 1/2(p)(V2^2 - V1^2) + p\int_1 (dV/dt)dS + R(v)$$

(5-2)

where V1 is the peak velocity proximal to the valve, V2 is the velocity distal to the valve, p is the density of blood, and S is the distance over which the flow accelaration takes place. The first term represents the convective acceleration, the second term represents the flow acceleration, and the third term represents the contribution due to viscous friction. The term for flow acceleration is negligible except in high acceleration states as in valve opening or closure. The term for viscous friction, R(v) is also omitted as the ultrasonic beam should be directed to the center of the flow to measure the peak velocity. The effects of viscous friction are not significant in the center of flow but must be considered when examining flow proximal to the vessel or chamber walls.

The equation may then be re-written, leaving out the terms for flow acceleration and viscous friction:

$$P1 - P2 = 1/2 \ (p)(V2^2 - V1^2)$$

(5-3)

If V2, the velocity distal to the obstruction, is assumed to be much greater than V1, V1 may be eliminated from equation 5-3. This is a reasonable assumption in cases where the obstruction is localized to one site, as in valve stenosis.

Equation 5-3 may then be re-written:

$$P1 - P2 = 1/2(p)(V2)^2$$

(5-4)

The constant for the density of blood, denoted as p, is 1060kg/cubic m. Half of this value (1/2p) is then 530 kg/cubic m. This value is stated in units of kg/cubic m, and the pressure drop calculated using these units would be expressed in nts/sq m. This must be converted to mm Hg, since these are the units of presssure utilized in angiography. The conversion is:

$$1 \text{ nt/sq m} = .0075 \text{ mm Hg}$$

So (1/2)p in units of mm Hg is (530)(.0075) or 3.975 mm Hg. This value may be rounded off to 4.0 and inserted into equation 5-4:

$$P1 - P2 = 4 (V2)^2$$

(5-5)

V2 represents the maximum flow velocity distal to the obstruction, and may be replaced by the term Vm:

$$P1 - P2 = 4 (Vm)^2$$

(5-6)

Equation 5-6 is known as the modified or simplified Bernoulli equation. The clinical utility of using confinuous wave Doppler ultrasound to assess the pressure gradient has been well established (1, 2, 4). The greatest source of error lies in the underestimation of the peak flow velocity when a parallel alignment to the interrogated flow is not acheived. When the peak velocity is underestimated, the peak pressure gradient determined by the modified Bernoulli equation will be lower than the actual gradient.

An overestimation of the peak velocity and the presssure gradient will result when an erroneously large angle is assumed to exist between the ultrasonic beam and the interrogated flow. There is no reliable way to ascertain the beam-to-flow angle since the flow is not parallel to the vessel or chamber walls, and the flow is three-dimensional. The best method of obtaining the true peak flow velocity is to use the audio signal to guide the beam into a parallel alignment with the blood flow. An audio signal which contains mostly high frequencies indicates a good alignment to flow, and the recorded flow velocity curve will have a well-defined envelope. Using this technique, continuous wave Doppler ultrasound may be used to determine the pressure gradients across stenotic valves, prosthetic valves, and ventricular septal defects.

It should be noted that the modified Bernoulli equation yields a simultaneous peak pressure gradient, while the catheterization peak gradient represents a peak-to-peak gradient. Variations in heart rate and cardiac output must also be considered when the Doppler-derived pressure gradient is compared to the catheterization gradient.

Aortic Stenosis

Doppler ultrasound is valuable in assessing the severity of aortic stenosis. By using continuous mode to record the aortic flow velocity curve, it is possible to noninvasively estimate the mean transvalvular gradient and the peak simultaneous pressure gradient. Several transducer positions should be used in the examination of aortic flow in order to ensure that the peak flow velocity is recorded. The jet in aortic stenosis is eccentric and one can not predict which position on the chest wall will results in an optimal

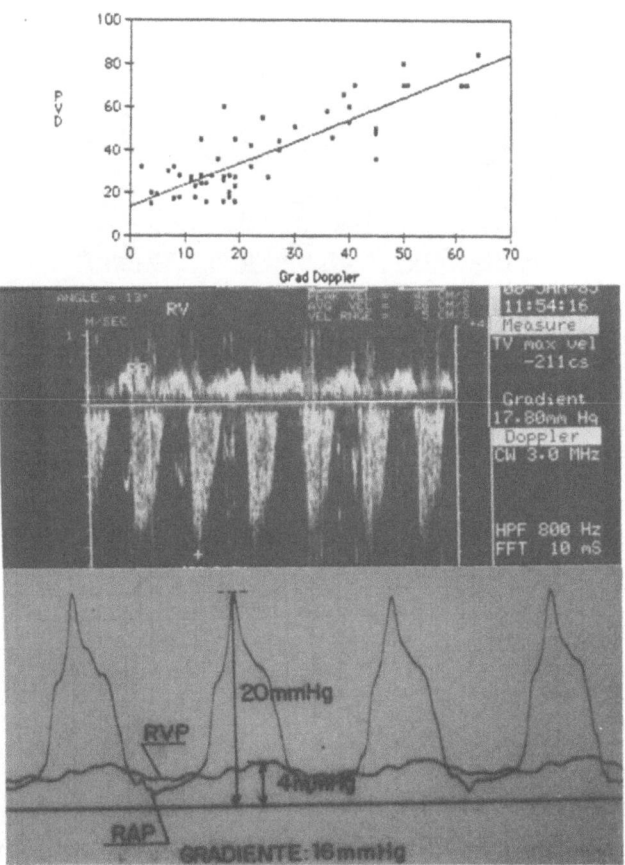

Fig 5-1. A. Correlation between the Doppler estimated gradient and the invasively estimated right ventricular-right atrial gradient in a series of 55 measurements in open-chested dogs. The right ventricular pressure was altered by pulmonary artery banding and volume loading. (Grad Doppler = Doppler-estimated gradient, RVD = invasively meadured right ventricular-right atrial gradient). B. The continuous mode recordng of tricuspid flow; the instantaneous peak gradient is estimated to be 17.8 mm Hg. C. The invasively measured peak to peak gradient is 16 mm Hg.

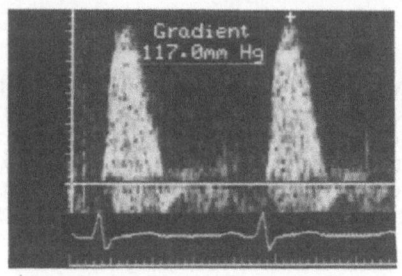

Fig. 5-2 . Continuous mode recording from the right parasternal window in a patient with severe aortic stenosis. The maximal velocity is 5.4 m/s, and the peak gradient is 117 mm Hg.

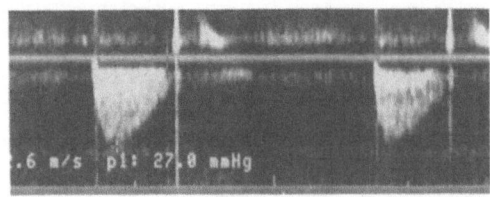

Fig. 5-3 . Continuous mode recording from the apical window in a patient with mild aortic stenosis. The maximal velocity is 2.6 m/s, corresponding to a peak outflow gradient of 27 mm Hg. The spikes for valve opening and closure are clearly recorded in the spectral trace. The flow velocity curve peaks and declines rapidly; this is a finding consistent with the presence of a mild obstruction.

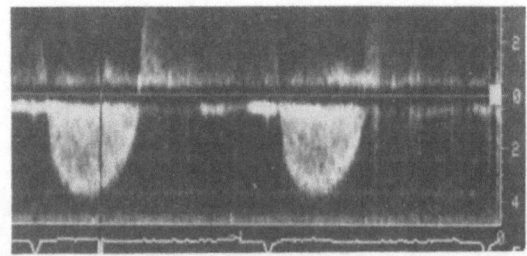

Fig.5- 4 Continuous mode recording form the apical window in a patient with severe aortic stenosis. The peak velocity is 3.8 m/s, and the peak gradient is approximately 58 mm Hg. Nevertheless, the peak velocity declines slowly towards end systole, and the rise time to the peak is prolonged. This indicates the presence of severe obstruction.

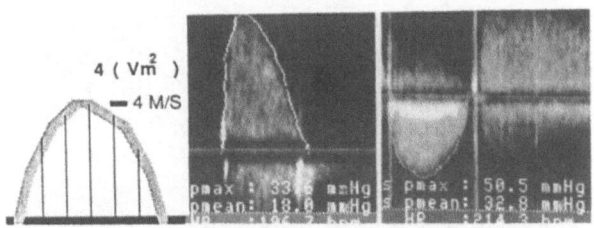

Fig. 5-5. The mean gradient is calculated by measuring the peak velocity at 5 or more intervals along the flow velocity curve, calculating the peak gradient at those points, and then obtaining the average value. The value of the peak gradient is influenced by the cardiac output, and patients with severe obstruction and reduced cardicac output will have a low peak gradient. The mean gradient is more sensitive an indicator of severity. In cases of reduced output, the peak gradient may be low but the mean Doppler-derived gradient will be relatively high.

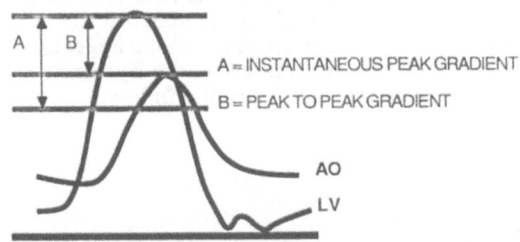

Fig. 5-6. Measurement of the peak gradient in aortic stenosis. The peak transvalvular gradient measured at catheterization is a peak to peak gradient (arrow B), which is a value that does not exist physiologically. The Doppler derived peak gradient is a peak simultaneous gradient (arrow A). A systematic overestimation will occur when comparing the Doppler peak gradient to the catheterization gradient, although the difference between the two values is less in moderate to severe aortic stenosis.

V_2 ONLY	V_1 INCLUDED	V_1 DIFFERENCE	% ERROR
12 mmHg (1.8 m/s)	6.2 mmHg	6.7mmHg(1.3m/s)	52 %
36mmHg (3.0 m/s)	29 mmHg	6.7mmHg(1.3m/s)	19 %
100mmHg(93 m/s)	93 mmHg	6.7mmHg(1.3m/s)	7 %

Fig. 5-7. The effect of neglecting V1 when V1 is 1.3 m/s is calculated in the setting of mild, moderate, and severe obstruction. With increasing severity, the percent error resulting from the exclusion of V1 in the gradient calculation decreases significantly. In this example, the mild obstruction is represented by a peak flow velocity (V2) of 1.8 m/s, the moderate obstruction is represented by a peak flow velocity of 3.0 m/s, and the severe obstruction is represented by a peak flow velocity of 5.0 m/s.

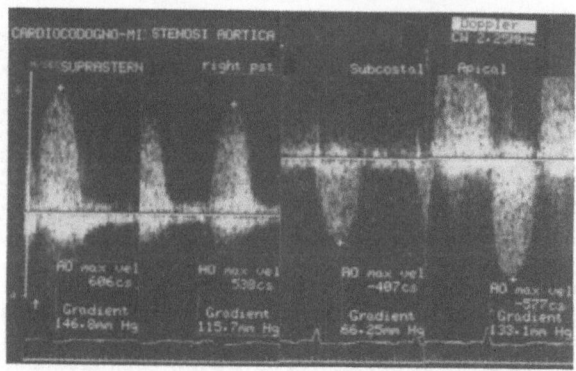

Fig. 5- 8. In aortic stenosis, several transducer positions should be used when attempting to acheive a parallel alignment with the stenotic jet. These four recordings of aortic flow in the same patient were made from the positions indicated on the spectral traces (Suprastern = suprasternal, Right pst = right parasternal). Although the spectral envelope appears to be well-defined from each position, the value of the peak flow velocity varies markedly. In this example, the highest peak velocity (6.06 m/s) was recorded from the suprasternal window.

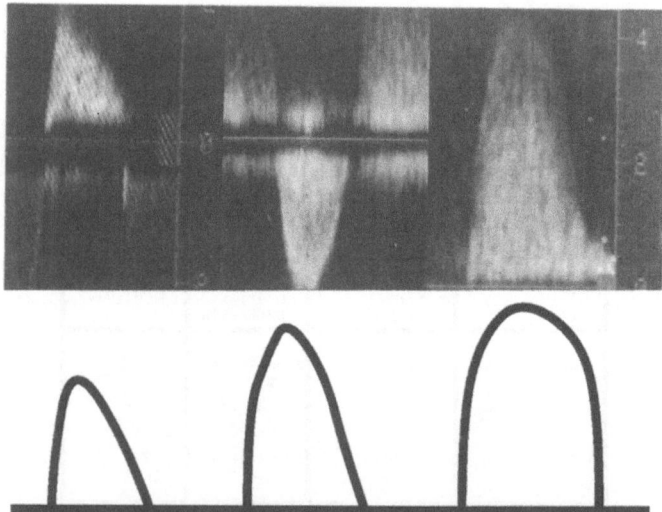

Fig. 5- 9. Pressure time course. The rise time to peak velocity in aortic stenosis should be considered when assessing severity, especially in cases of reduced cardiac output. These three aortic flow patterns were recorded in patients with mild (left), moderate (middle) and severe (right) aortic obstruction. Note how the time interval required for the development of the peak velocity increases with the severity of the obstruction. The deceleration is also more prolonged in severe obstruction, resulting in a bullet-shaped contour of the flow velocity curve.

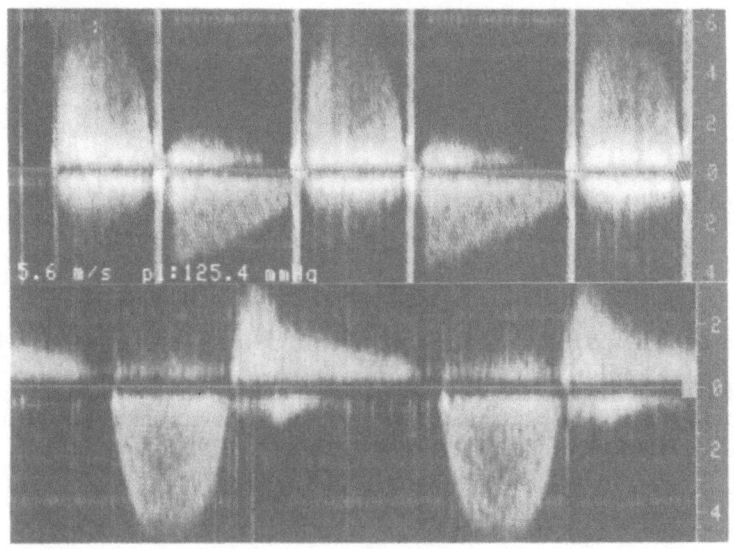

Fig .5-10. Continuous mode recordings of aortic flow in severe aortic stenosis recorded from the right parasternal window (top) and the apical window. The peak velocity recorded from the apical window is higher than that obtained from the right parasternal window . The aortic regurgitation was detected from the right parasternal window, and the apex . The variability of the jet direction in aortic stenosis makes it impossible to predict which imaging window will yield the clearest flow velocity curve and the highest peak velocity.

recording of the high frequencies in the flow signal. Often the right parasternal position provides the best access to the stenotic jet, and the spectral trace of aortic flow has a clearly delineated envelope. In some cases, the apical or subcostal recordings of aortic flow provide the best alignment to the jet. By relying upon the audio signal, the transducer angulation can be changed slightly until a signal with mostly high frequencies is heard. A recording of the flow velocity curve should then be made. In cases of congenital aortic stenosis, the suprasternal window frequently provides the best beam-to-flow alignment.

The simultaneous peak pressure gradient is estimated by applying the modified Bernoullii equation (2-5). An increased flow velocity may be recorded in high output states or when moderate to severe aortic insufficiency is present. If the peak velocity is high due to increased cardiac output, the left ventricular ouflow velocity will be high as well. Increased flow velocities will be recorded across all the other valves. In cases of aortic insufficiency, the increased peak velocity reflects the increased volume of flow. More blood must be ejected in systole to compensate for the regurgitant volume. The presence of a valvular obstruction is established when the flow velocity increases rapidly at the level of the aortic orifice. Calculation of the mean pressure gradient is important in aortic stenosis. The peak velocity will be sustained in a severe obstruction, and the estimated mean gradient will be high.

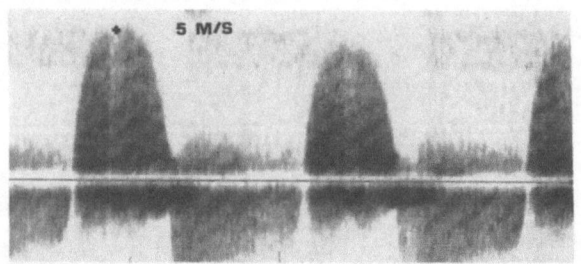

Fig. 5-11. Continuous mode recording of aortic flow from the right parasternal window in severe aortic stenosis.   like the previous example, the regurgitation could be clearly recorded from the right parasternal window. The peak flow velocity is 5.0 m/s, corresponding to a peak transvalvular gradient of 100 mm Hg. The rise time to the peak velocity is increased and the maximum velocity declines slowly, indicating that a severe obstruction is present.

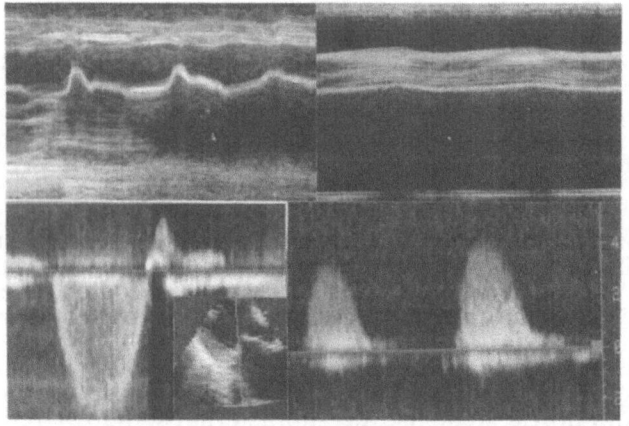

Fig. 5-12. Using the apical transducer position the continuous wave Doppler is swept from the mitral valve to the aortic valve . The TM sweep is aldo displayed

Aortic Stenosis - Factors to consider

1) Peak Gradient and mean gradient
2) Pressure time course
3) Is regugitation detected in the descending aorta ?
4) Aortic insufficiency pressure halftime and deceleration slope

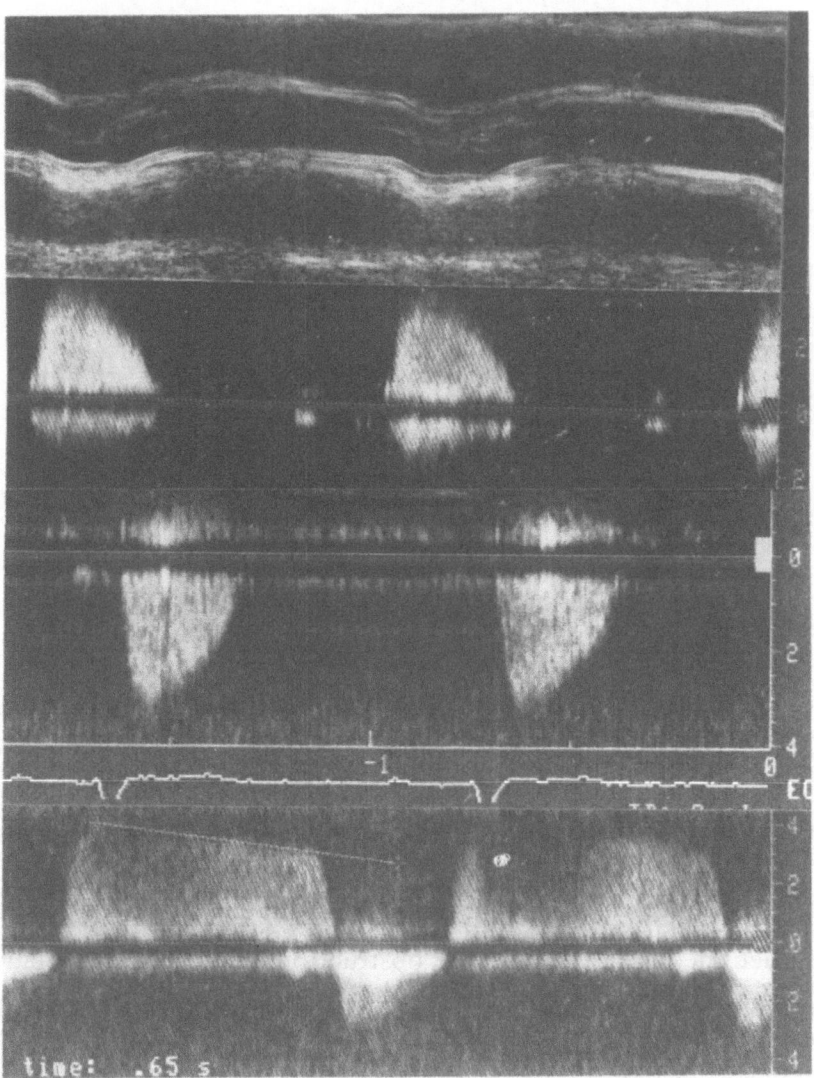

Fig. 5-13. Moderate aortic stenosis. A. The M-mode recording of the aortic valve demonstrates reduced cusp separation and thickened aortic cusps. B. Continous mode recording of aortic flow from the right parasternal window. The peak velocity is 3.6 m/s, corresponding to a peak gradient of approximately 52.3 mm Hg. C. Continous mode recording of the aortic flow from the apical window. The maximal flow velocity in this trace is approximately 3.2 m/s. D. With a slight change in angulation, aortic regurgitation was recorded from the apex, although it was not detected from the right parasternal window. The regurgitant signal was weak, indicating that the regurgitation was mild. The aortic regurgitation half time (650 ms) indicates the left ventricular end diastolic pressure is not elevated.

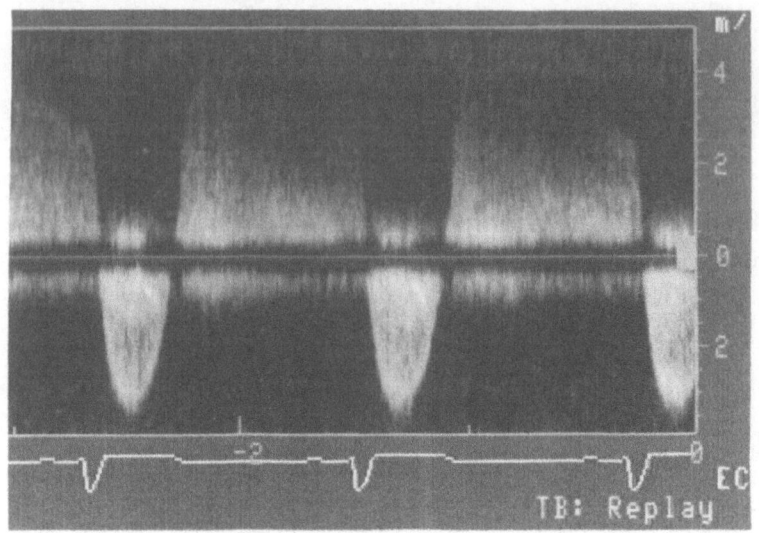

Fig.5-14.   Continuous mode recording of aortic flow from the apical window in a patient with moderately severe aortic stenosis and insufficiency.

If the maximal velocity is high but the left ventricular ejection time is short, the obstruction is less severe than an equivalent peak velocity with a long ejection time.

In cases of combined aortic stenosis and insufficiency, the peak velocity may be increased to compensate for the regurgitant flow volume. Consequently, the peak instantaneous pressure gradient may be difficult to interpret. A combined aortic stenosis and regurgitation of moderate severity may yield a peak pressure drop indicative of a more severe obstruction. However, calculation of the mean pressure gradient in such cases will enable one to differentiate between a severe obstruction and a moderate obstruction with regurgitation. The mean gradient in the combined lesion will be lower than the mean gradient in a severe obstruction. The maximal velocity will decline slowly in a severe obstruction, resulting in a relatively high mean gradient.

The spectral trace is more rounded in appearance in severe stenosis because of the delay in the development of the peak flow velocity. The contour of the aortic spectral trace in severe stenosis has been described as bullet-shaped due to the prolongation of the development of the peak velocity and the slow decline of the peak flow velocity.

Estimation of the Aortic Valve Area

Estimation of the aortic valve area with Doppler techniques is possible, and several methods have been proposed. One method is based upon the principle that the stroke volume measured at each of the cardiac valves should be the same. The aortic valve area can therefore be estimated from the stroke volume measured at another sampling site:

$$AVA = \frac{SVnd}{(\overline{Vmn})(ET)}$$

where AVA is the aortic valve area, SVnd is the stoke volume measured across a nondiseased valve, Vmn is the aortic mean velocity, and ET is the left ventricular ejection time. The aortic mean velocity can be obtained by planimetering the aortic flow velocity curve. The ejection time is measured directly from the Doppler recording of aortic flow. The success of this method depends upon the maintenance of a constant heart rate during the examination, and the accuracy of the Doppler-derived stroke volume measured at the nondiseased valve. The stroke volume at the nondiseased valve is calculated with the following equation:

$$SVnd = (VTI)(A)$$

where VTI is the velocity time integral of the nondiseased flow velocity curve and A is the cross-sectional area of the nondiseased valve. If there is a variation in heart rate during the examination, the stroke volume measured at the nondiseased valve can not be assumed to be equal to the stroke volume at the aortic valve.

A second method is based upon the continuity equation, which states that flow across a cross=section in a closed circuit must be equal to the flow measured at another given cross-section. This equation may be applied in the setting of aortic stenosis to derive the orifice area. Flow in the left ventricular outflow tract must equal the aortic flow:

$$V_{lv} A_{lv} = V_{ao} MA_{ao}$$

(5-6)

where V_{ao} and V_{lv} represent the peak velocity recorded in the aorta and left ventricular ouflow tract, respectively. The peak velocity in the outflow tract should be measured at a distance of about 1.0 cm below the aortic valve to avoid the prestenotic region of increased velocity. Either high pulse repetition frequency or pulsed mode may be used to measure the outflow velocity. A_{lv} is the left ventricular outflow tract area, and MA_{ao} is the maximal aortic orifice area. The left ventricular outflow area is estimated from the outflow tract diameter measured in the two-dimensional image. The diameter should be estimated at the same level from which the pulsed Doppler recording was obtained. Rearranging:

$$MA_{ao} = [V_{lv} A_{lv}] / V_{ao}$$

(5-7)

Because the value of the pressure gradient changes during left ventricular ejection, it is helpful to derive a mean aortic valve area (Aao)

$$VTI_{lv}\ A_{lv} = VTI_{ao}\ A_{ao}$$
(5-8)

where VTI(lv) and VTO(ao) represent the velocity time integrals of the left ventricular outflow tract and the aorta, respectively. Rearranging:

$$A_{ao} = (\overline{VTI}_{lv}\ A_{lv}\ ) / VTI_{ao}$$
(5-9)

AORTIC VALVE AREA

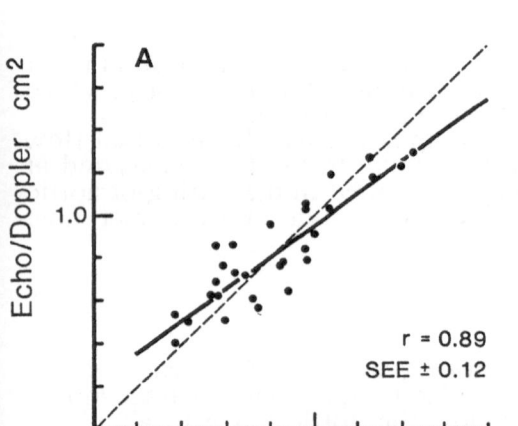

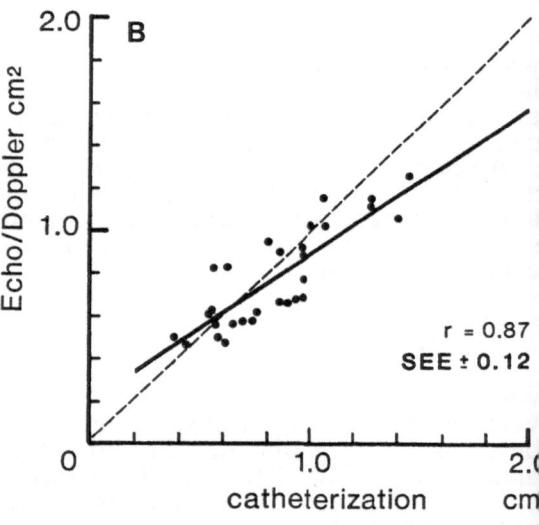

Fig.5-15 A . The data of Skjaerpe et al (personal communication) showing the statistical correlation between the aortic valve area calculated by Doppler technique using the peak flow velocities in the continuity equation, and the aortic valve area estimated from the Gorlin formula. Figure 5-15 B. The data of Skjaerpe et al showing the statistical correlation between the aortic valve area calculated by Doppler techniques and the invasively derived aortic valve area. The cardiac output was estimated by Fick's method, and the aortic valve area was estimated by application of the Gorlin formula. Noninvasive results are based on integration of the velocity curves.

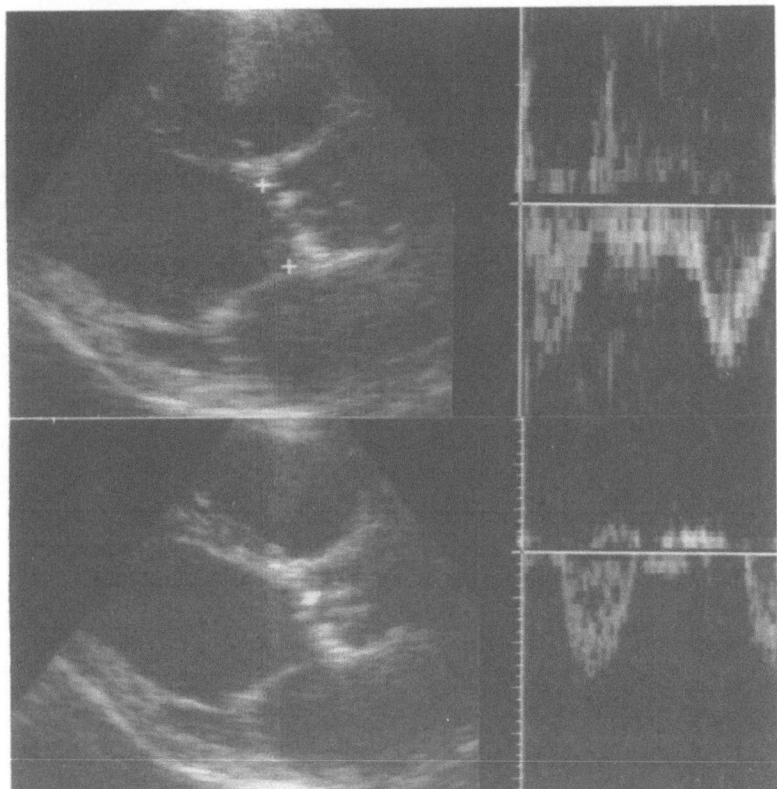

Fig.5-16 . Aortic stenosis in a patient with a low cardiac output. Due to the presence of reduced output, the continuity equation was used to estimate the aortic valve area. Top left. The diameter of the left ventricular outflow tract was 2.52 cm. Top right. The left ventricular ouflow was interrogated from the apical window and the peak ouflow velocity was approximately .42 m/s. Bottom left. Parasternal long axis view of the aortic valve. Bottom right. Continuous mode recording of aortic flow from the apical window. The peak velocity was slightly over 3.0 m/s, corresponding to a peak gradient of 37 mm Hg. By application of the continuity equation, the aortic valve area was estimated to be 0.7 sq cm. The cardiac output was estimated to be 2.42 l/min/sq m with Doppler techniques, while the output measured during catheterization was 2.9 l/min/sq m.

Good correlations with invasive estimates of aortic valve area have been reported by Skjearpe and coworkers using both derivations of the continuity equation. The value of the orifice area obtained by this method will not be affected by the presence of aortic insufficiency or decreased left ventricular function.

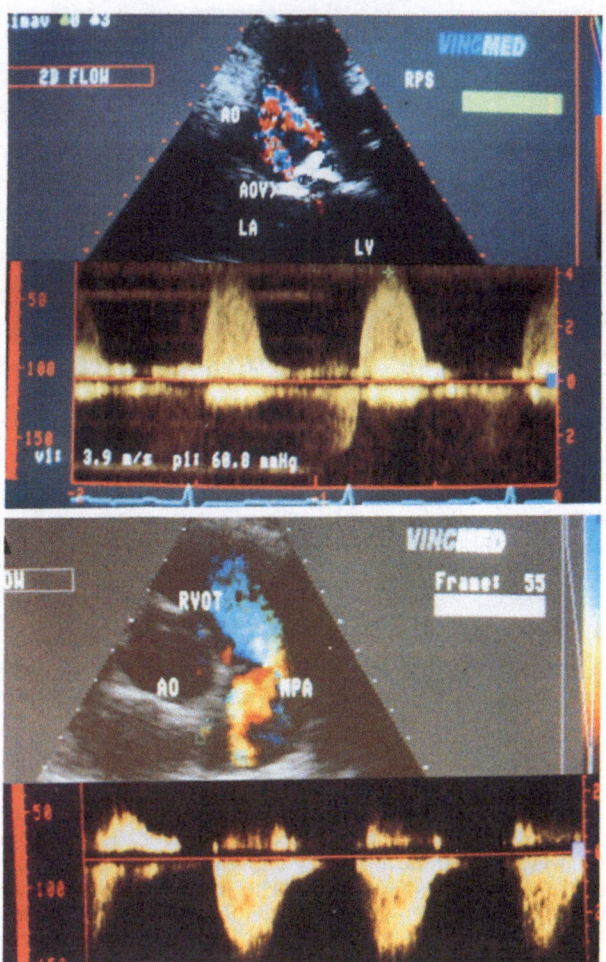

Fig. 5-17 . Color flow imaging in stenotic lesions. Although the flow imaging mode is two-dimensional whereas flow is three dimensional, the color flow display often allows one to select the best position for flow interrogation with continuous mode. Top. Aortic stenosis. The mosaic pattern seen in the color flow display represents the stenotic jet. Note the eccentricity of the jet and the change in jet direction after the jet strikes the aortic wall. In this case, the best window for recording the aortic flow was the right parasternal window. Bottom. Pulmonary stenosis. Using a different color scheme, the pulmonary flow in a patient with pulmonary obstruction was examined from a parasternal short axis view. The blue bolus of flow represents right ventricular outflow, while the aliased yellow-orange flow represents the flow past the obstruction. Using continuous mode, the pulmonary flow was interrogated from a low parasternal position.

Mitral Stenosis

The jet in mitral stenosis can usually be interrogated with continuous wave Doppler ultrasound from the apical window. The investigation can also be performed with high pulse repetition frequency mode. Due to the presence of moderately increased flow velocities and high signal strengths, high pulse repetition frequency mode can be applied with acceptable results.

The Bernoulli equation can be utilized to calculate the peak diastolic gradient, but a mean gradient should also be calculated. One may estimate the mean gradient by measuring the maximal velocity at several points on the flow velocity curve, calculating the gradient at each point, and then obtaining the mean diastolic gradient (3 , 5). Changes in heart rate or cardiac output will alter the value of the mean and peak gradient.

Another method of estimating the severity of the obstruction is to calculate the pressure halftime. The pressure halftime is the period of time required for the peak diastolic pressure to decrease to half its initial value. This parameter is not significantly affected by changes in heart rate or cardiac output, and is easy to estimate. Once the peak velocity has been measured, the value of the pressure halftime velocity can be obtained by dividing the peak velocity by $\sqrt{2}$. The time interval from the peak velocity to the pressure halftime velocity, or pressure haltime, is then measured. Hatle et al have shown that the normal range for the pressure halftime is 20-60 ms. When mild obstruction is present, the pressure halftime ranges from 100-200 ms. Moderate obstruction is indicated when the pressure halftime lies between 200-300 ms, and sever obstruction is indicated by a pressure halftime greater than 400 ms. Slightly prolonged pressure halftimes of 60-120 ms are frequently found in a nonobstructed valve when significant mitral regurgitation exists. The measurement of the pressure halftime is made on the passive filling component of the flow velocity curve regardless of the amplitude of the atrial component.

Hatle et al have described a method of calculating the mitral orifice area from the estimated pressure halftime using the following empirical formula:

$$MVA = 220/PH$$

where MVA is the mitral valve area in sq cm and PHT is the pressure halftime. When the cardiac rhythm is irregular, at least five beats should be measured and the mean value of the pressure halftime used to estimate the orifice area. (Fig. 5-41)

Friart and coworkers compared the Hatle method of estimating the valve area to the standard two-dimensional method. The reproducibility was superior with the Hatle method, and the inter-observer variability was reduced. Bosiljanoff and

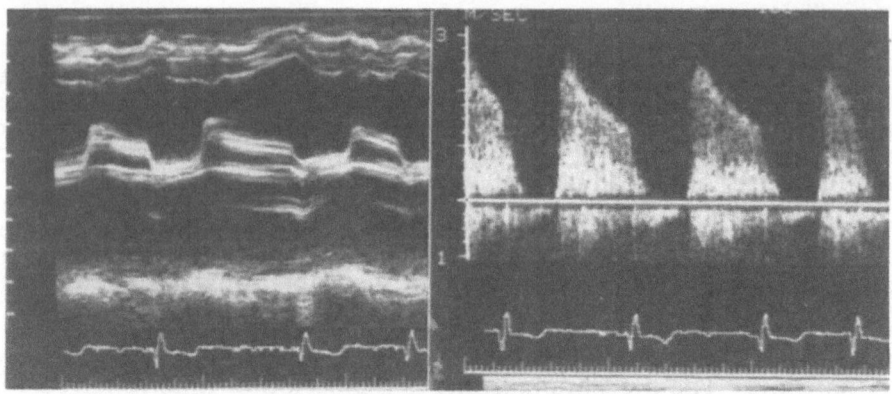

Fig. 5-19 . Severe mitral stenosis. Right. Continuous wave recording of transmitral flow from the apical window. The peak velocity is 2.5 m/s, and the peak diastolic gradient is 25 mm Hg. The average pressure half time is 300 ms. Left . The M-mode recording of the mitral valve shows the characteristic thickened appearance of the mitral leaflets and reduced EF slope.

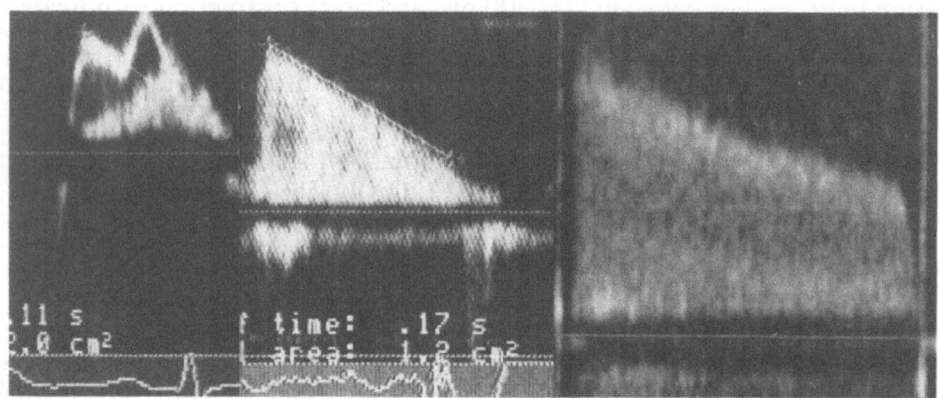

Fig. 5-20 . Mitral flow patterns in mild (A), moderate (B), and severe (C) mitral stenosis. Patient A is in sinus rhythm, the peak flow velocity is 1.25 m/s, and the pressure half time is 120 ms. In patient B, the peak velocity is 1.5 m/s, and the average pressure half time is 200 ms. In patient C, the peak velocity, the peak velocity is also 1.5 m/s. However, the average pressure half time is 300 ms. The peak flow velocity and the Doppler-derived gradient can change appreciably with heart rate and cardiac output. The pressure half time changes less with variations in these parameters, although a slight beat to beat difference may be noted. When the cardiac rhythm is regular, 3 to 5 halftime measurements should be made and averaged.

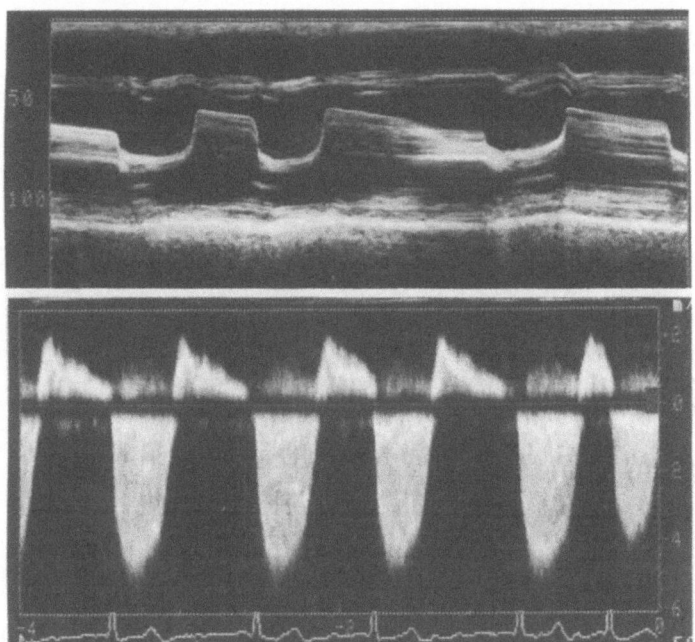

Fig. 5-21 . Severe mitral stenosis with insufficiency. The continuous wave recording of transmitral flow from the apical window. The peak velocity is 2.0 m/s, and the peak diastolic gradient is 16 mm Hg. The average pressure half time is 250ms. Bottom. The M-mode recording of the mitral valve shows the characteristic thickened appearance of the mitral leaflets and reduced EF slope.

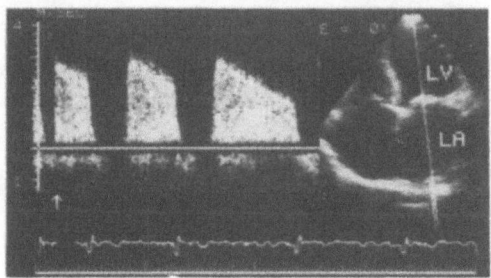

Fig. 5-22. Continuous mode recording of mitral flow in a patient with moderately severe mitral stenosis. The peak flow velocity is 3.0 m/s, and the Doppler-derived peak gradients is 36 mm Hg, Because this patient is in atrial fibrilation a uniphasic flow pattern is recorded. The atrial flow component is ignored when calculating the pressure half time (TG1/2) which in this case is 250 ms. The estimated orifice area is 0.88 sq cm.

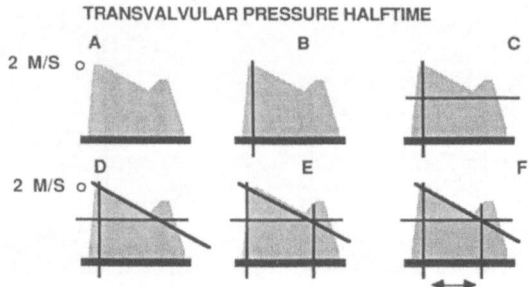

TRANSVALVULAR PRESSURE HALFTIME

Fig. 5-23 . Calculation of the Pressure Half Time
A. The peak velocity of the passive filling component is measured.
   (2.0 m/s in this example).

B. The pressure half velocity y, is obtained by dividing the peak velocity by the square root
   of 2.
   y = peak velocity / 1.4
C. A horizontal line is drawn at the point of the pressure half.
D. The time interval required for the peak velocity to decrease to
   the pressure half velocity is the pressure half time.
E. The pressure half time is indicated by the black arrows.
   The lower panel is an example of an actual halftime measurement in a moderately severe
   stenosis.

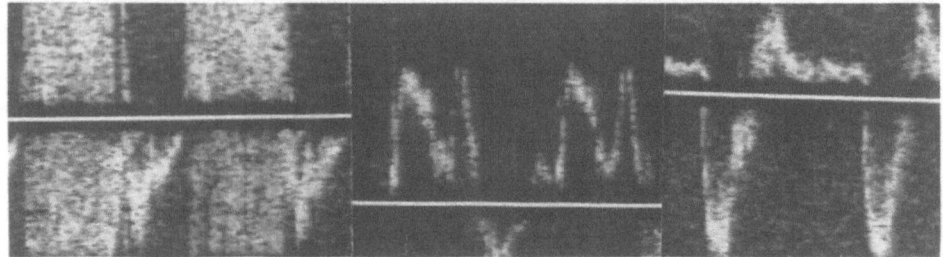

Fig. 5-24. Mild mitral stenosis and aortic insufficiency. A. Pulsed mode recording from the apical window. A small sample volume is used to record the regurgitant flow behind the aortic valve. The regurgitant flow signal is quite intense from this position. B. Pulsed mode recording of mitral flow from the apex. The mitral flow velocity curve appears normal in configuration, but the average pressure half time is slightly prolonged (110 ms). C. Pulsed mode recording of flow in the descending aorta from the suprasternal window. The reversed diastolic flow represents the regurgitation. A high pass filter setting of 400 Hz has been selected so that none of the regurgitant flow signal is unintentionally filtered out.

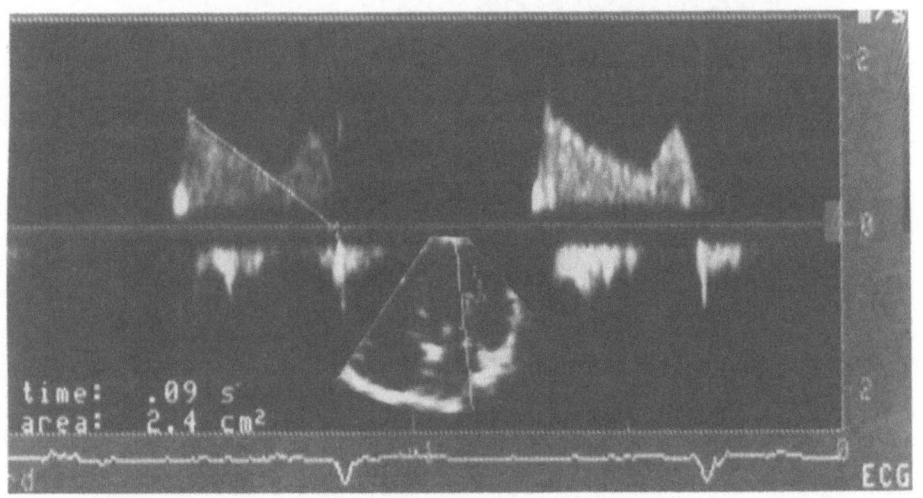

Fig. 5-25. Continuous mode recording of mitral flow in a patient with mild mitral stenosis. The peak flow velocity is 1.75 m/s, and the Doppler-derived peak gradients is 12 mm Hg. Because this patient is in sinus rhythm, a biphasic flow pattern is recorded. The atrial flow component is ignored when calculating the pressure half time which in this case is 90 ms. The estimated orifice area is 2.4 sq cm.

coworkers demonstrated a close linear correlation between the Doppler-derived values for mitral valve area and the invasively derived valves (r =0.96) in their study of 100 mitral stenosis patients.

Color flow analysis demonstrates a characteristic flow pattern in mitral stenosis. The mitral jet tends to flow along the posterior wall of the left ventricle, curving at end-diastole into the outflow tract. Occasionally multiple jets will be seen emanating from the stenotic orifice. Flow mapping has been proposed as a means of directly delineating the mitral orifice. From the short-axis view, the mitral flow at the orifice level could be planimetered and the flow area calculated. At this time, the efficacy of this method has not been established. Improper use of the flow gain in color flow analysis may result in the over or underestimation of the orifice area using this technique. The pressure halftime technique of estimating the orifice area is well-established and easy to implement.

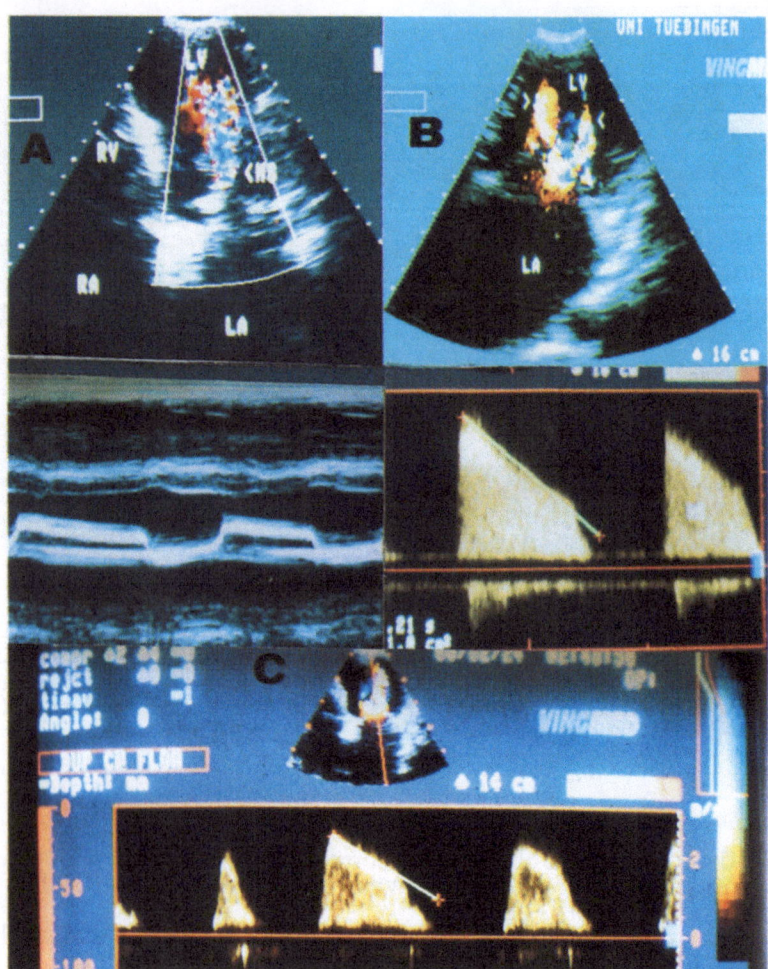

Fig. 5-26. Color flow imaging in mitral stenosis. A. Color flow display of the stenotic jet from the apical window using the red/blue color assignment. The mosaic pattern seen is characteristic of stenotic flows. The M-mode recording of the mitral valve demonstrates the thickened appearance of the mitral leaflets. B. Color flow display of mitral flow in another patient with mitral stenosis using the rainbow color assignment . A twin jet may be seen emanating from the mitral orifice. To obtain an accurate continuous mode recording of the mitral flow, the ultrasonic beam must be aligned with one of the mitral jets. The average pressure halftime measured from the continuous mode trace is 200 ms, indicating that moderately severe obstruction is present. C. Mixed modality assessment of mitral stenosis. Once an adequate color flow display of the stenotic jet has been obtained, the continuous mode cursor is aligned with the visualized jet. The audio signal is then used to guide the continuous wave beam into a parallel alignment with the three dimensional jet.

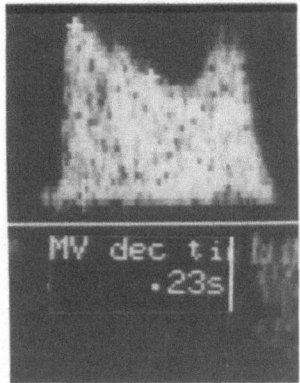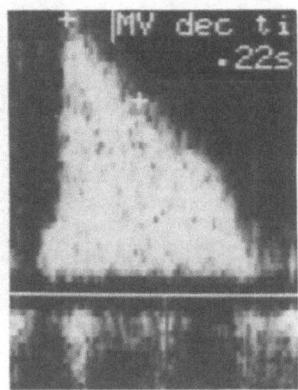

Fig. 5-27 . The peak gradient is not a reliable indicator of severity in mitral stenosis because it is influenced by the cardiac output and the presence of mitral regurgitation. The pressure half time, in contrast, is less affected by changes in these parameters. The peak gradient in A is approximately 16 mm Hg, whereas the peak gradient in B is 36 mm Hg. The pressure halftimes in both traces are nearly the same: 230 ms in A, 220 ms in B.

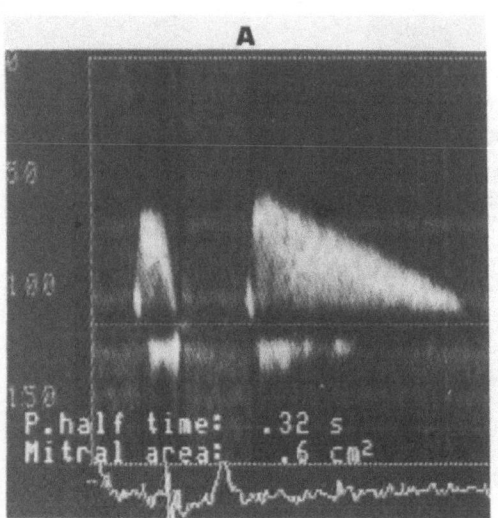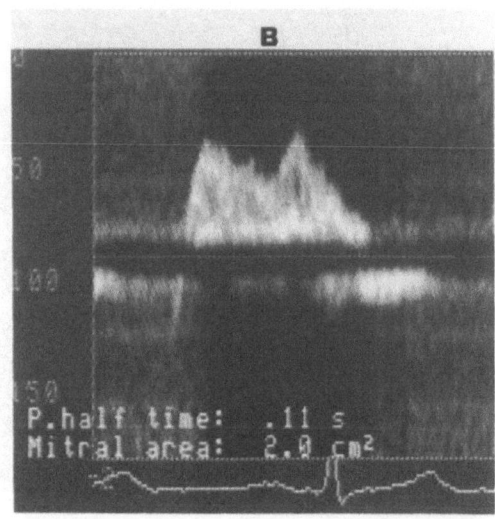

Fig. 5-28 . The peak diastolic gradient in recording A is nearly identical to that in recording B, hence the peak gradients are almost the same. The pressure half time in A (320 ms) however, is much more prolonged than that in B (110 ms). Severe obstruction is present in patient A, and the estimated mitral orifice area is 0.69 sq cm. Only mild obstruction is present in patient B; the estimated mitral orifice area is 2.0 sq cm.

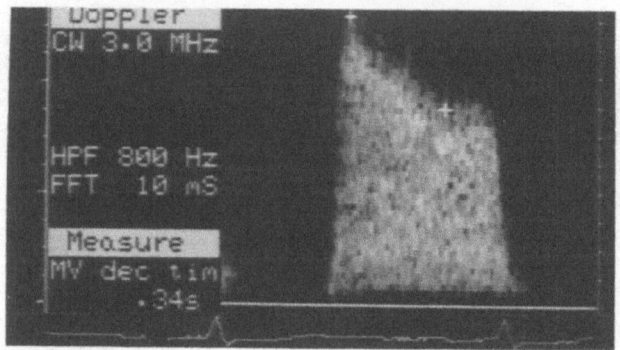

Fig.5-29. Severe mitral stenosis. The slow decline of the peak velocity in this continous mode recording of mitral flow indicates that the mean gradient is high, and the pressure halftime is prolonged. In this case, the pressure half time is 320 ms, and the estimated orifice area is 0.65 sq cm.

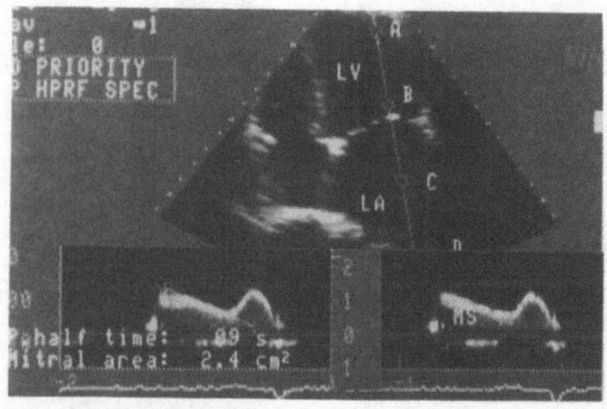

Fig.5-30. High pulse repetitiion frequency recording of mitral flow in a patient with mitral stenosis. The positions of the four range gates are indicated in the four chamber view. Range gate B, at a level slightly downstream from the mitral annulus, is the primary sample volume. Due to the large interrogation depth, the mitral flow was aliased when recording with pulsed mode. High pulse repetition frequency mode was then utilized to record the mitral flow and thereby resolve the peak velocity of 1.6 m/s. The average pressure half time is 90 ms, indicating the presence of mild obstruction.

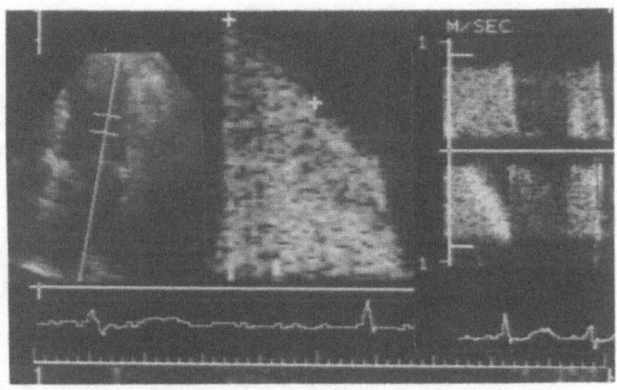

Fig. 5-31. Pulsed mode recording of mitral flow in mitral stenosis. The mitral flow signal has wrapped around to the other side of the baseline, and the peak of the flow velocity curve can be seen superimposed within the aliased spectral trace. The continous mode recording of the mitral flow in which the peak velocity of 2.5 m/s is resolved. The average pressure half time is 220 ms, corresponding to an orifice area of 1.2 sq cm.

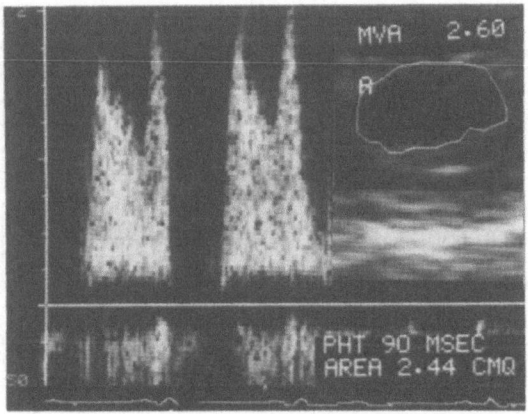

Fig. 5-32. The two-dimensional versus the Doppler method of estimating the mitral valve area. Top. Planimetry of the short axis view of the mitral area; the calculated area is 2.60 sq cm. In technically difficult patients, it may be time consuming to obtain an adequate two-dimensional view of the mitral orifice. Bottom. Continuous wave recording of mitral flow from the apical window. The average pressure half time (PHT) is 90 ms, corresponding to a mitral valve area of 2.44 sq cm. The Doppler estimation of mitral valve area is rapid and reliable. It is possible to obtain a Doppler recording of mitral flow even in technically difficult patients.

105

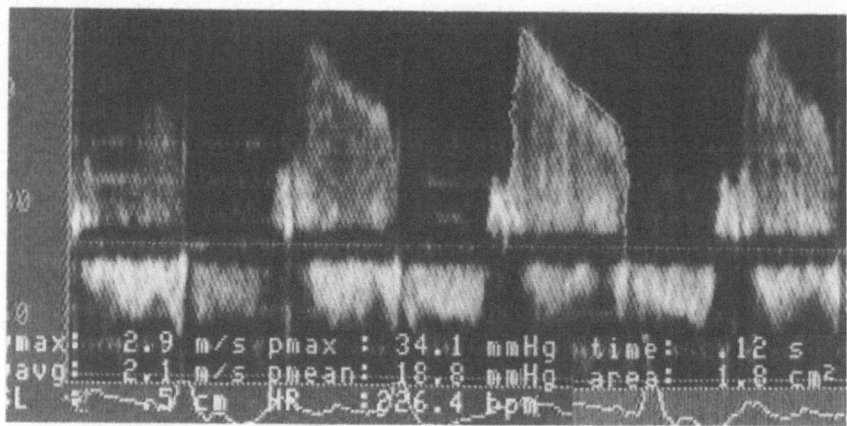

Fig. 5-33. Top. The mean gradient may be calculated manually as described in the text, or it may be estimated on line by planimetry of the flow velocity curve. In this continuous mode recording of the mitral flow, the mean gradient is approximately 19 mm Hg. Bottom. The pressure half time measured in the same patient is 120 ms.

$$\frac{220}{PHT} = MVA$$

A)	60 MS	3.6 CM^2	NORMAL
B)	100 MS	2.2 CM^2	MILD
C)	200 MS	1.1 CM^2	MODERATE
D)	300 MS	.73 CM^2	SEVERE

Fig. 5-34 . The empirical formula for estimating the mitral valve orifice area from the pressure half time. A pressure half time less than 60 ms is found in most normal mitral flow patterns.

106

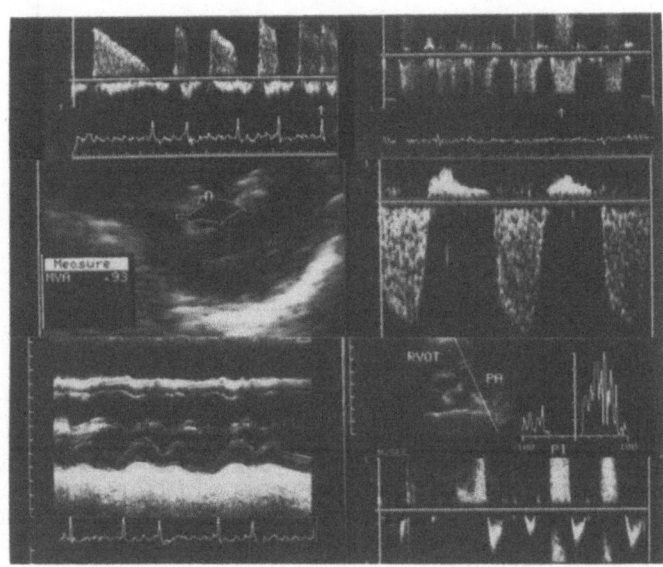

Fig. 5-35 . Mitral stenosis and pulmonary hypertension. A. Continuous mode recording of mitral flow. The peak velocity is moderately elevated and the average pressure half time is 225 ms. The Doppler-derived mitral orifice area is .97 sq cm. B. The planimetered mitral orifice area from the two-dimensional image is 0.93 sq cm. C. The M-mode recording demonstrates the presence of thickened mitral leaflets. D. Tricuspid insufficiency was detected with pulsed mode from the apical position. E. Continuous mode recording of tricuspid flow. The regurgitant peak velocity is 3.4 m/s, corresponding to an estimated systolic pulmonary artery pressure of 46 mm Hg. F. Pulsed mode recording of the mild pulmonary insufficiency detected from the parasternal window.

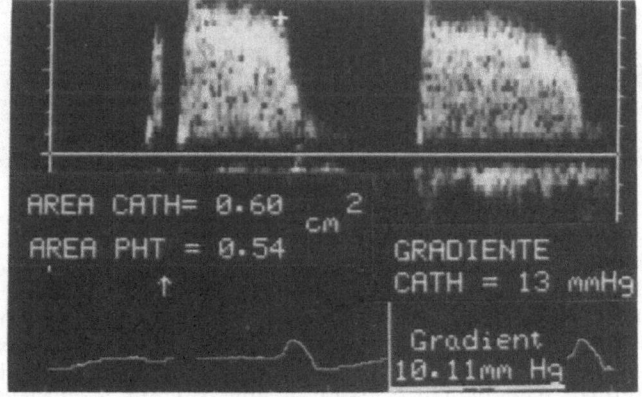

Fig. 5-36 . Top. Severe mitral stenosis. The Doppler-derived mitral valve orifice area (AREA PHT) was estimated to be 0.54 sq cm. The orifice area measured at catheterization was 0.60 sq cm.

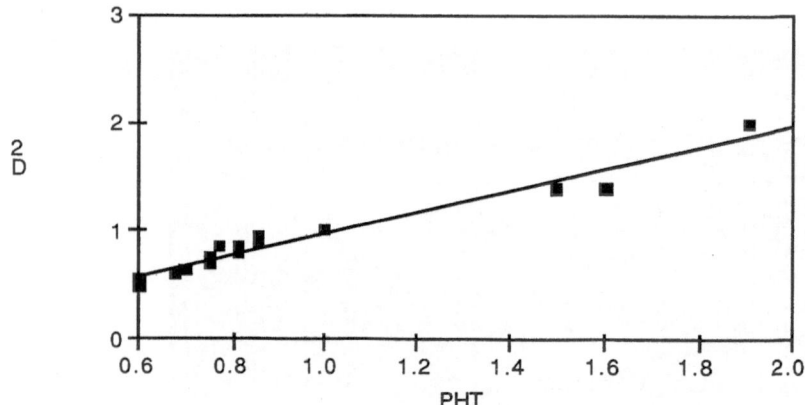

Fig. 5-37 . In a small study group (15 patients) we compared the mitral valve area (MVA) measured by direct planemetry of the 2D echo defined MVA and that measured by the pressure halftime method (PHT) . This study demonstrates a good correlation between the methods when both studies are of acceptable quality (which established one of the criteria for the selection of the patient population .

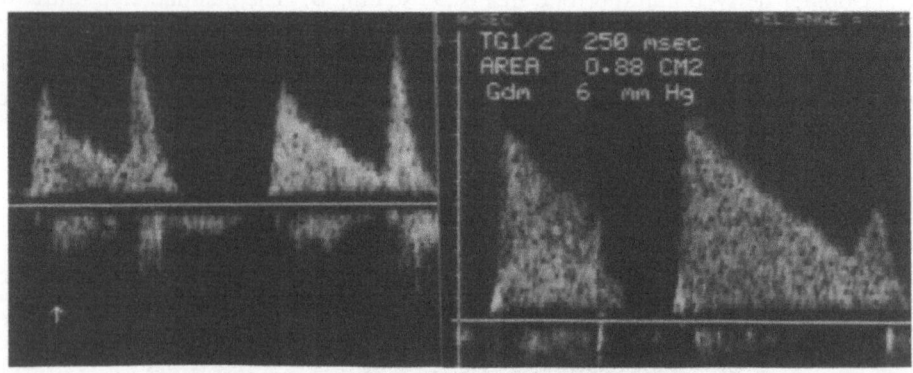

Fig. 5-38 . Continuous mode recording of mitral flow in a patient with moderately severe mitral stenosis. The peak flow velocity is 2.0 m/s, and the Doppler-derived peak gradient is 16 mm Hg . Because this patient is in sinus rhythm, a biphasic flow pattern is recorded. In figure B Continuous mode was used to measure mitral flow in a patient with moderately severe mitral stenosis. The peak flow velocity is 2.25 m/s, and the Doppler-derived peak gradients is 20 mm Hg. This patient is also in a sinus rhythm, a biphasic flow pattern is recorded. The atrial flow component is ignored when calculating the pressure half time even when it is a higher velocity than the initial filling period, as in example A . The pressure halftime is 250 ms. The estimated orifice area is 0.88 sq cm.

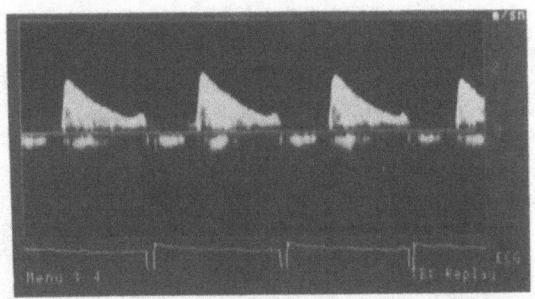

Fig. 5-39 .Mild mitral stenosis. Continuous wave recording of transmitral flow from the apical window. The peak velocity is 2.0 m/s, and the peak diastolic gradient is 16 mm Hg. The average pressure half time is 110ms.

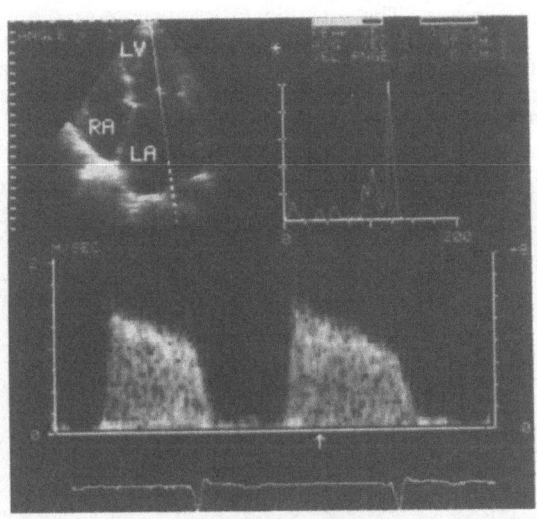

Fig.5-40 . Continuous mode recording of mitral flow in a patient with mitral stenosis. The peak flow velocity is 1.5 m/s, corresponding to a peak diastolic gradient of 9.0 mm Hg. The average pressure halftime is 310 ms, and the estimated valve area is 0.70 sq cm. The power spectrum taken at the point indicated by the vertical arrow below the baseline is plotted on the right side of the display. A narrow band of high velocity signals is seen, confirming a parallel alignment with the mitral jet. The lower velocity signals in the power spectrum originate from blood flow within the left ventricle and the left atrium.

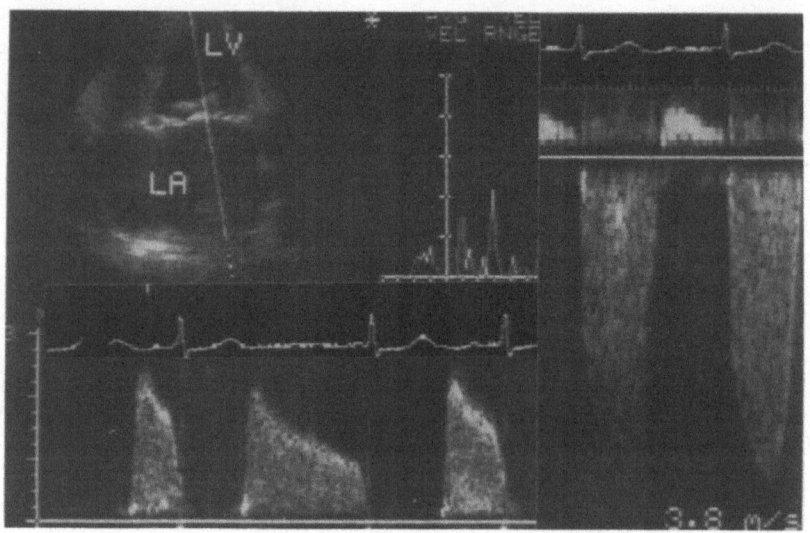

Fig. 5-41. Mitral stenosis with pulmonary hypertension. Left. Continuous mode recording of mitral flow from the apical window. The peak diastolic pressure gradient is approximately 20 mm Hg. The average pressure halftime is 160 ms, corresponding to an estimated valve area of 1.3 sq cm. Right. Continuous mode recording of the tricuspid regurgitation in the same patient. The peak regurgitant flow velocity is 3.8 m/s. Applying the Bernoulli equation, the peak systolic pulmonary artery pressure is estimated to be 58 mm Hg.

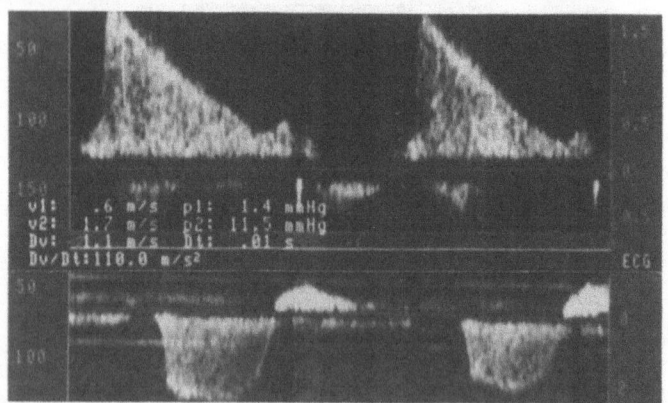

Fig.5-42. Mitral stenosis without pulmonary hypertension. Top. Continuous mode recording of mitral flow from the apical window. The peak diastolic pressure gradient is approximately 16 mm Hg. The average pressure halftime is 170 ms, corresponding to an estimated valve area of 1.2 sq cm. Bottom. Continuous mode recording of the tricuspid regurgitation in the same patient. The peak regurgitant flow velocity is 2.25 M/S . Applying the Bernoulli equation, the peak systolic pulmonary artery pressure is estimated to be 20 mm Hg.

Tricuspid Stenosis

Tricuspid stenosis is an infrequently encountered lesion which almost invariably coexists with mitral stenosis. Simultaneous measurement of the right atrial and right ventricular pressure is needed in order to demonstrate a right ventricular-right atrial gradient at catheterization. The continuous mode recording in cases of tricuspid stenosis is similar to the recording in mitral stenosis, although the peak velocity is usually lower in tricuspid stenosis. The value of the peak velocity may show a marked increase with inspiration. The peak diastolic gradient and the mean gradient should also be estimated.

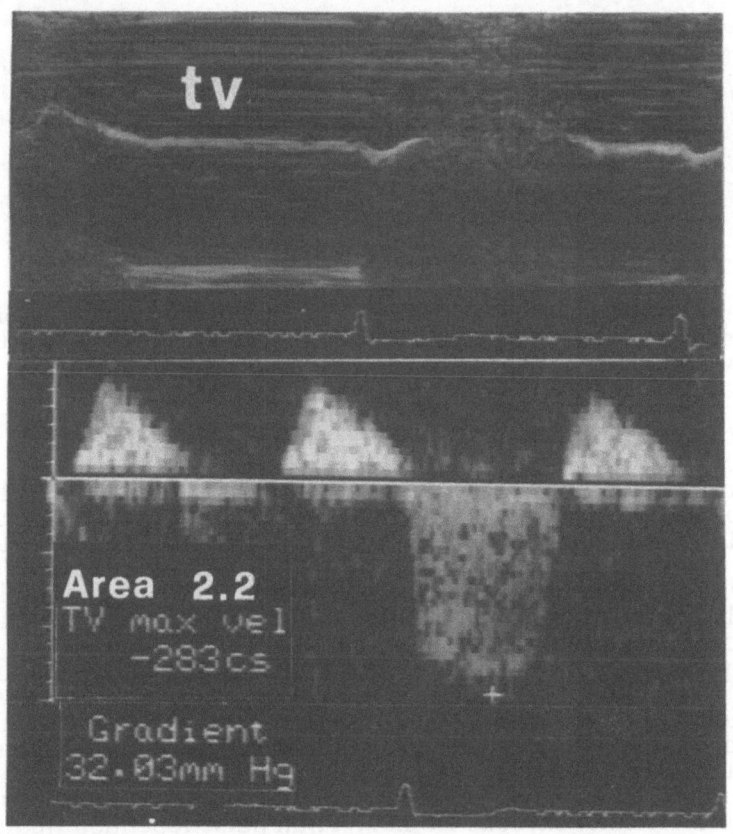

Fig. 5-43. Tricuspid stenosis and regurgitation. The m-mode findings include a fusion of the leaflets with a restriction of motion, as in mitral valve stenosis. The peak velocityof the regurgitation is 2.8 M/S , yeilding a peak gradient of 32. mm Hg. The pressure half time was used to calculate a valve area of 2.2 cm2

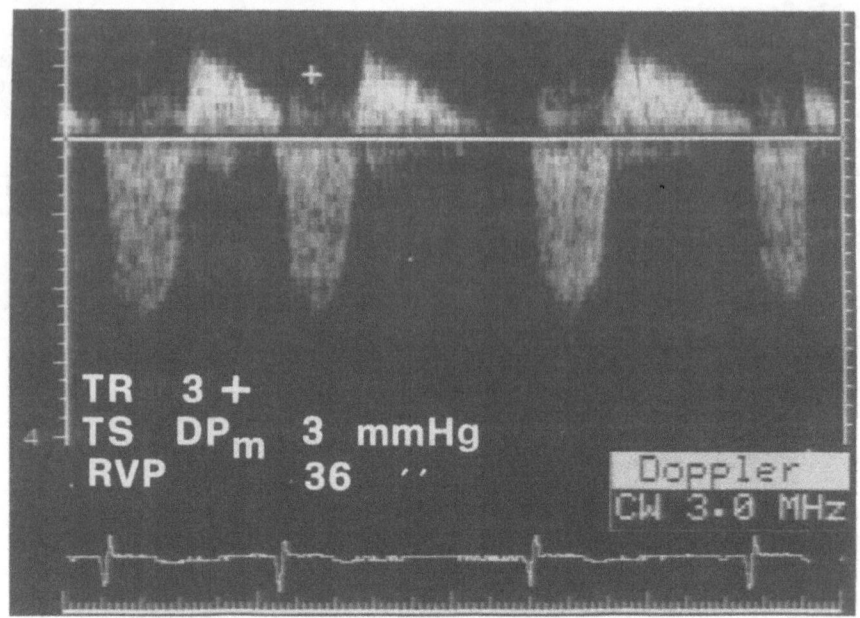

Fig.5-44. Tricuspid valve annuloplasty. Continuous mode recording of tricuspid flow from the apical window. The peak regurgitant flow velocity is 2.4 m/s < and the tricuspid insufficiency was graded 3+ by pulsed Doppler flow Mapping techniques.

Pulmonary Stenosis

The stenotic jet in pulmonary stenosis is usually interrogated from a left parasternal or subcostal imaging window. The peak frequencies in the jet can be recorded with continuous mode, and pulsed mode can be used to determine the site of the obstruction. By listening to the audio signal, the transducer angulation can be altered slightly so that a parallel or nearly parallel alignment to flow is acheived. The peak and mean systolic gradient should be calculated by application of the modified Bernoulli equation.

When infundibular and valvular stenosis coexist, a characteristic pattern is recorded in the pulmonary artery. There is a superimposed flow of lower velocity which has a late systolic peak; this flow represents the flow through the infundibulum. Using pulsed mode, the infundibular flow can be separated from the flow distal to the pulmonary valve. To calculate the transvalvular gradient, the peak infundibular velocity should be included in the Bernoulli equation when the infundibular velcoity exceeds 1.0 m/s. High pulse repetition frequency mode can usually be applied to measure the peak flow velocity in pulmonary stenosis.

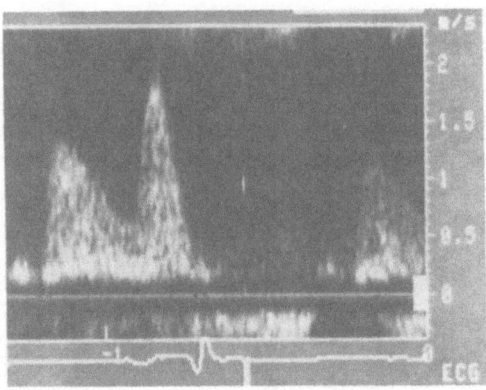

Fig. 5-45. Tricuspid stenosis . Continuous mode recording of tricuspid flow from the apical window. The peak flow velocity is 1.5 m/s, (the atrial flow is neglected) corresponding to a peak diastolic gradient of 9mm Hg. The average pressure halftime is 150 ms .

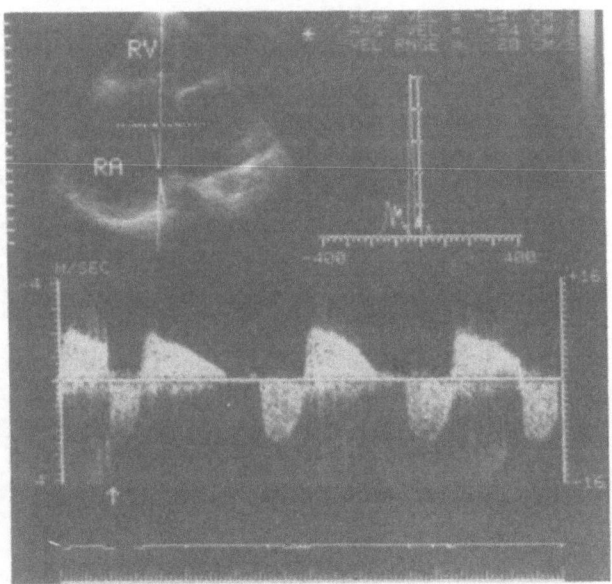

Fig.5-46. Tricuspid stenosis and regurgitation. Continuous mode recording of tricuspid flow from the apical window. The peak flow velocity is 2.0 m/s, corresponding to a peak diastolic gradient of 16 mm Hg. The average pressure halftime is 210 ms. The maximum regurgitant flow velocity is 2.0 m/s, indicating the presence of normal systolic pressure in the pulmonary artery.

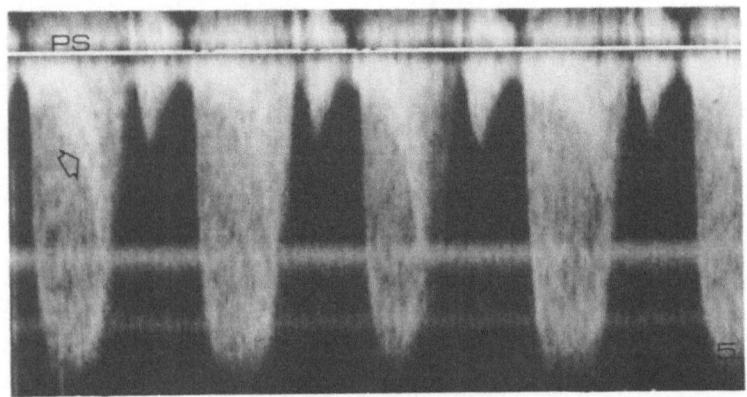

Fig.5-47 Severe pulmonary stenosis. Continuous mode recording of pulmonary flow from the parasternal window. The peak velcotiy is 5.0 m/s, and the peak systolic gradient is 100 mm Hg. The infundibular flow trace is super-imposed on the valvular flow trace . It is often helpful to turn the patient in an extreme left lateral position to access the best examination window.

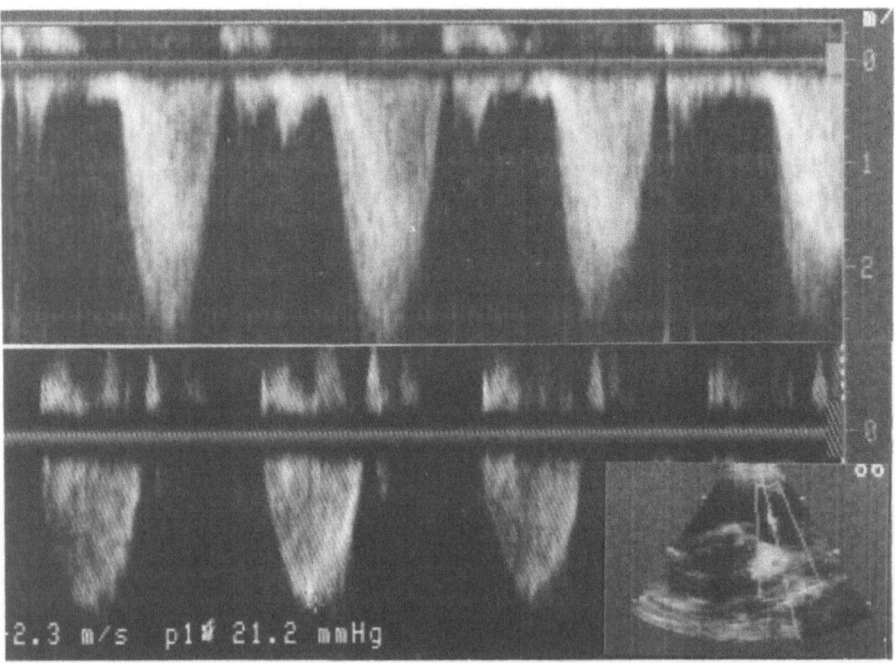

Fig. 5-48. Continuous mode recording of pulmonary flow in a patient with mild pulmonary stenosis. The peak velocity is 2.9 m/s, and the peak systolic gradient is 34 mm Hg. The flow velocity measured before the obstruction was high , 2.3 m/s, yeilding a pressure of 21 mm Hg . The corrected gradient was the product of the peak pressure minus the pre-stenotic flow pressure, in this case 13 mm Hg.

A low parasternal position is most often used to record the jet velocities in adults. In younger patients, the subcostal window usually provides a better alignment with the jet, resulting in the recording of a higher maximal velocity. As in aortic stenosis, it is difficult to predict which transducer position will provide the highest quality flow velocity trace. Color flow imging may initially be utilized to provide spatial orientation of the stenotic jet.

Increased flow velocities as well as spectral broadening will be detected when valvular obstruction is present. However, increased velocity alone does not indicate the presence of stenosis, nor does the appearance of a disturbed flow pattern. Infundibular stenosis or a large ventricular septal defect may create turbulence in the right ventricular outflow tract and in the main pulmonary artery. Pulmonary flow velocity may be increased due to the existence of a left-to-right shunt. Moderate to severe pulmonary regurgitation may also be the cause of increased forward flow velocity in the pulmonary artery. Obstruction at the valvular level produces a characteristic audio signal and flow velocity curve.

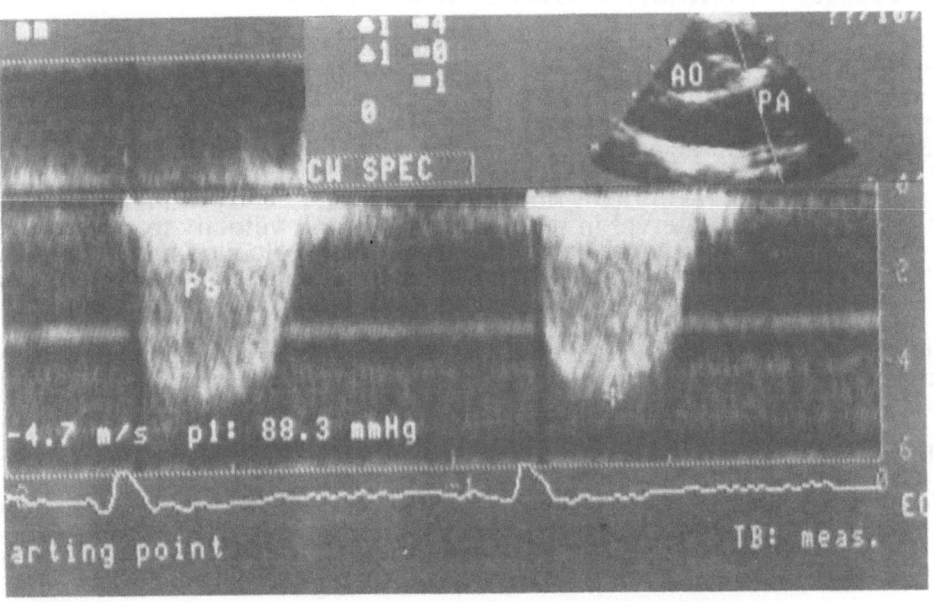

Fig. 5-49. Severe pulmonary stenosis. Continuous mode recording of pulmonary flow from the parasternal window. The peak velcotiy is 4.7 m/s, and the peak systolic gradient is 88.0 mm Hg.The subvalvular increase in flow velocity can be appreciated in the 2 m/s velocity range.

Aortic Insufficiency

The echocardiographic findings in hemodynamically significant aortic insufficiency include left ventricular dilatation and hypertrophy. Fluttering of the anterior leaflet of the mitral valve may be recorded if the regurgitant jet is oriented towards the mitral leaflets. While the echocardiographic findings of left ventricular dilatation and hypertrophy are indicative of a significant incompetence, such findings are detected at a late stage in the course of the disease. The presence of a diastolic mitral valve flutter is a specific but not sensitive finding in aortic insufficiency, and provides no indication of severity.

Doppler echocardiography allows one to semi-quantify the severity of the aortic insufficiency. Using conventional pulsed mode or color flow mapping, the regurgitant flow can be mapped in the left ventricle as in angiography. The width and extension of the regurgitant flow may be used to estimate the degree of incompetence. This technique is known as flow mapping. (6 ,7 ,9 ,10 ,11) A patient with aortic insufficiency can be followed with serial Doppler studies, and a semi-quantitative assessment of severity can be made at the time of the examination. Using this approach, the decision to replace the aortic valve can be made before the onset of left ventricular failure.

The Pressure Halftime in Aortic Insufficiency

The presure halftime is an accurate means of assessing the severity of mitral stenosis. More recently, this parameter has been applied in the evaluation of aortic insufficiency. Continuous mode is used to record the regurgitant flow signal, most often from the apical window. Parallel alignment with the regurgitant jet is essential in order to accurately record the peak flow velocities. The pressure halftime of the regurgitant flow signal is calculated in the same manner as in mitral stenosis. The peak regurgitant flow velocity is divided by $\sqrt{2}$, and the pressure halftime is the time interval in required for the peak velocity to decrease to the pressure half velocity. If the maximum regurgitant velocity is not recorded, the pressure halftime measurement will not be accurate. The envelope of the aortic insufficiency signal can be difficult to obtain. An independent Doppler transducer is sometimes used to track these high velocity but low intensity signals.

Hatle and coworkers showed that pressure halftimes tended to decrease with increasing severity of aortic incompetence. They found that pressure halftimes less than 250 ms indicated the presence of severe insufficiency.

Color Flow Mapping in Aortic insufficiency

Color flow analysis provides another method od evaluating the severity of aortic insufficiency by enabling one to measure the regurgitant jet width. The left ventricular outflow width is also measured, and a ratio of the jet width to the outflow width calculated. This ratio increases with greater degrees of

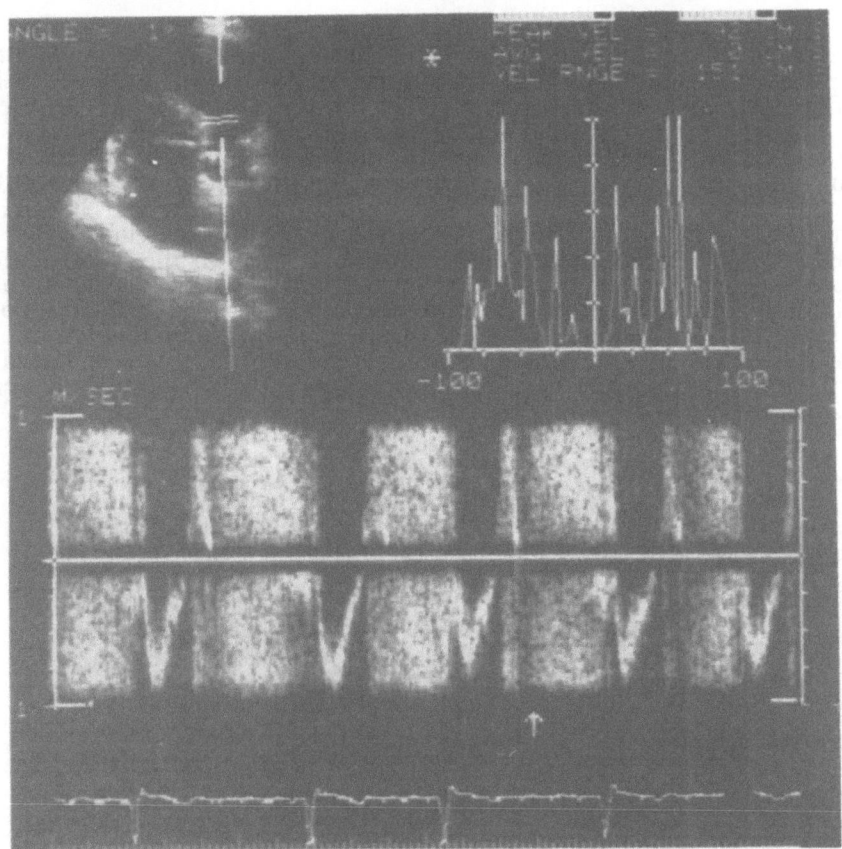

Fig. 5-50 . A modified five chamber view is obtained, and the sample volume is positioned in the left venrtricular outflow tract. The systolic flow below the baseline represents the left ventricular outflow. The aliased diastolic flow recorded from the time of aortic valve closure until aortic valve re-opening represents the regurgitant flow. Using flow mapping techniques, this insufficiency was graded as moderate when the left ventricular function was taken into consideration. The spike which occurs approximately after the onset of the regurgitant flow represents the movement of the mitral valve through the sample volume. The power spectrum (top right) indicates that the intensity of the aliased flow signal is quite strong. a large volume of blood is moving in the regurgitant jet, hence the intense signal. when the aortic insufficiency is flow mapped from the apex, one ahould be aware of the potential for range ambiguity. As the range gate is set at a shallower depth, the pulse repetition frequency increases if anoptimized pulse repetition frequency mode is automatically implemented. This results in the possibility of recording a range ambiguous signalif the sample volume and the flow jet remain in alignment.

117

incompetence. Since the flow velocity in the regurgitation is not of interest in this application, a non-parallel transducer position is utilized. Either a parasternal long-axis or short-axis view of the left ventricle can be selected in order to measure the jet and outflow width.

Perry and coworkers (56) have shown that the ratio of the jet area to the left ventricular outflow area is more sensitive in the prediction of severity than the width ratio. Short-axis views of the left ventricular ouflow and the regurgitant flow are used to determine the area. However, if the jet width or jet area is measured too far beneath the aortic valve, the severity of the regurgitation will be underestimated. The reason is that the jet appears to be larger in the color flow display at this level due to the presence of flow eddies. To avoid overestimation, the measurements should be made at a level immediately beneath the aortic valve. Another source of error is sample contamination by flow in the elevational plane. The use of a concentrically focused beam can help minimize such an error.

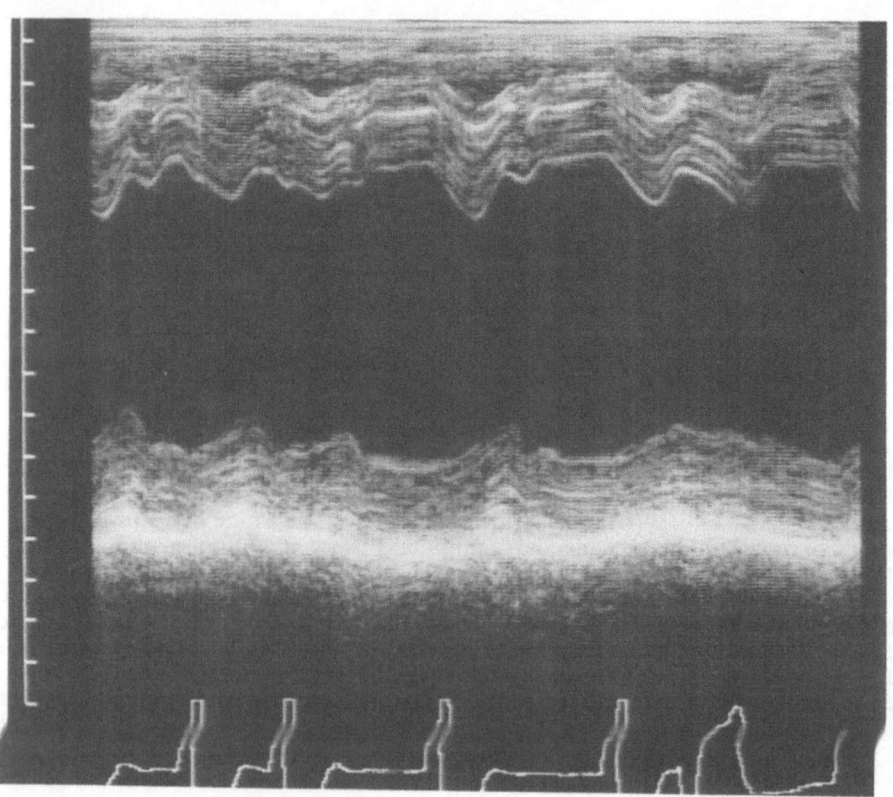

Fig. 5-51 . M-mode recording of the left ventricle in aortic insufficiency.

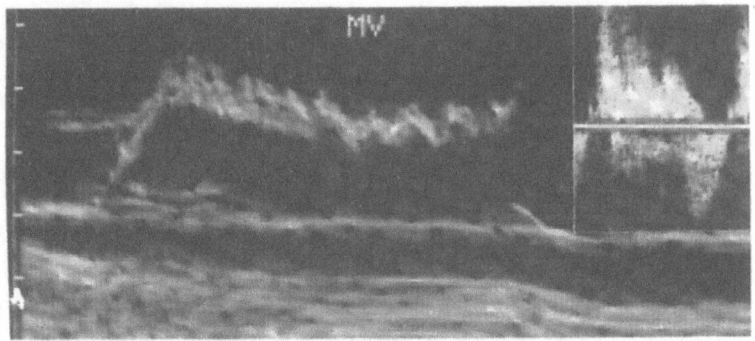

Fig.5-52. A. Continuous mode recording of aortic insufficiency recorded from the apical window. The high velocities in the regurgitant flow signal may be difficult to record; this is partially due to the relatively highintensity of the low velcotiy signals. B. The M-mode recording of the mitral valve demonstrates the presence of valve flutter. C. Fluttering of the anterior mitral leaflet recorded with a slow sweep speed.

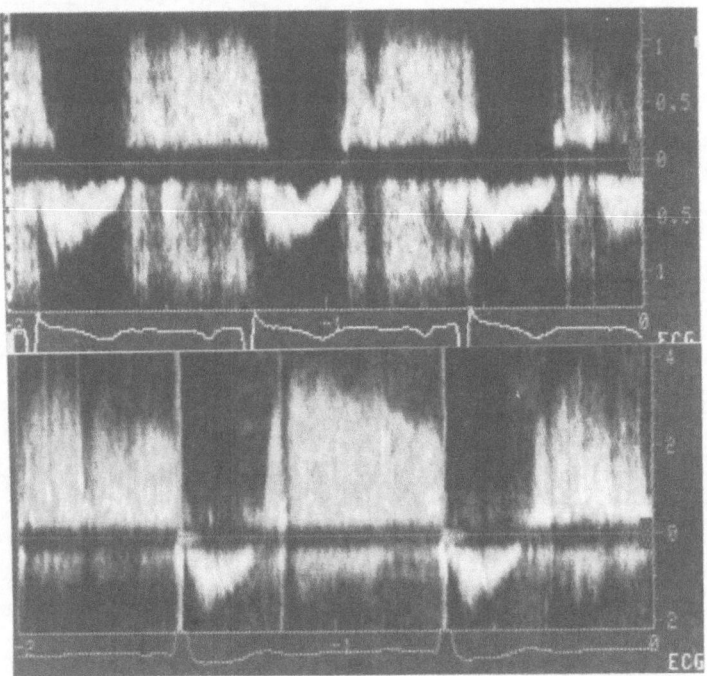

Fig. 5-53. Moderately severe aortic insufficiency. A. Pulsed mode recording from the apical window made with an independent Doppler transducer. The sample volume is placed 4.0 cm behind the aortic valve. B. Continuous mode recording in the same patient. Note the relatively high intensity of the regurgitant flow signal.

119

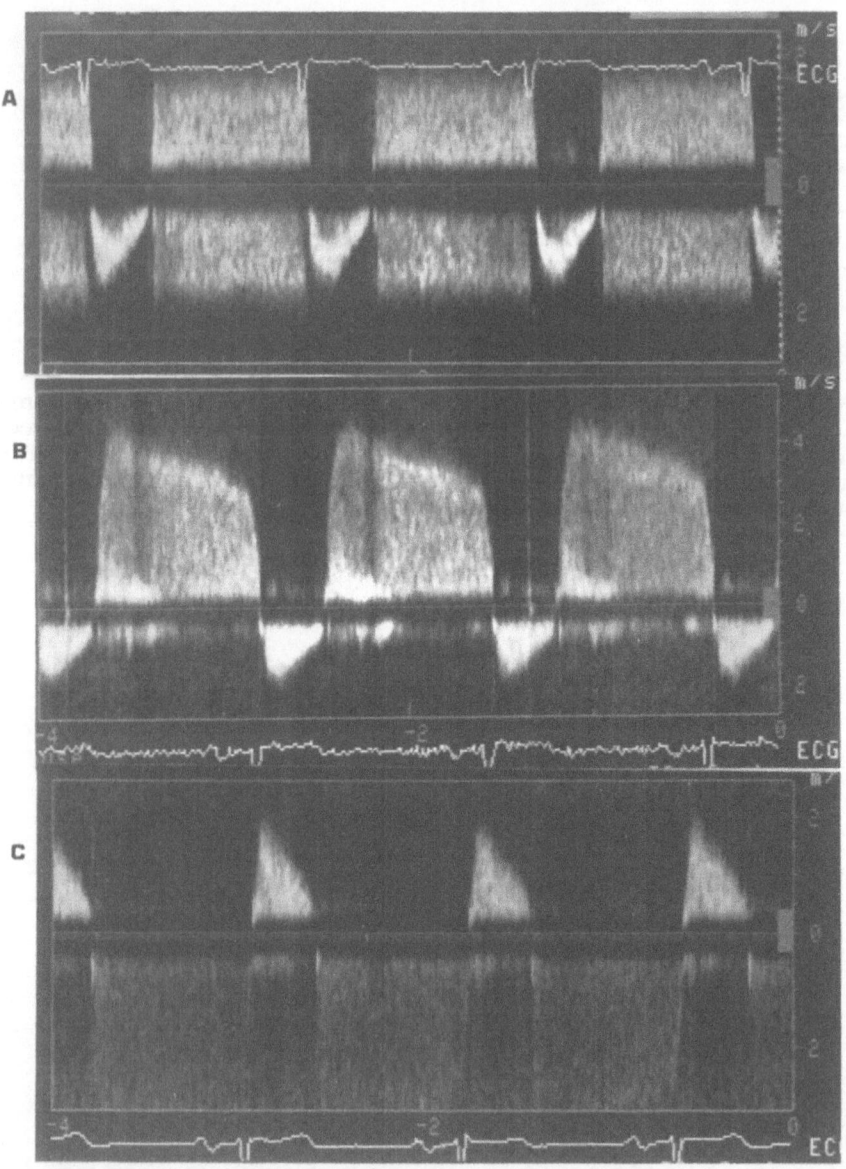

Fig. 5-54 . Moderate aortic insufficiency. A. Pulsed mode recording from the apex with the sample volume placed 3.0 cm behind the aortic valve. B. Continuous mode recording from the same position. C. Continuous mode recording of aortic flow from the right parasternal window. The forward flow velocity is higher than that obtained from the apex, but the regurgitant flow signal is barely recorded.

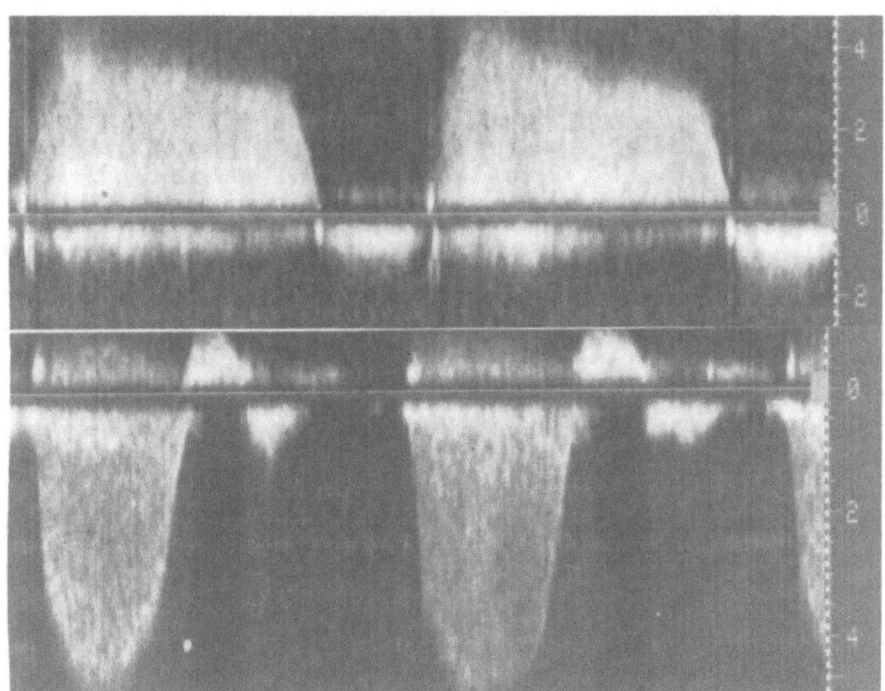

Fig. 5-55. Aortic insufficiency (A) and mitral insufficiency (B) recorded with continuous mode from the apical window in the same patient. By angling the transducer superiorly, the aortic regurgitation was recorded. With inferolateral angulation, the mitral regurgitation was interrogated. The bottom recording (B) demonstrates a trace of the systolic mitral regurgitation flow after mitral closure and before aortic valve opening .

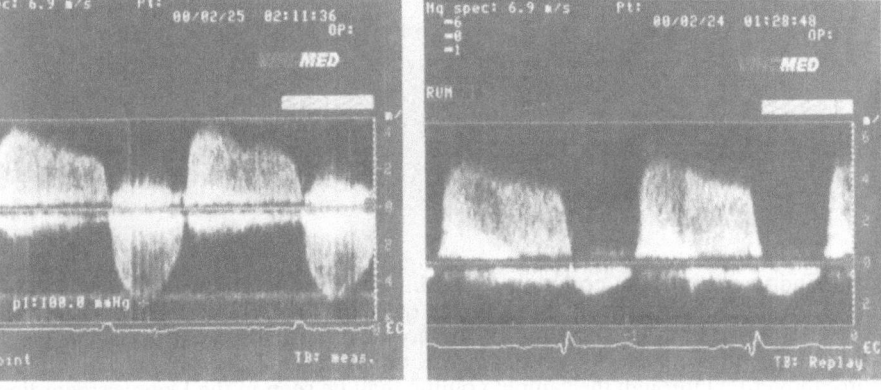

Fig. 5-56. The CW mode recording in two patients with aortic insufficiency, from the apical position. The first recording is from a patient with a coexistant stenosis. The second is from a patient with pure regurgiation. In both examples the pressure halftime is greater than 500 ms , indicating a normal end diastolic LV pressure.

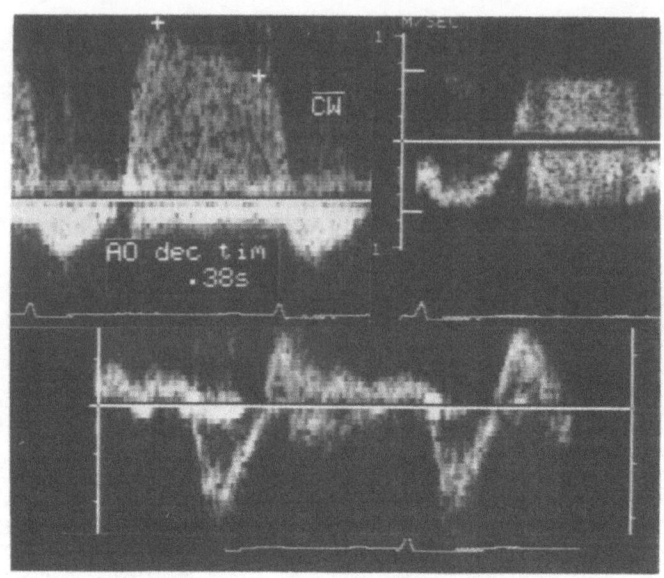

Fig. 5-57. Moderate aortic insufficiency. A. Continuous mode recording from the apical window; the pressure half time of the regurgitant flow signal is 380 ms. B. Pulsed mode recording of the regurgitant flow signal recorded 3.0 cm behind the aoric valve. C. Pulsed mode of flow in the descending aorta recorded from the suprasternal window. The reversed diastolic flow represents the regurgitation.

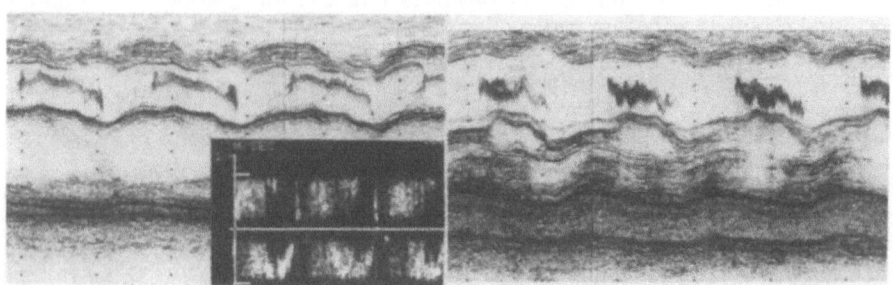

Fig. 5-58 . Endocardititis is a common cause in aortic insufficiency. Top. The M-mode recording of the aorta demonstrates the presence of shaggy echoes on the aortic valve leaflets. Bottom insert. Pulsed mode recording of the aortic insufficiency with the sample volume placed in the left ventricular outflow tract directly behind the aortic valve. The effects of the vegetations' movement through the sample volume may be seen in the Doppler recording; there are intense signals within the regurgitant flow signal followed by areas of signal dropout. A high pass filter of 800 Hz was used to reduce some of this motion artefact.

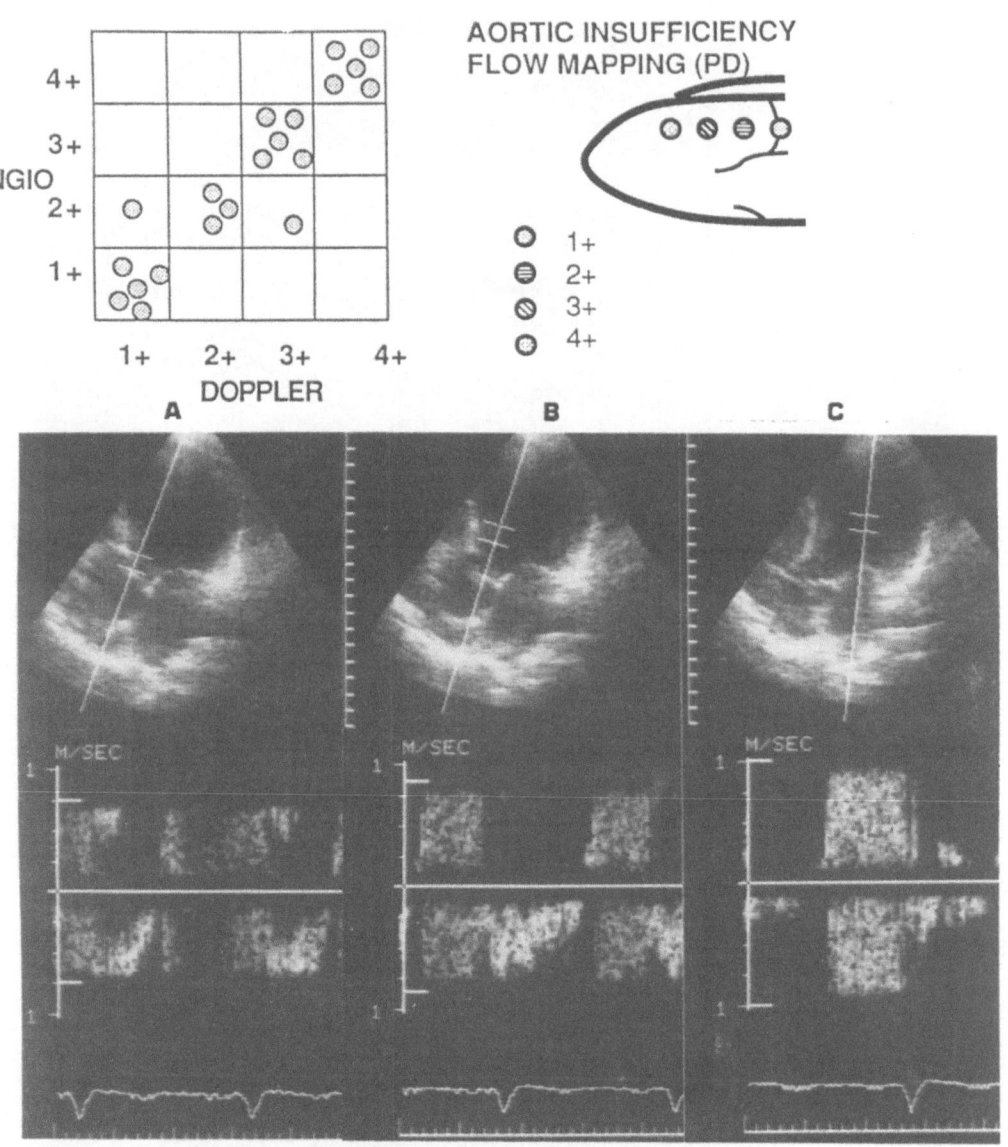

Fig. 5-59. Flow mapping in aortic insufficiency. In order to assess the severity of aortic insufficiency, pulsed mode may be used to determine the regurgitant flow extension into the left ventricle. The greater the regurgitant flow extension, the more severe the insufficiency. The intensity of the regurgitant flow signal and the left ventricular function should also be considered when grading the severity of the regurgitation. The results obtained by angiography and pulsed Doppler flow mapping techniques compared well in this pilot study on a small patient population.

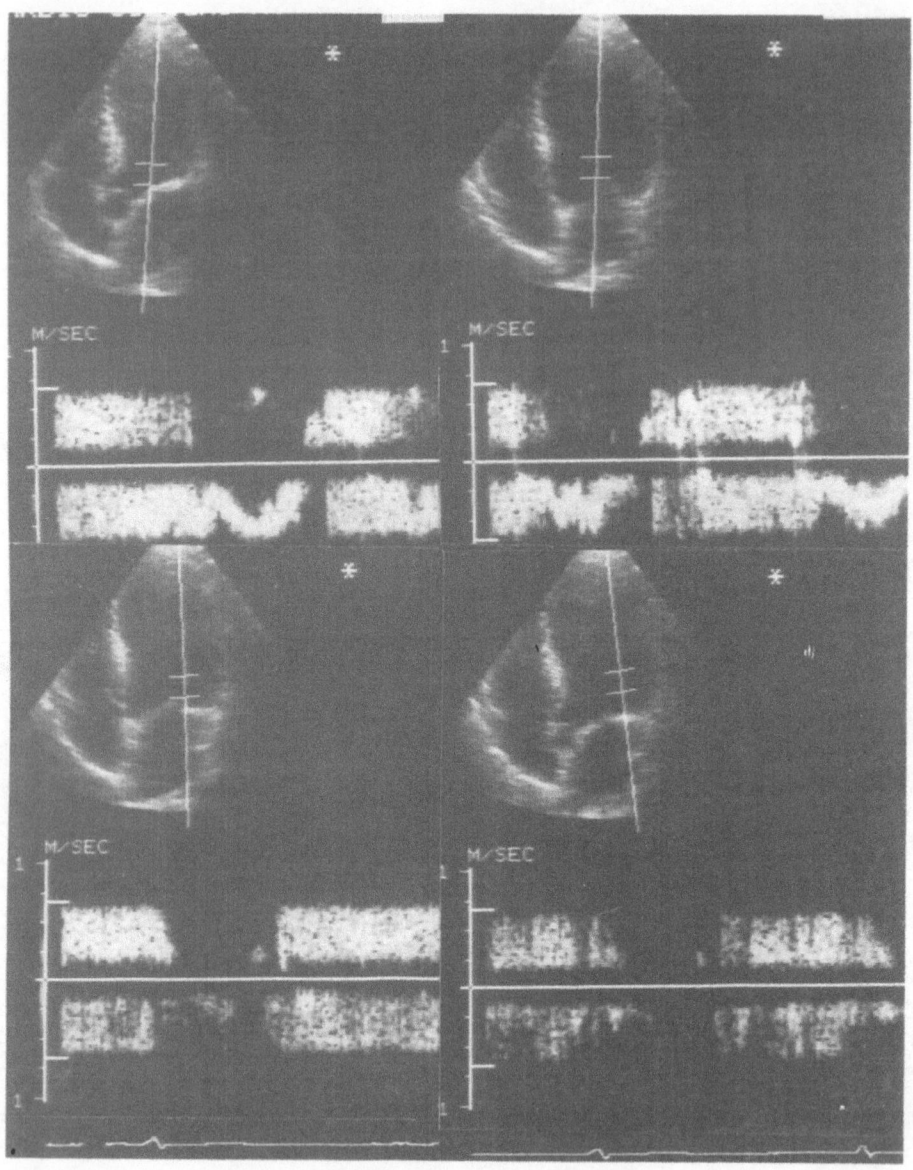

Fig. 5-60 . Flow mapping in aortic insufficiency. In order to assess the severity of aortic insufficiency, pulsed mode may be used to determine the regurgitant flow extension into the left ventricle. The greater the regurgitant flow extension, the more severe the insufficiency. The intensity of the regurgitant flow signal and the left ventricular function should also be considered when grading the severity of the regurgitation.

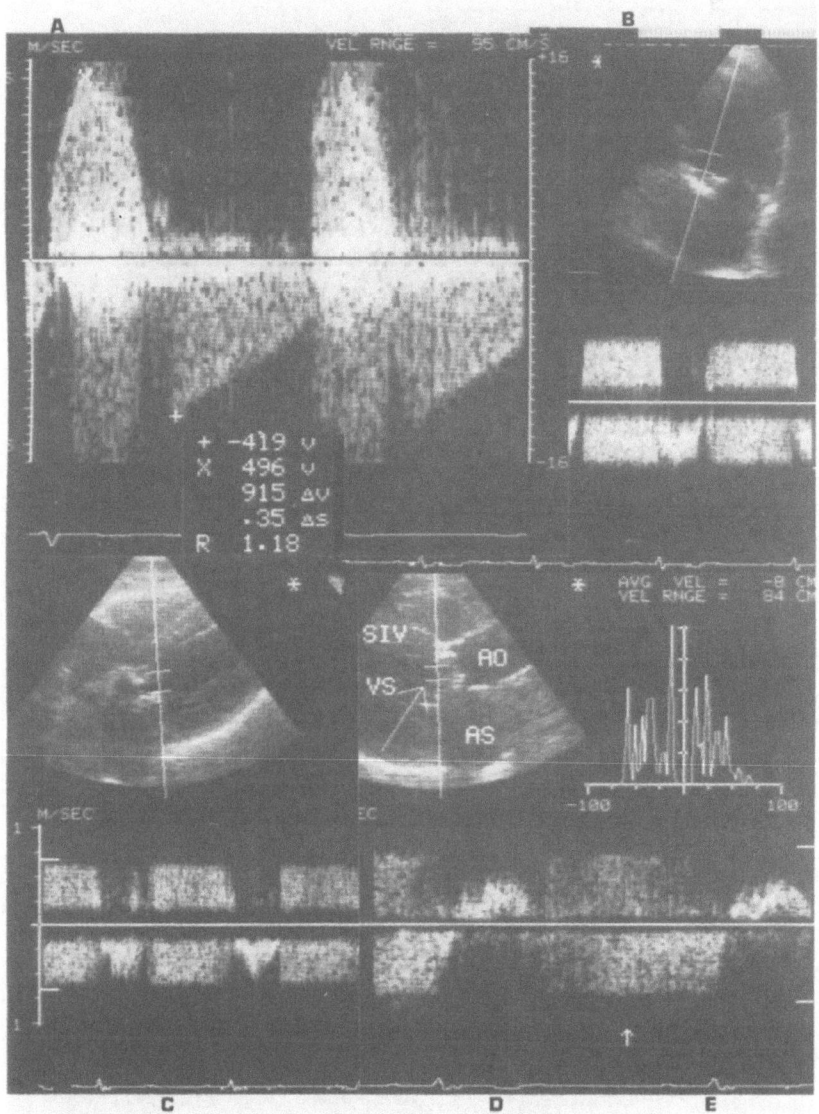

Fig.5-61. Moderate aortic insufficiency. A. Continuous mode recording from the right parasternal window. In order to adequately record the regurgitant signal from this position, the receiver gain had to be increased. B. Pulsed mode recording of the regurgitation from the apical position. C. Pulsed mode recording from the subcostal position. D. Pulsed mode rcording from the parasternal position. Note that the strongest intensity of the regurgitant flow signal in pulsed mode is from the apical window.

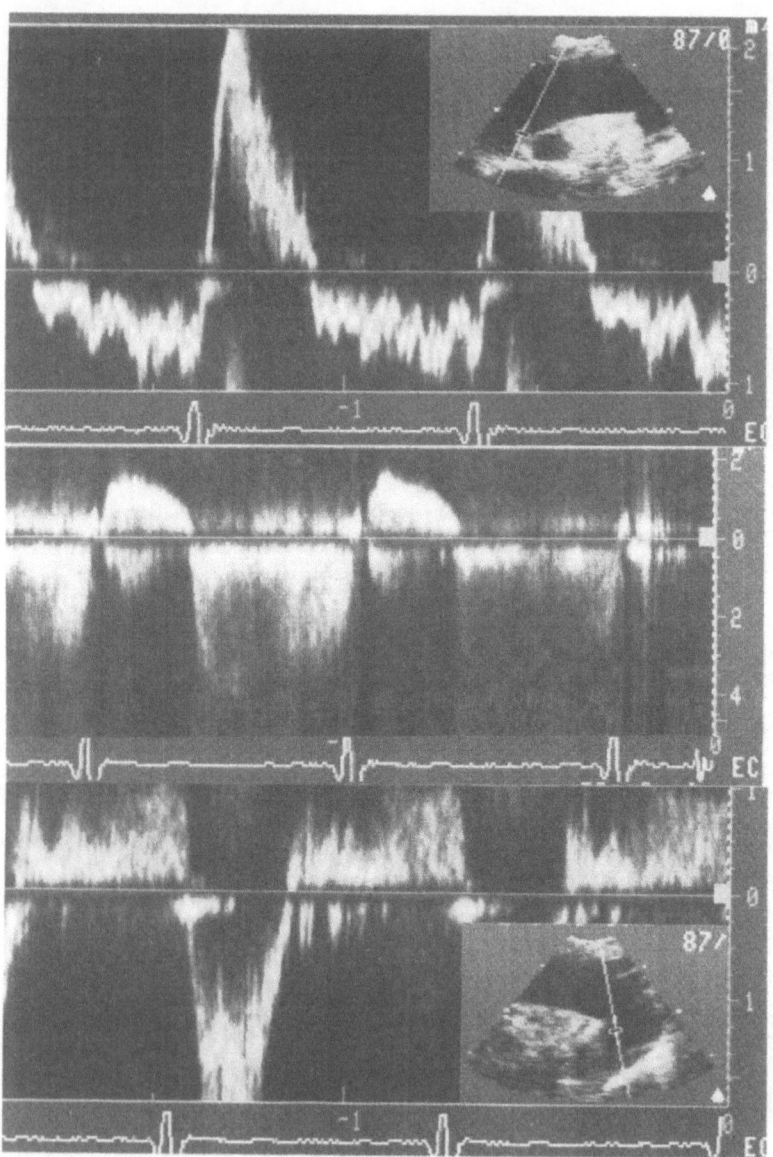

Fig.5-62. Pulsed and continuous wave Doppler interrogation of the ascending and descending aorta in a patient with severe aortic regurgitation. Top . Pulsed Doppler recording from the ascending aorta , the diastolic regurgitant flow is clearly demonstrated. Middle . The continuous wave recording from the same transducer position . The high velocity jet of the aortic regurgitation is detected . Bottom . Pulsed Doppler recording from the descending aorta , the regurgitation is seen as flow towards the transducer in diastole.

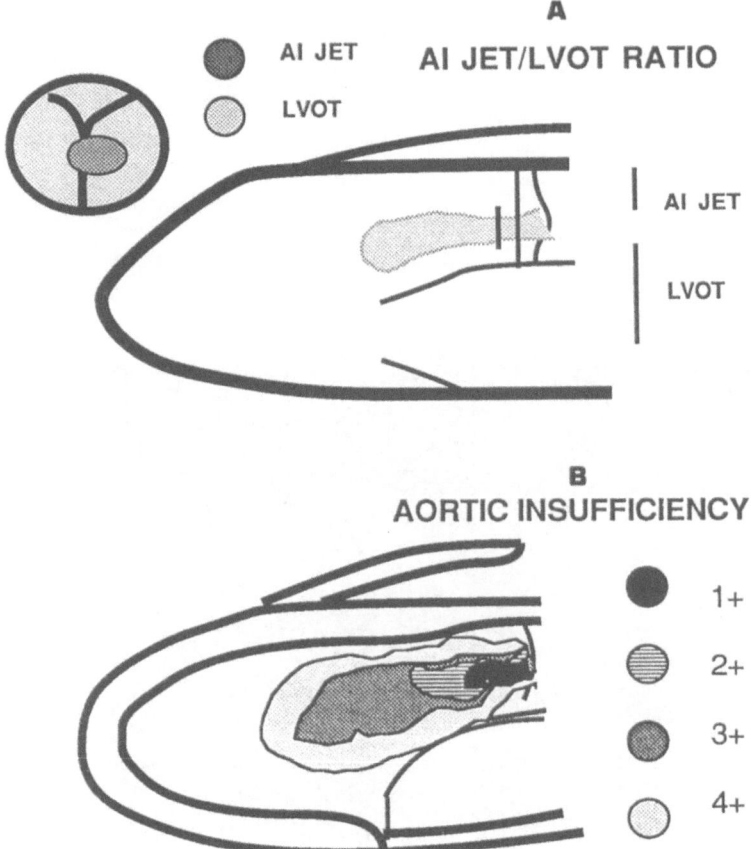

Fig.. 5-63 . Top . The ratio of the aortic jet width to the left ventricular outflow tract width can be calculated from the color flow display of left ventricular outflow. These measurement should be made approximately 1.0 cm beneath the aortic valve to avoid overestimation of the jet width. In a similar mannner, the ratio of the regurgitant jet area to the outflow area can be estimated from the short axis view of the aortic root. Bottom . Color flow imaging can also be used to estimate the regurgitant jet extension into the left ventricular cavity. A modified parsternal long axis view may be used when flow mapping with real time Doppler ultrasound. Angulation of the scan plane is necessary to ensure that the maximal jet extension has been obtained because the flow varies in three dimensions. Left ventricular function should also be considered when flow mapping with color flow imaging.

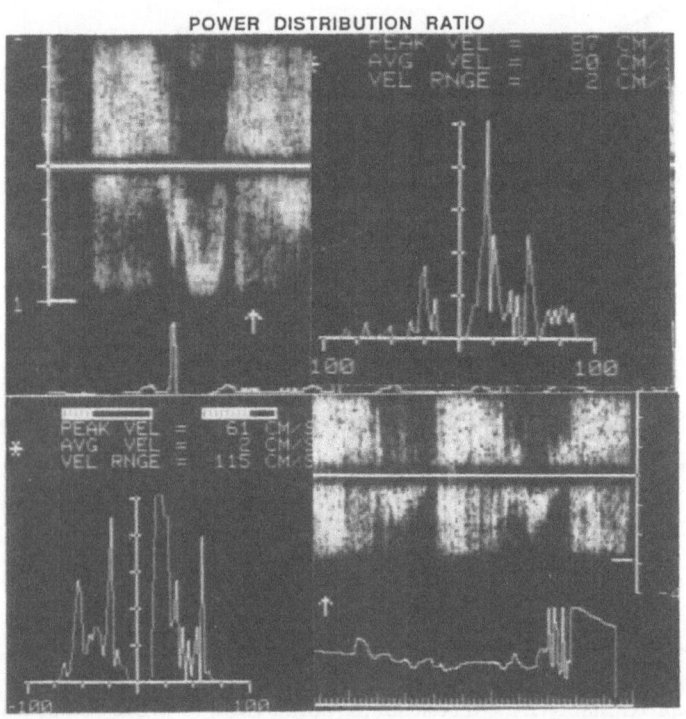

Fig. 5-64 . The structure of a regurgitant jet will remain organized further into the retrograde chamber with a larger incompetence . When a small regurgitation is sampled at the tip of the open mitral valve leaflet , and a spectra by spectra analysis of the Doppler shifted signals power distribution is obtained , a high amplitude low velocity / low amplitude high velocity signal is noted . Middle . The signal in a large regurgitation is characterized by a high amplitude low velocity / high amplitude high velocity signal . This is due to the more organized structure of the regurgitant jet at a point distal to the incompetence . Top. A ratio between the averaged low velocity power and average high velocity power was calculated . The power distribution within the interrogated signal was demonstrated to bear a relationship to the angiographic grade of severity in a limited study. (1-5)

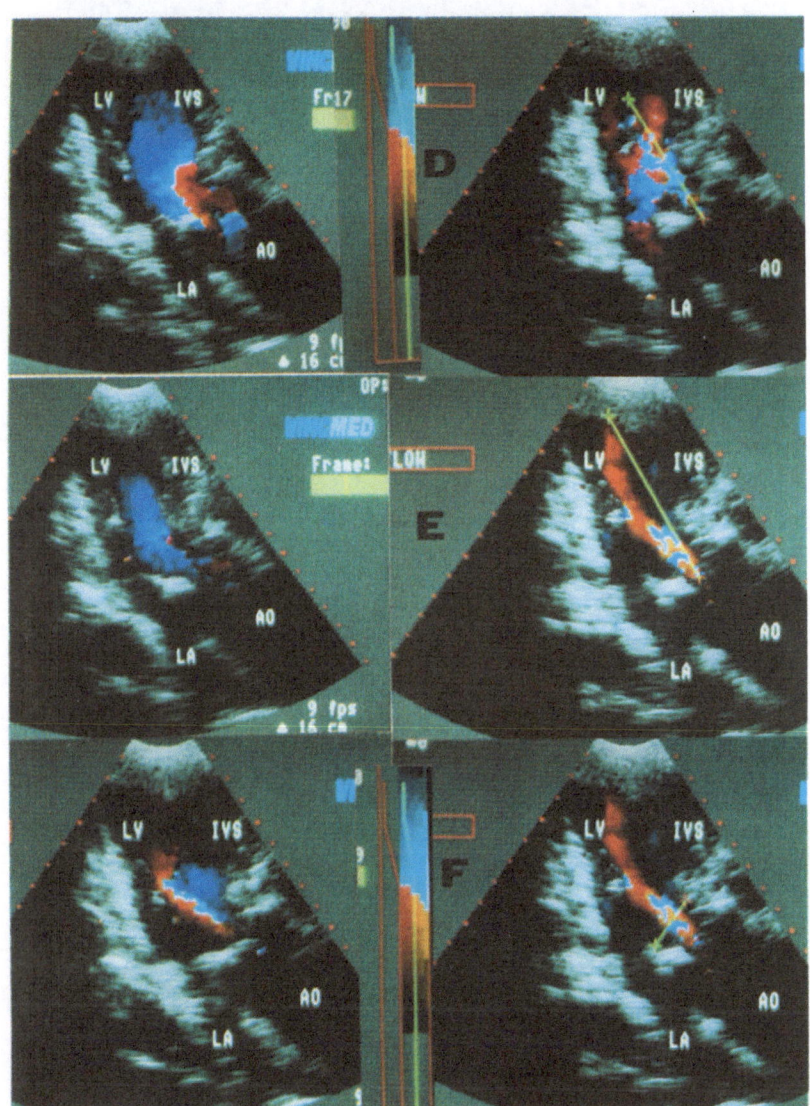

Fig. 5-65 . Severe aortic Insufficiency recorded from an apical long axis view. A. In mid-systole, the left ventricular outflow is visualized as a blue bolus. The center of flow has exceeded the Nyquist value, and color aliasing is seen at a level immediately beneath the aortic valve. B. In late systole, the outflow velocity has decreased and aliasing is no longer seen. C. In early diastole, the regurgitant jet is seen originating from the aortic orifice. D. The typical mosaic pattern assigned to high velocity jets is seen by mid-diastole. E. The jet extension to the apex of the left ventricle is detected in this still frame. F. The ratio of the jet width to the outflow width was estimated to be 0.60.

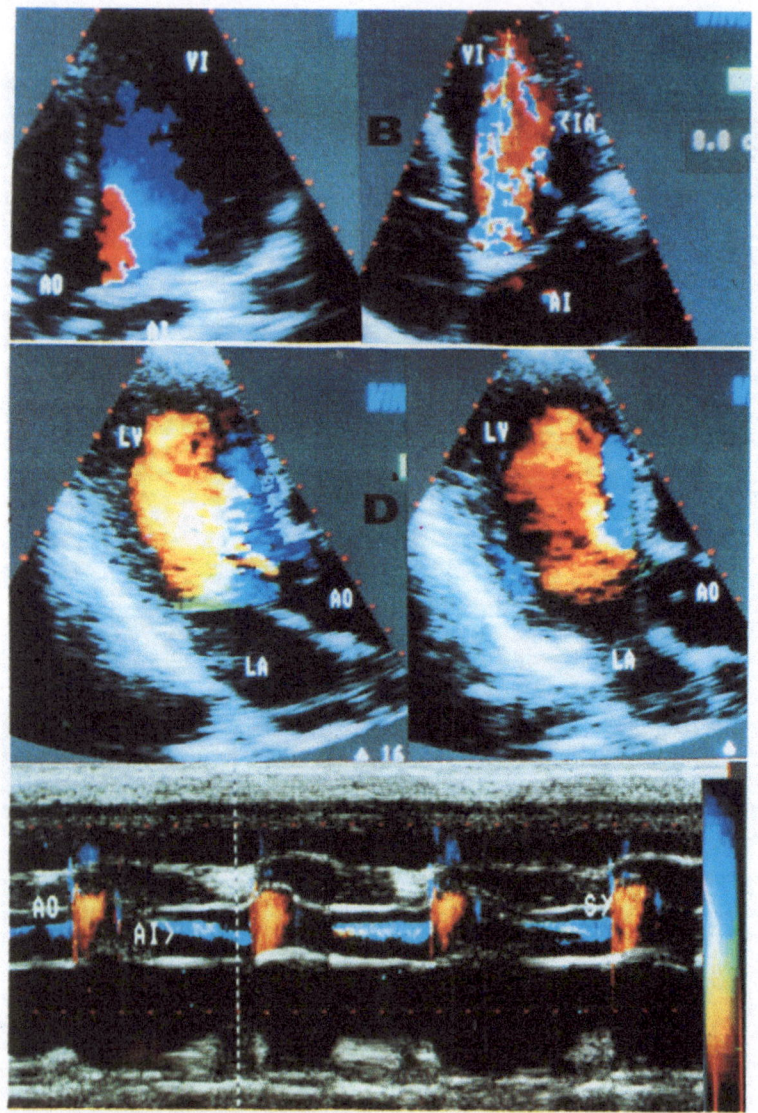

Fig. 5-66. Color Flow mapping in Aortic Insufficiency. The flow mapping technique described for conventional pulsed mode is subject to several limitations related to the lack of spatial reference. The problem of mitral flow contamination of the aortic insufficiency signal occurs with color flow imaging as in pulsed mode. However, the mitral flow signal is more readily recognized in the flow imaging mode when compared to pulsed mode.

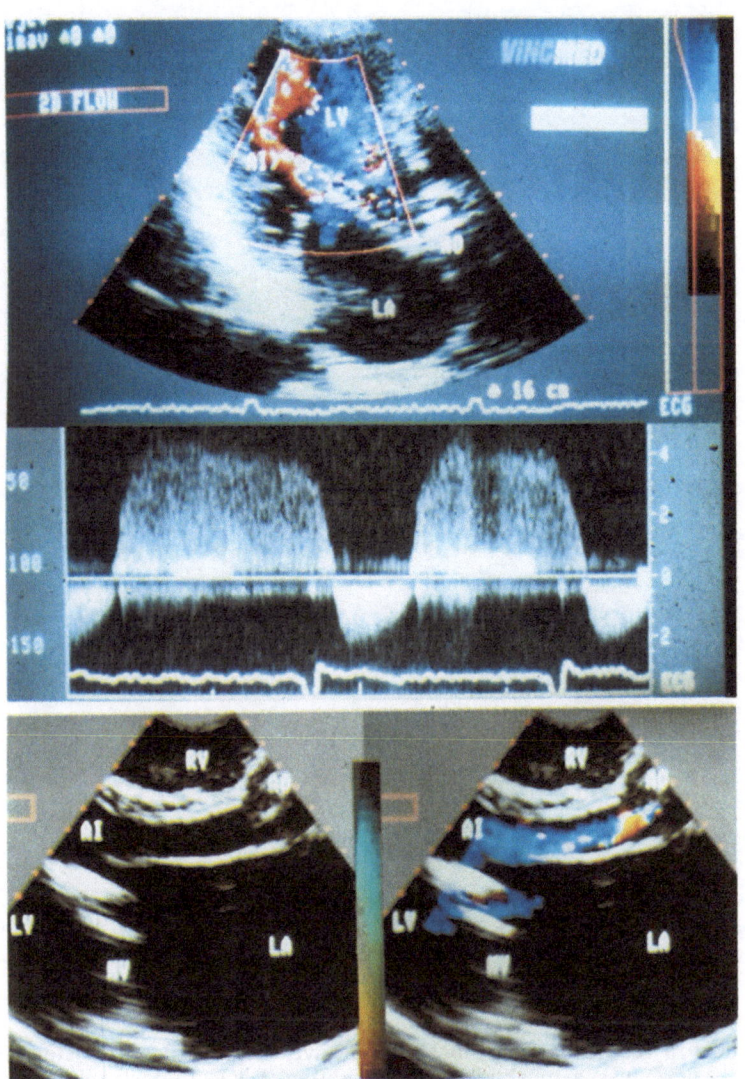

Fig. 5-67 Severe aortic insufficiency recorded in two different patients with color flow mapping. Top. In this case, the regurgitant jet is displayed as a mosaic pattern colored predominantly in red. Left ventricular filling is displayed in shades of blue. The continuous mode recording of the aortic regurgitation is also shown. Bottom. The aortic regurgitation visualized from the parasternal long axis view is displayed predominantly in shades of blue, since the jet moves away from the transducer in this view. The jet width is nearly 80% of the outflow tract width, indicating that a significant regurgitation is present.

131

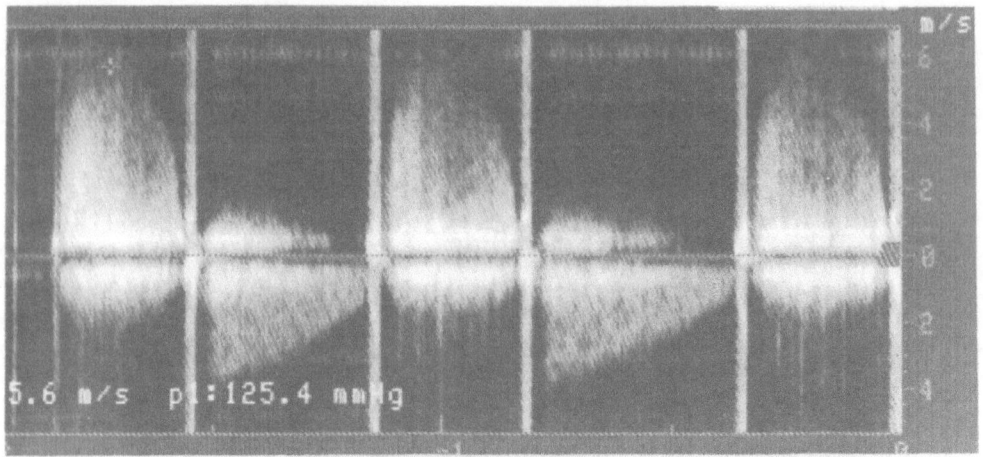

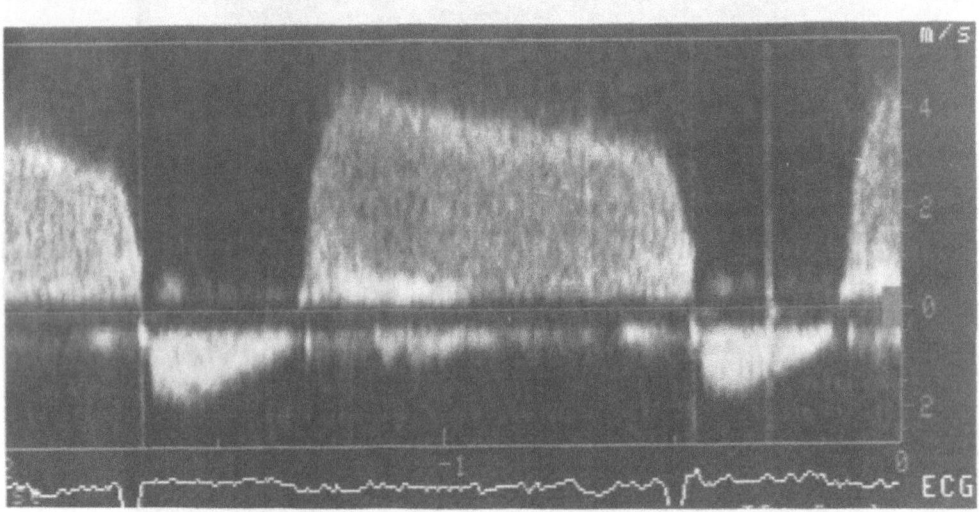

Fig. 5-68. The top recording is from a patient with a severe aortic stenosis and 2 + regurgitation . There was a marked left ventricular (LV) hypertrophy , and the rapid deceleration slope of the systolic flow component reflects the effect on (LV) compliance . The second study was recorded from a patient with pure regurgitation . The (LV) end diastolic pressure is normal , and a long pressure halftime is obtained (650 ms) . The end diastolic peak flow velocity reflects the pressure drop between the aorta and left ventricle . Therefore if the end diastolic LV pressure is high the Ao/LV gradient will be low and the regurgitant jet velocity will also be low . After the initial onset the regurgitant flow peak velocity falls off rapidly, resulting in a decreased halftime and deceleration slope.

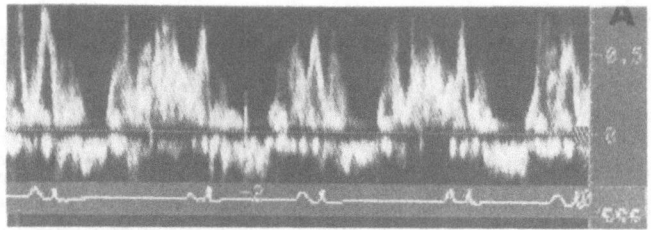

Fig. 5-69 . Moderately severe aortic insufficiency. Pulsed mode recording from the apical window. The regurgitant flow signal is mixed with the signal from the left ventricular inflow. The biphasic flow pattern from the mitral valve is super-imposed on the aortic regurgitation recording . The timing of valve opening and closing , and the onset of flow may be used to seperate these two flows .

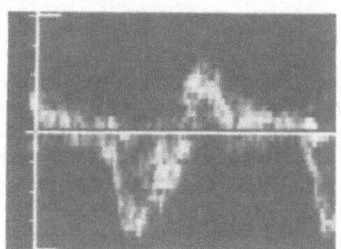 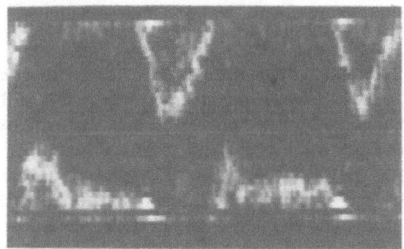

Fig. 5-70. This flow was obtained from the suprasternal notch position with pulsed Doppler. The sample volume was positioned in the descending aorta and both the systolic outflow and the diastolic regurgitation were sampled. The systolic component is shown at the top and the regurgitant flow is displayed at the bottom, with the dual channel recording in the center.

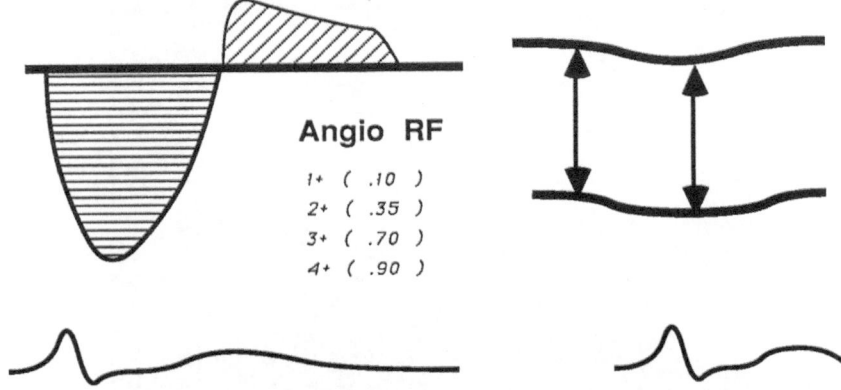

Fig.5-71. The regurgitant fraction can be measured by planimetry of the systolic and regurgitant flows in the descending aorta so that a ratio of the regurgitant flow velocity integral to the forward flow velocity integral can be calculated. The comparable angiographic values are listed. Some groups have corrected for changes in the aortic root dimensions during the cardiac cycle. The example on the bottom demonstrates the ultrasonic information required to measure this parameter.

133

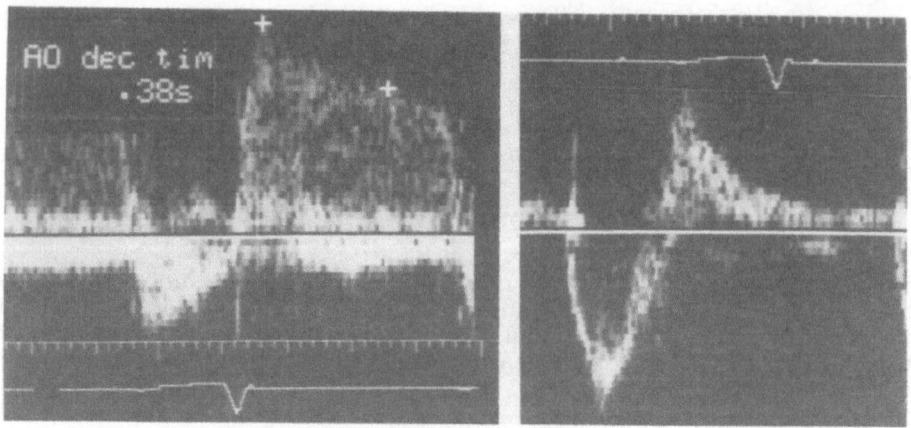

Fig.5-72. Aortic regurgitation recorded from the apical transducer position with continuous wave Doppler (A). The pressure half time measured was 380 ms. The pulsed Doppler grading of the regurgitation by flow mapping technique was 3+ , and the shortened halftime indicated that a significant regurgitation was present. (B). Pulsed Doppler was used to interogate flow in the descending aorta in the same patient. The presence of a relatively high amplitude diastolic regurgitant flow signal supports the finding of a moderately severe regurgitation.

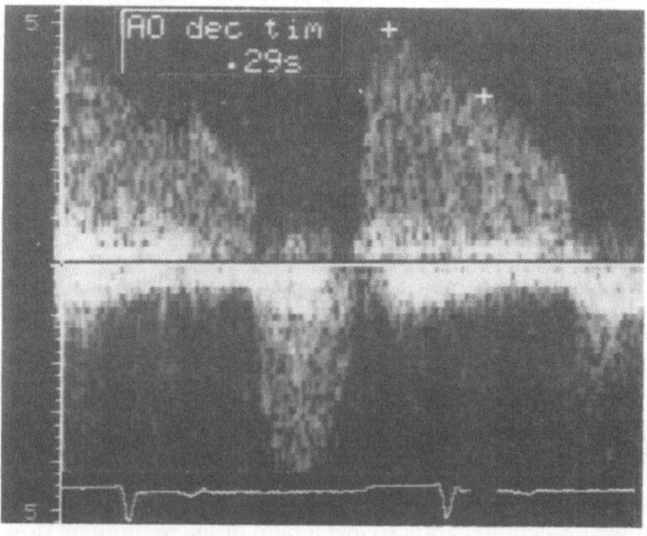

Fig.5-73. Aortic regurgitation recorded from the apical transducer position with continuous wave Doppler . The average pressure half time measured was 290 ms. The pulsed Doppler grading of the regurgitation was 3+, and the decreased halftime indicated that an increased left ventricular end diastolic pressure was present.

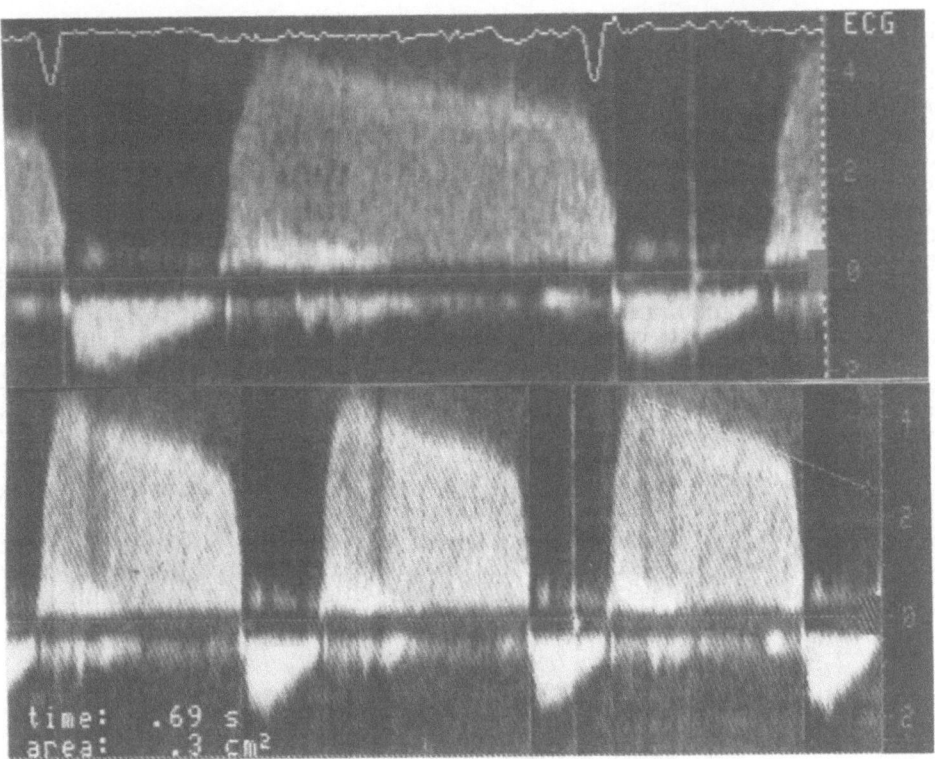

Fig.5-74. Aortic regurgitation recorded with continuous mode from the apical transducer position. The systolic outflow velocity is increased and the diastolic flow towards the transducer represents the regurgitant flow. The top panel was recorded at a sweep speed of 100 mm/s and the lower panel was recorded at a sweep speed of 50 mm/s. In order to measure time intervals, it is often helpful to increase the sweep speed. The pressure half time in this case is 690 ms , which indicates that the left ventricular end diastolic pressure is not elevated.

Aortic Insufficiency - Factors to Consider
1. Flow mapping grade.
2. Is there an increase in left ventricular outflow velocity?
3. Is the regurgitant flow signal detected in the ascending and descending aorta? Does it persist throughout diastole?
4. Left ventricular function and diastolic dimensions.
5. Left ventricular posterior wall and septal thickness (determined from the M-mode recording).

Mitral Insufficiency

The pulsed mode technique of flow mapping can be applied in the assessment of mitral insufficiency. The apical transducer position is used, and the sample volume is placed in the left atrium behind the mitral annulus. When the regurgitant flow signal is detected, a systolic aliased signal will be recorded. The sample volume is then moved further back into the left atrium in an attempt to follow the regurgitant flow. When a severe incompetence is present, the regurgitant signal may be detected at the atrial wall near the entrance of the pulmonary veins. The jet width is estimated by sweeping the sample volume laterally at various depths. In general, the greater the flow width and extension, the more severe the incompetence.

An apical transducer position may be used but often an intermediate position between the apex and the sternum can facilitate the examination. The distance between the probe and the regurgitant flow is decreased, and the flow signal may be stronger than that recorded from the apex. The jet in mitral insufficiency is often eccentric,and is directed towards the left atrial wall. Due to the jet eccentricity, the intermediate transducer position provides a better alignment to the regurgitant flow. If the regurgitant signal is very intense, the regurgitation may be considered to be at least moderate in severity. A smaller sample volume can be used in flow mapping to improve the spatial resolution. This provides a more precise definition of the regurgitant flow extension, although the signal-to-noise ratio of the signal is decreased. Agrading scale which may be used to interpret the flow mapping results.

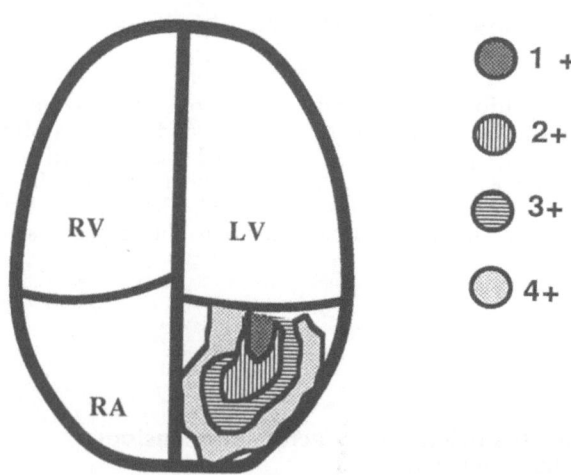

Fig.5-75. Flow mapping in mitral insufficiency. Pulsed mode recordings of the regurgitant flow signal are tracked into the left atrium from the level of the mitral annulus , flow further back in the left atrium indicates a more severe insufficiency .one should note the audio signal intensity as it is related to the amount of blood which is leaking into the left atrium.

While the flow mapping technique represents a semi-quantitative approach to grading mitral regurgitation, the examination can be time -consuming. In the presence of left ventricular dilatation, the increased depth of interrogation results in a very poor signal strength even when an intermediate transducer position is used. Patient movement may cause erroneous localization of flow. When reduced ventricular function coexists with mitral insufficiency, the flow mapping results may be equivocal. In order to supplement the flow mapping examination, continuous mode may be used to determine the orientation of the regurgitant jet. The relative intensity of the forward mitral flow and the regurgitant flow can be compared in the continuous wave recording. When moderate to severe incompetence is present, the forward flow velocity across the mitral valve may be increased. The increased velocity reflects the increased forward flow needed to compensate for the regurgitant volume. The mitral peak velocity will be disproportionately increased when compared to the flow velocities across the non-diseased valves.

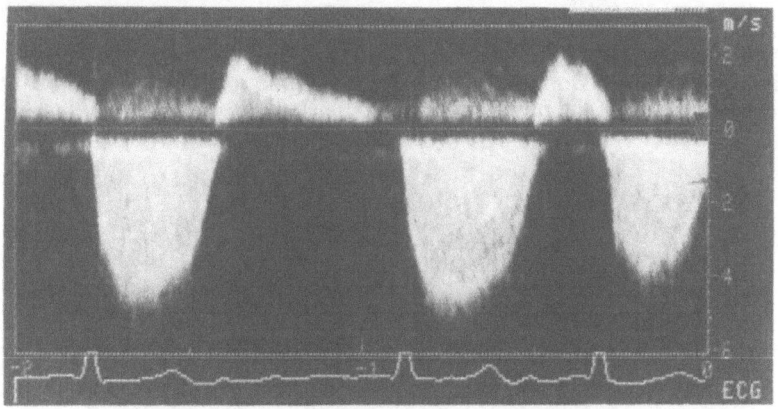

Fig. 5-76. Mitral insufficiency is often found in the setting of mitral stenosis. In this case the forward diastolic flow velocity 2 M/S and the systolic regurgitant flow velocity is 5,7 M/S. The regurgitant Doppler signal is quite strong in comparison to the diastolic signal strength suggesting a more severe insufficiency.

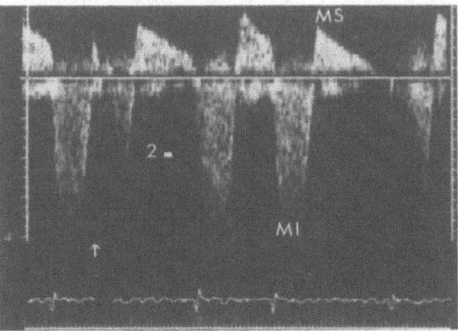

Fig.5-77. This study is also from a patient with mitral stenosis and regurgitation. Note that the regurgitant signal strength is weak in comparison with the diastolic flow signal.

137

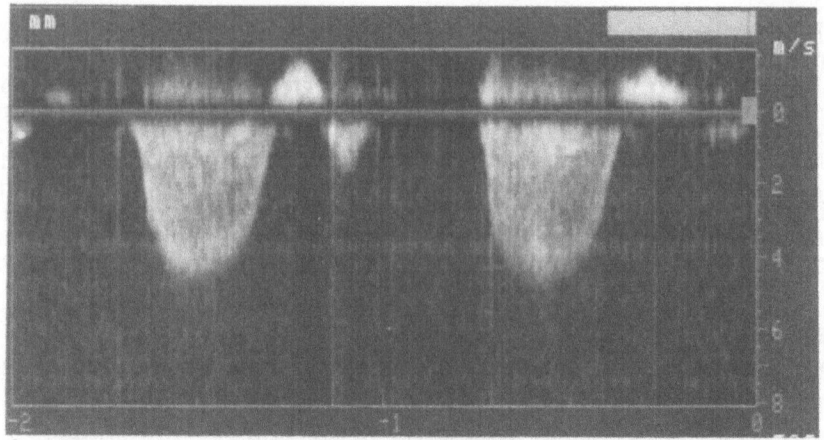

Fig.5-78. This study is from a subject without mitral stenosis (pressure half time = 90 ms) and a 2+ regurgitation by pulsed Doppler flow mapping techniques. The onset of the regurgitation coincides with the closure of the mitral valve and persists until valve opening.

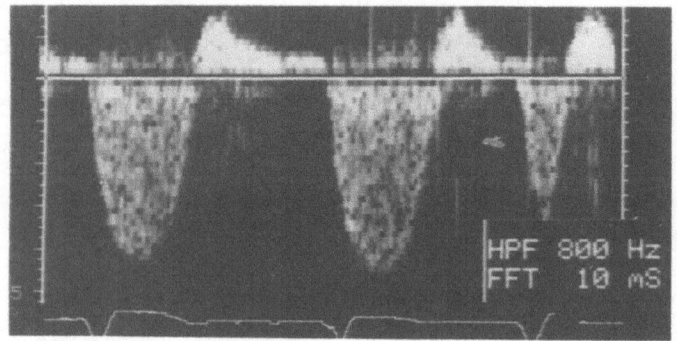

Fig.5-79. This study is from a subject with a mild mitral stenosis (pressure half time = 130 ms) and a 2+ regurgitation by pulsed Doppler flow mapping techniques. The onset of the regurgitation coincides with the closure of the mitral valve and persists until mitral valve re-opening. The signal intensity is stronger in this study than in the previous study, though the extension of flow was approximately the same in both studies. The imaging windows were better in this patient. One must consider the technical difficulty involved in obtaining the Doppler information when evaluating regurgitant flow extension.

Color Flow Analysis in Mitral Insufficiency

Color flow mapping in mitral insufficiency involves the use of several transducer positions in order to record the regurgitant jet from different incident angles. The jet dimensions may vary markedly in different imaging planes, and by recording the jet from multiple positions, the true jet extension into the left atrium can best be estimated.

DETECTION OF MITRAL REGURGITATION BY PULSED DOPPLER

58 POS	3 FALSE NEG
4 FALSE POS	40 NEG

SENSITIVITY : 95 %
SPECIFICITY : 91 %

N = 105

Fig.5-80. Early work by Sgalambro and coworkers demonstrated very good sensitivity and specificity in detecting mitral insufficiency.

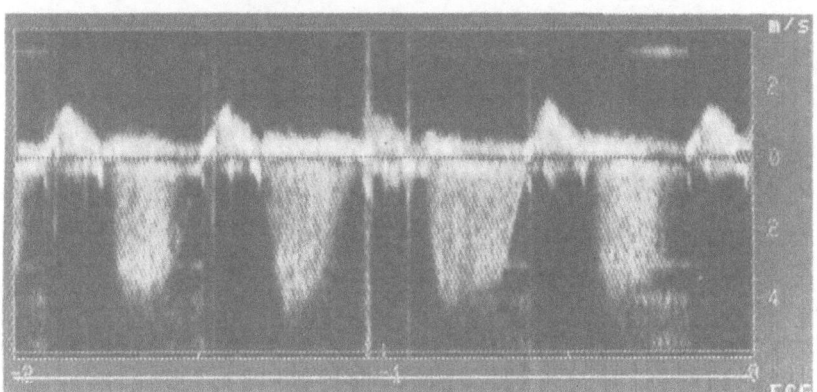

Fig. 5-81. Mitral regurgitation after commissurotomy. Continuous mode recording of the mitral flow in a patient following commissurotomy. The forward flow velocity is approximately 1.5 m/s and the pressure half time is normal. The mitral regurgitation was estimated to be moderate (2+) with flow mapping techniques.

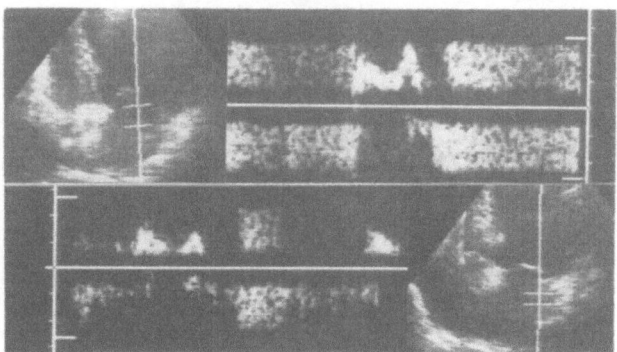

Fig. 5-82 . Mild (2+) mitral insufficiency recorded in a patient following an anterior myocardial infarction. Pulsed mode recordings of the regurgitant flow signal at the level of the mitral annulus (top), and at the level 2 cm behind the annulus.

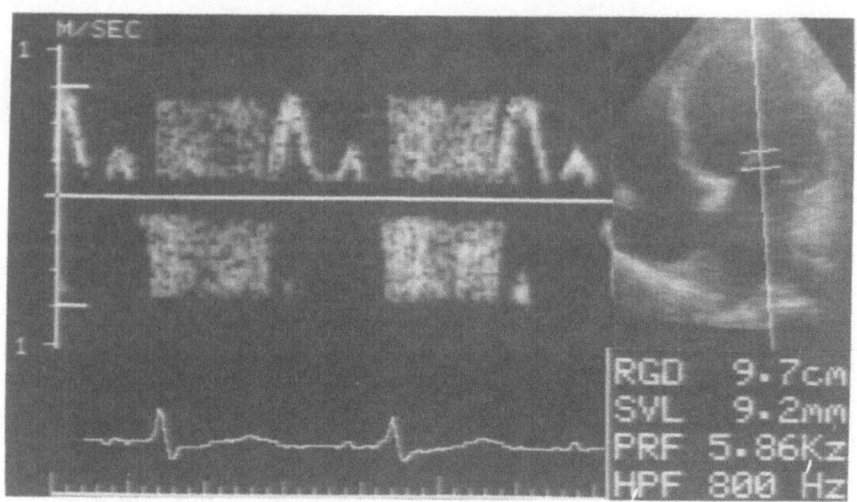

Fig. 5-83 . Mitral insufficiency recorded in a patient following an anteroseptal infarct. The pulsed mode interrogation of the left atrium indicated that the regurgitant flow signal was restricted to the level of the mitral annulus. The insufficiency was therefore graded as mild.

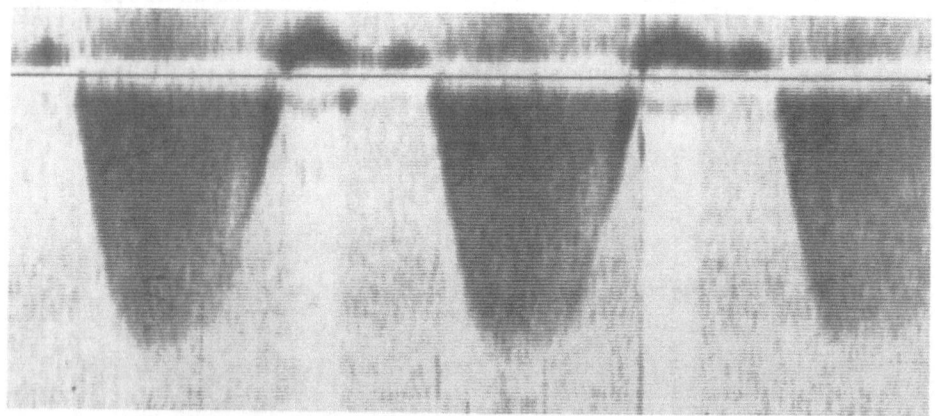

Fig.5-84. This 5.5 m/s flow was obtained in a patient with pure mitral insufficiency. Continuous wave Doppler is well suited for the initial evaluation of the heart because of the large "sample volume" size. This permits one to sweep the Doppler beam through the cardiac chambers without concern for the radial sample volume position. Pulsed Doppler can then be used for flow localization.

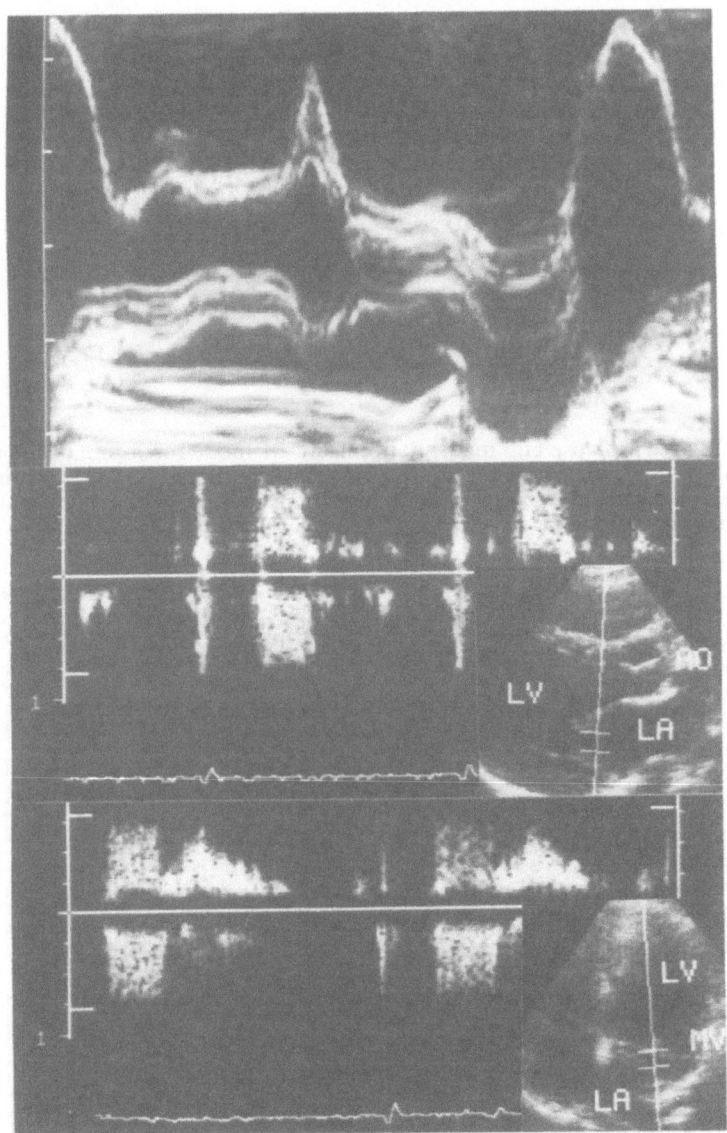

Fig. 5-85. Mitral valve prolapse and regurgitation. Top. M-mode recording of the mitral valve showing the late systolic buckling of the mitral leaflets. Center. Pulsed mode recording from the parasternal window of the mitral regurgitation. The regurgitant flow signal is only detected in mid- to end-systole when the valve is prolapsing. Bottom. Pulsed mode recording of the mitral regurgitation from the apical window showing the same regurgitant flow pattern. The line of mitral valve closure is clearly recorded, followed by an absence of flow until mid-systole.

141

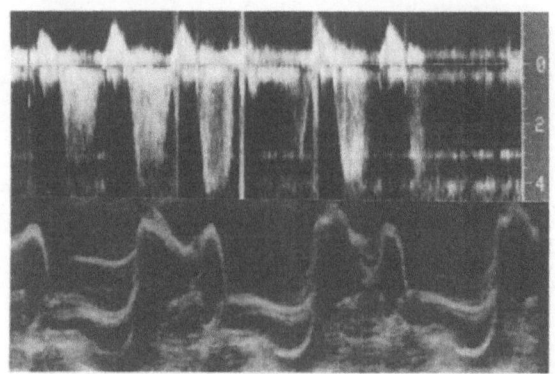

Fig. 5-86. Mitral valve prolapse and regurgitation.Left. M-mode recording of the mitral valve showing the holosystolic systolic buckling of the mitral leaflets. Right . Continuous wave recording from the parasternal window of the mitral regurgitation. The regurgitant flow signal is detected throughout systole .

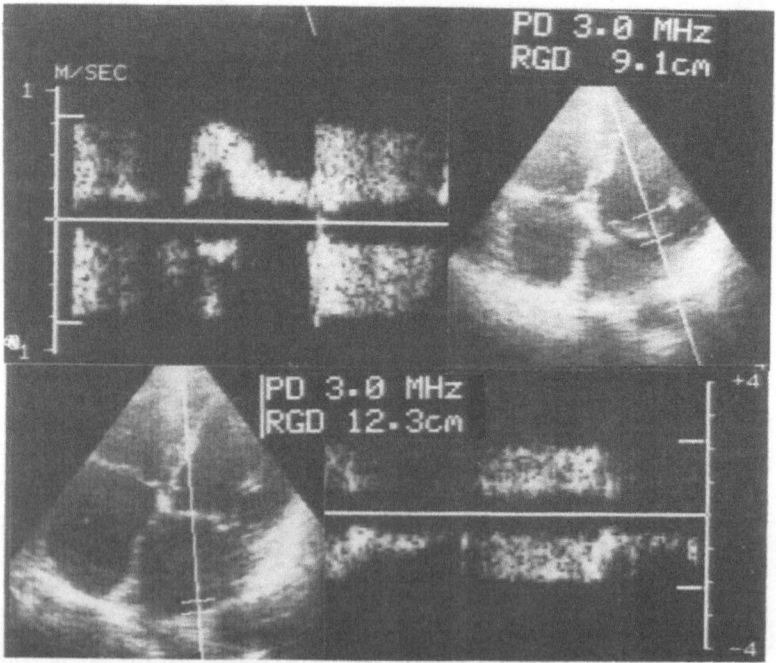

Fig. 5-87 . Flow mapping in another case of severe mitral insufficiency. The regurgitant flow extends from the mitral annulus to the level of the entrance of the pulmonary veins. This represents a flow extension of nearly 6.5 cm. At the level of the pulmonary veins, the regurgitation is less intensely recorded, but this could be partially due to ultrasonic attenuation.

142

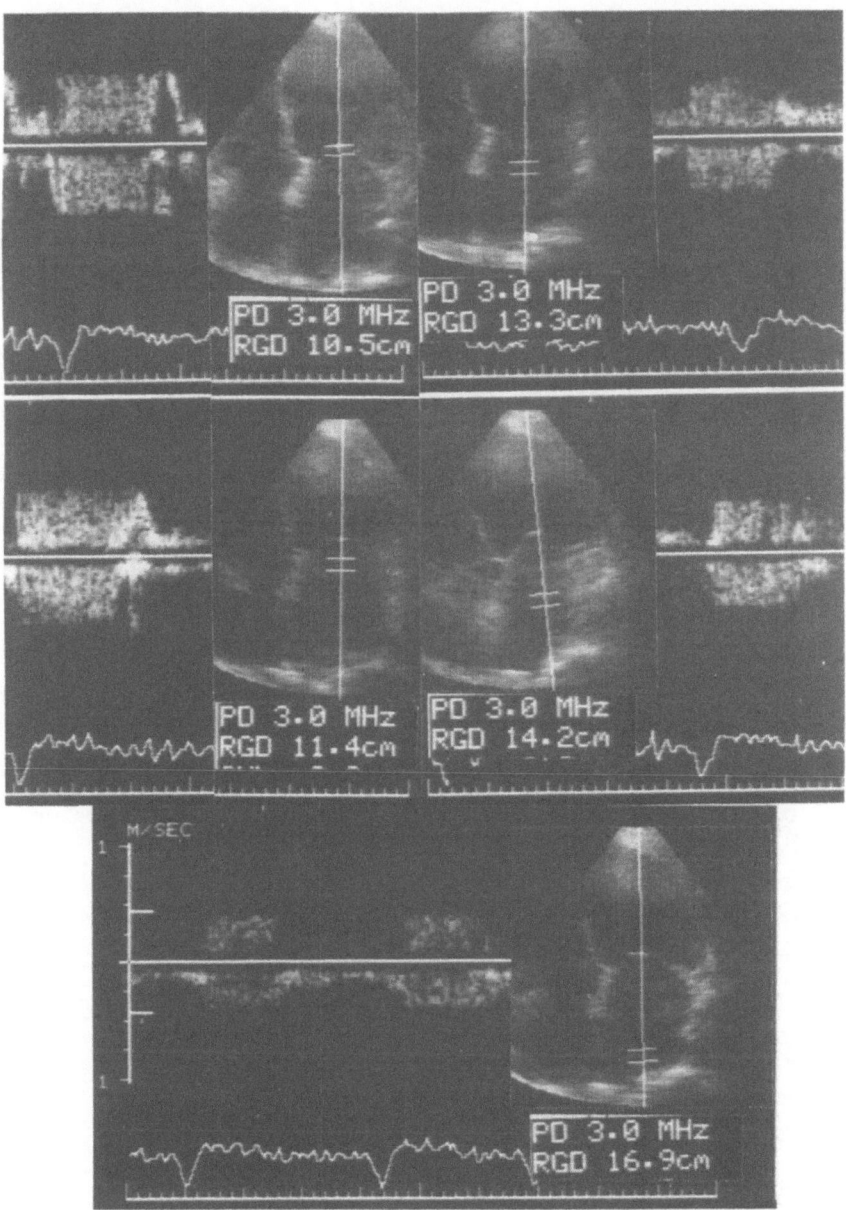

Fig. 5-88. Flow mapping in severe (4+) mitral insufficiency. Pulsed mode recordings of the regurgitant flow signal at the level of the mitral annulus (top), further back in the left atrium (center), and at the level of the pulmonary veins (bottom). Note the high intensity of the flow signal even in the last recording.

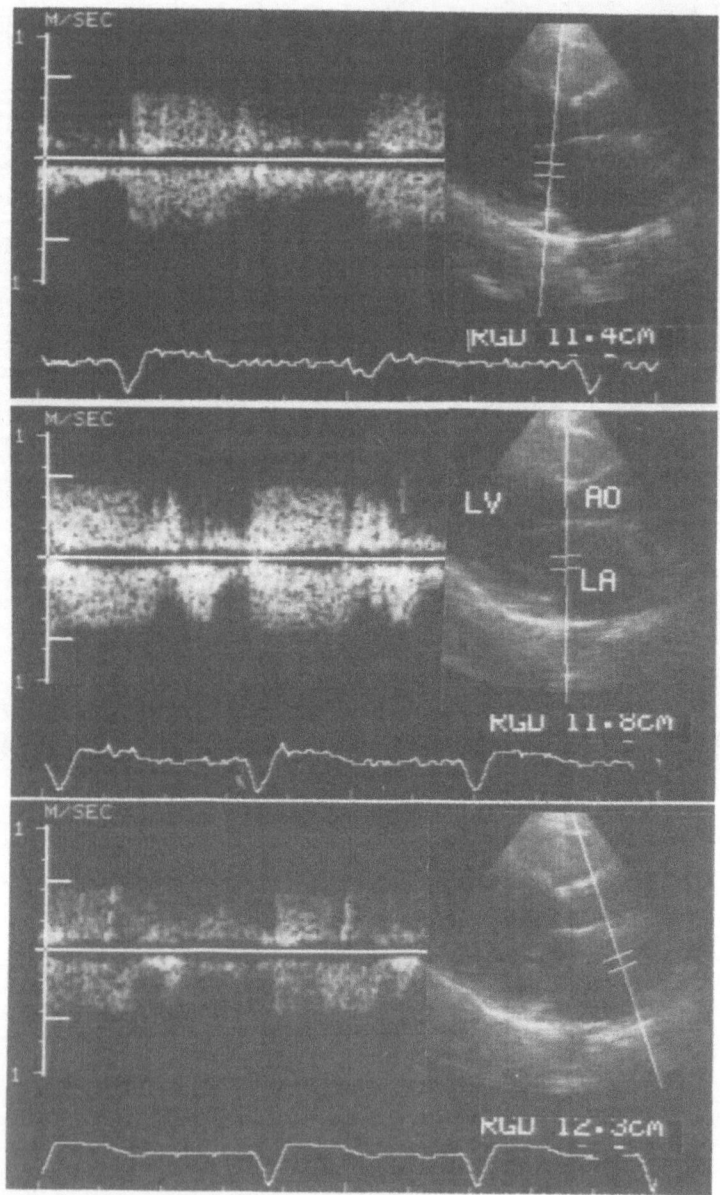

Fig. 5-89 . Flow mapping in mitral insufficiency from the parasternal window. The angle to the regurgitant flow may not appear to be optimal from the parasternal long axis view even if the jet is eccentric. However, the objective of the flow mapping procedure is only to establish the presence or absence of the regurgitant signal. In this example, the regurgitation extends 1.0 cm past the midpoint of the left atrium and is estimated to be moderate.

Miyatake and coworkers have used the regurgitant flow area as an indication of the severity . When the largest area of regurgitant flow has been located, the flow area is planimetered.

Flow extension can also be used to assess the severity of mitral incompetence. It is sometimes helpful to switch off the variance and use an unmodulated red/blue display when examining flow area or flow extension. Flow boundaries may be more clearly delineated when such a color scale is selected. The flow area or flow extension is still dependent upon several factors such as the left atrial pressure, left ventricular function, and left atrial geometry. Care must also be exercised with the instrument set-up. Improper use of the flow gain can result in the over- or under-estimation of the flow extension.

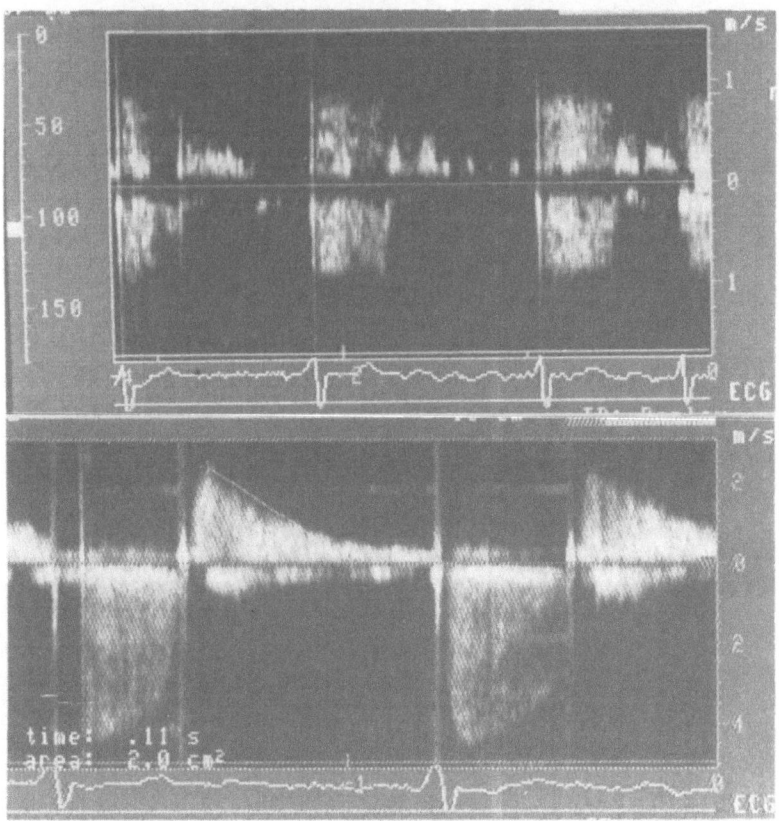

Fig. 5-90. Mitral regurgitation after commissurotomy. Continuous mode recording of the mitral flow in a patient following commissurotomy. The forward flow velocity is approximately 2.25 m/s with a pressure gradient of 20 mm Hg . The mitral regurgitation was estimated to be moderate by pulsed Doppler flow mapping techniques.

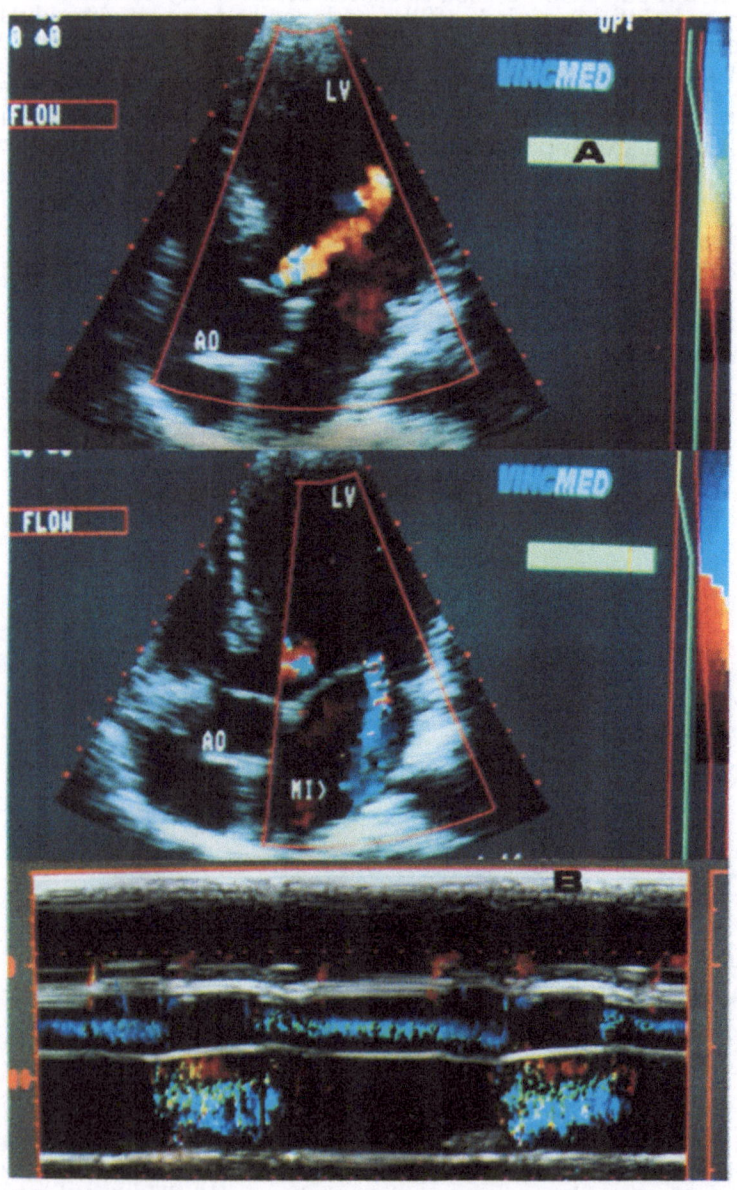

Fig. 5-91. Two dimensional color flow mapping in a patient with both mitral and aortic regurgitation (A and B). The temporal sequence of these flows is demonstrated by the clor T-M mode.

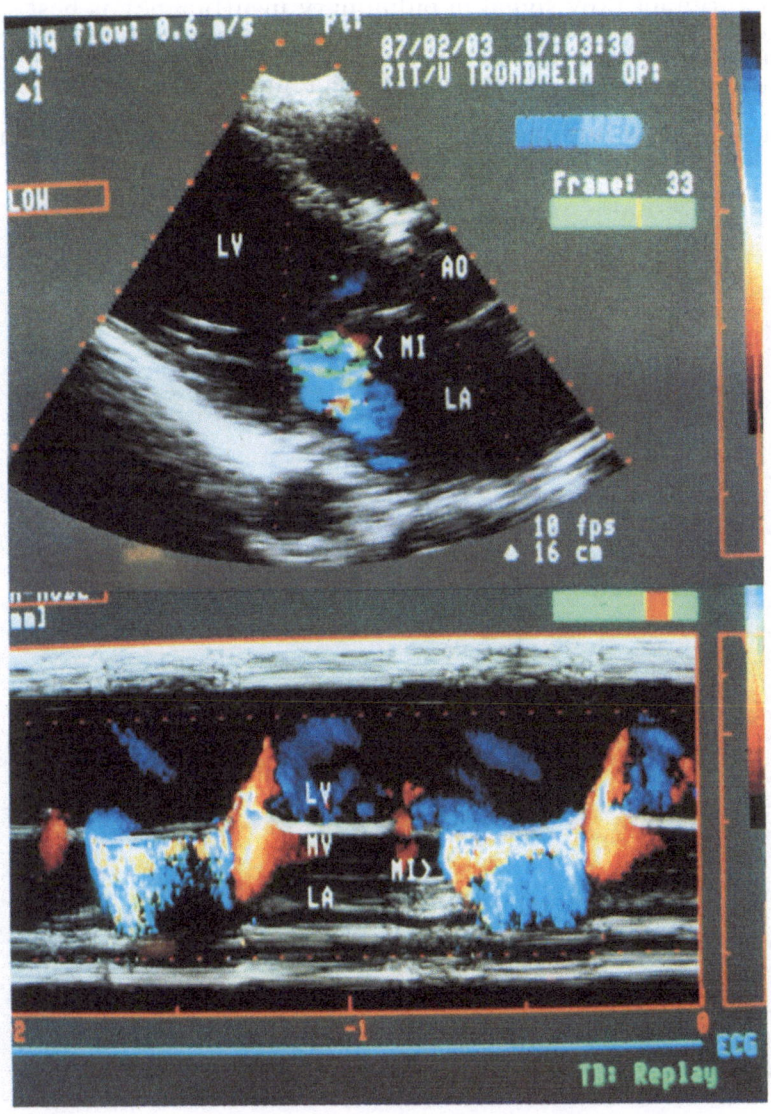

Fig. 5-92. This example was sampled from a low left parasternal notch position . The systolic regurgitant flow is noted to follow along the left atrial wall . The color T-M mode obtained from this position demonstrates the temporal sequence of flow events , the regurgitant flow is the mosaic color pattern seen in the left atrium in systole .

Pulmonary Insufficiency

The regurgitant flow signal in pulmonary insufficiency is best sampled from the parasternal or subcostal window. Using pulsed mode, the sample volume is placed in the right ventricular outflow tract proximal to the pulmonary valve. When searching for the presence of the regurgitant signal, one may initally increase the size of the sample volume to improve the signal-to-noise ratio. Mapping of the regurgitant flow extension into the right ventricular outflow tract yields a qualitative assessment of the degree of incompetence.

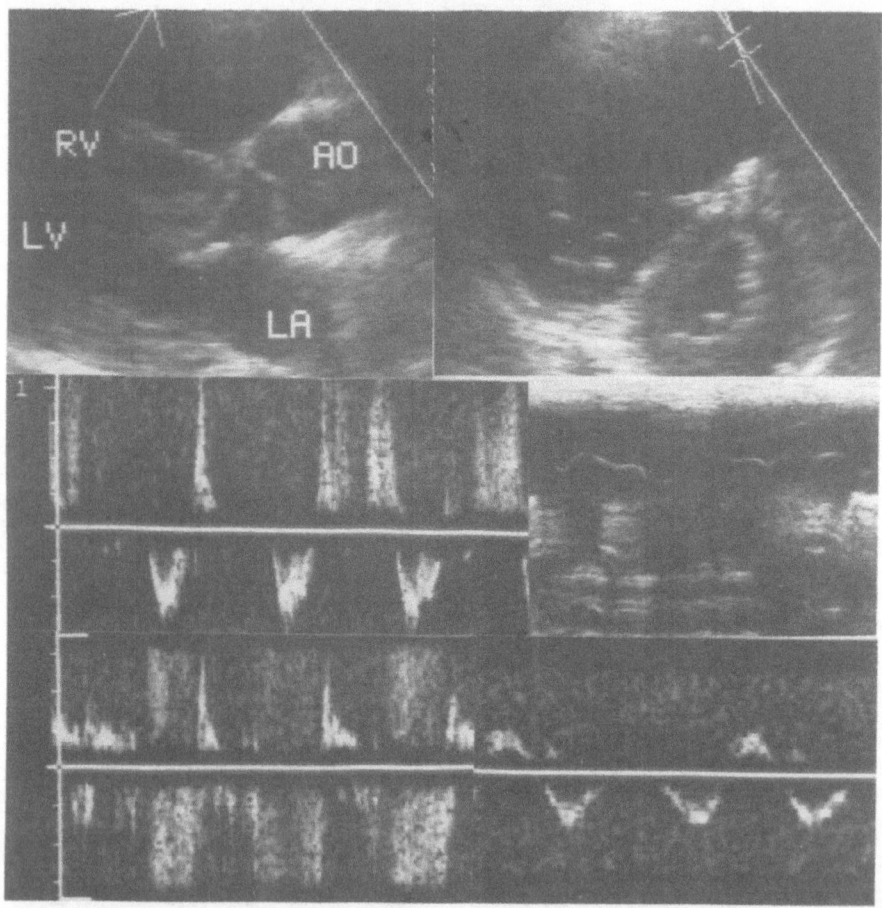

Fig. 5-93. Top. Parasternal long axis (left) and short axis (right) views in a young adult with pulmonary hypertension. Note the enlarged right ventricle and the flattened appearance of the septum. Middle. Pulsed mode recording of the mild pulmonary insufficiency present. The regurgitant flow signal was too weak to be optimally recorded with continuous mode. The M-mode recording of the pulmonary valve demonstrates the absence of an A wave. Bottom. Mild tricuspid insufficiency was also detected with pulsed mode (left). The pulsed mode recording of hepatic vein flow (right) appeared to be normal.

If the regurgitation is only detected behind the pulmonary valve cusps, it is graded as mild. The regurgitant signal intensity should be considered as it is directly related to the regurgitant volume. In a mild pulmonary insufficiency, the signal intensity will be weak. It may be difficult to record the flow signal throughout diastole. In severe pulmonary insufficiency, the flow will be detected with pulsed mode in a large portion of the right ventricular outflow tract, and the flow signal will be intense. Diastolic flutter of the pulmonary valve may interfere with the optimal recording of the regurgitation.

Continuous mode may be used to examine the relative intensity of the regurgitant flow signal as compared to the forward flow signal. The value of the regurgtiant velocity is not an indicator of severity but is determined by the diastolic gradient between the pulmonary artery and the right ventricle. The diastolic pressure in the pulmonary artery can therefore be estimated when the regurgitation is clearly recorded. There is a dip in the flow curve after atrial contraction due to the decreased pressure difference between the pulmonary artery and the right ventricle.

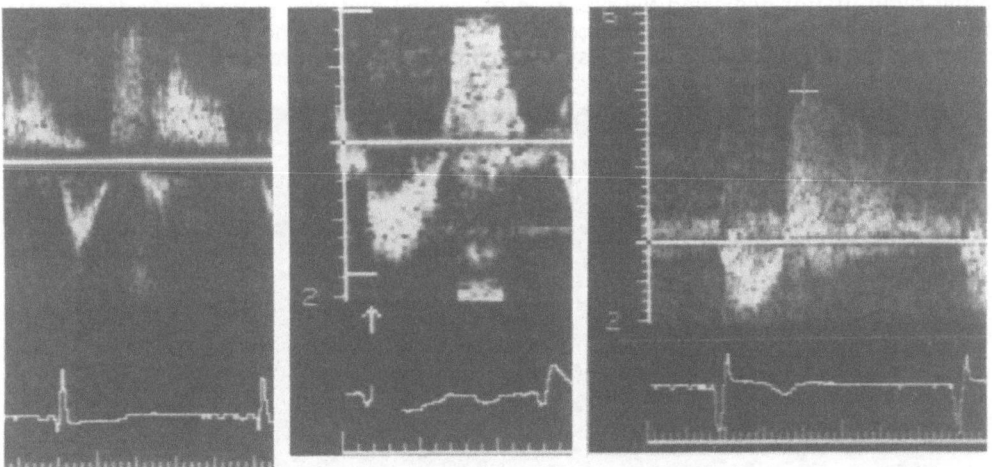

Fig. 5-94 . Three examples of pulmonary insufficiency are shown here. In the first trace, drop out of the regurgitant signal is caused by valve flutter. The low velocity of the regurgitant flow indicates a normal diastolic pulmonary artery pressure. The second trace is an example of a moderately severe regurgitation, with the regurgitant velocity decreasing rapidly. The diastolic pulmonary artery pressure in within normal limits. The third trace shows a mild pulmonary insufficiency with elevated diastolic pulmonary artery pressure; the peak regurgitant flow velocity is approximately 4.0 m/s.

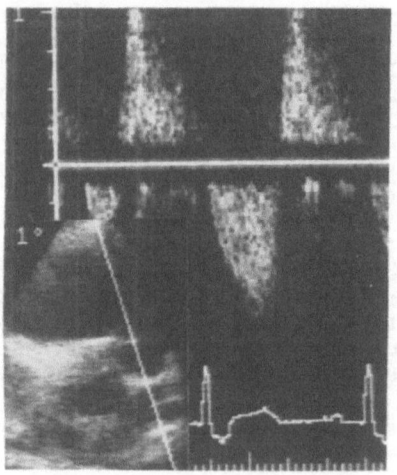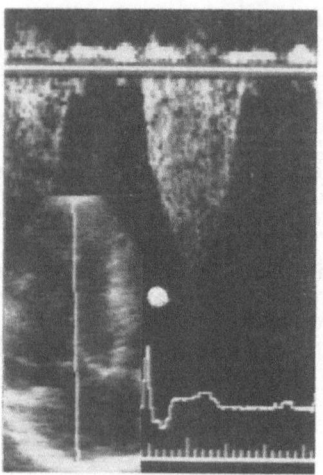

Fig.5-95. Left. Mild pulmonary insufficiency recorded from the parasternal window. The peak of the regurgitant flow velocity curve is not visible in this trace, but the maximal velocities in the regurgitation indicated the presence of normal diastolic pulmonary artery pressure. Right. Mild tricuspid insufficiency recorded from the paical window. The peak regurgitant velocity is 2.4 m/s, indicating that the systolic pulmonary artery pressure is normal.

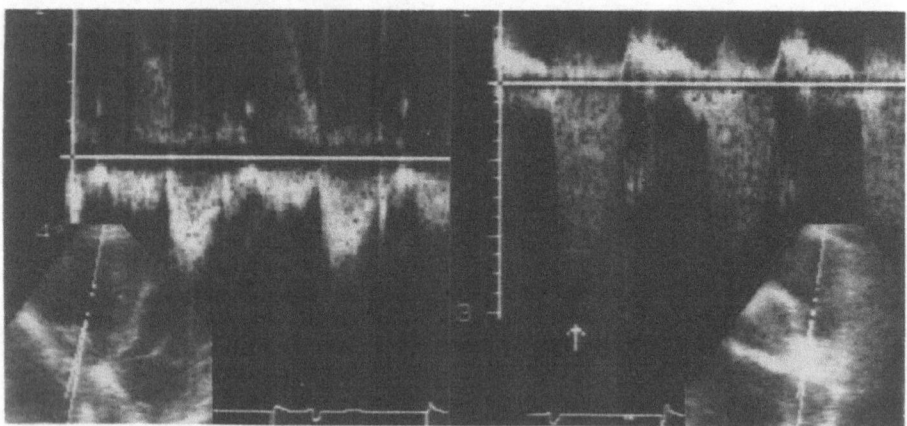

Fig. 5-96. Left. Physiological pulmonary insufficiency in a transplanted heart recorded with continuous mode from the parasternal window. The diastolic pressure in the pulmonary aretry is normal. Right. Physiological tricuspid insufficiency recorded from the apical window. The signal intensity is weak, but the peak regurgitant velocity of 2.5 m/s can still be ascertained. This confirms the presence of normal systolic pulmonary artery pressure. In our experience , a small amount of tricuspid and pulmonary insufficiency is not uncommon 2-3 weeks post-operatively in transplant patients.

When the pulmonary regurgitation is significant, a narrow bandwidth signal may be recorded in diastole and the peak regurgitant velocity declines quickly. No regurgitant flow may be recorded at end-diastole, indicating that the pressures in the pulmonary artery and right ventricle have equalized.

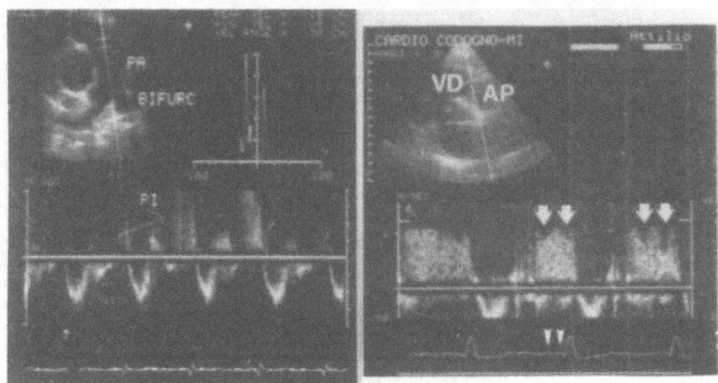

Fig.5-97 Physiological pulmonary insufficiency. Left. Frequently a positive diastolic flow can be recorded in the pulmonary artery of a normal subject (arrow). It is usually difficult to record this flow signal in early diastole, but the flow signal is easily detected in mid- to end-diastole. The flow signal is localized to a small area proximal to the pulmonary valve, and probably represents the presence of physiological insufficiency. Right. Pulmonary insufficiency in the presence of atrial flutter. Double dips (arrows) are seen in the regurgitant flow signal as a result of the atrial arrythmia. The pulmonary insufficiency itself is localized to a small area and is hemodynamically insignificant. The decreased reguigtant flow velocity following atrial contraction reflects the rise in the right ventricular pressure.

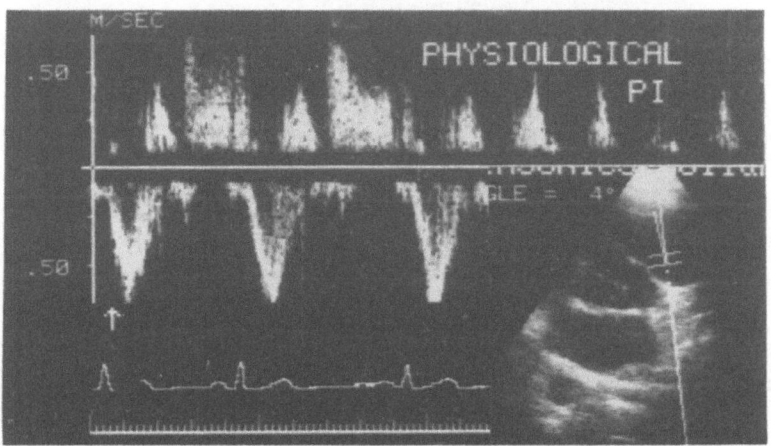

Fig.5-98 . Physiological pulmonary insufficiency recorded in a young adult. Note the signal drop out in early diastole.

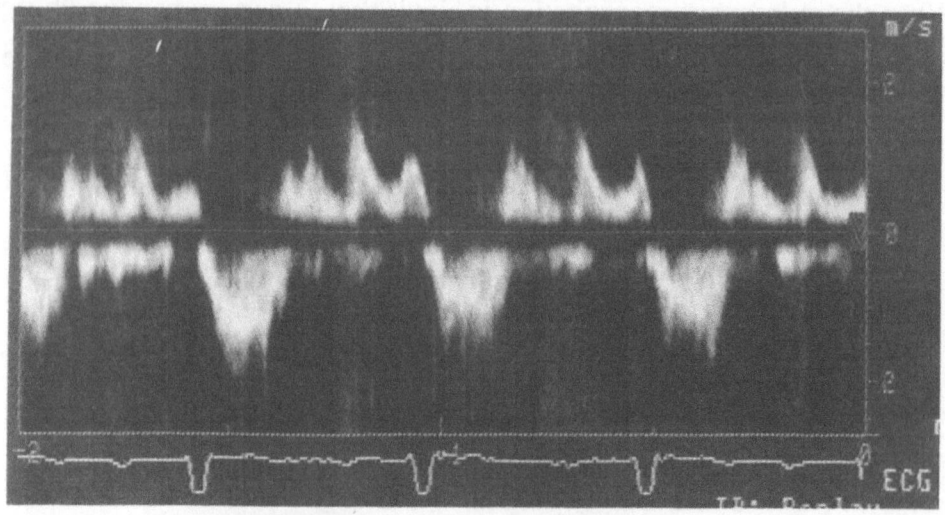

Fig.5-99 . Pulsed mode recording in pulmonary insufficiency. with an atrial septal defect.
Note the double notching of the diastolic flow curve .

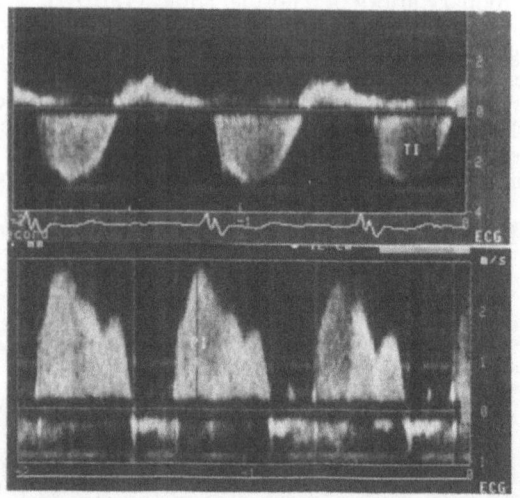

Fig.5-100 Pulmonary hypertension. Top. Continuous mode recording of tricuspid
regurgitation from the parasternal window. The peak regurgitant velocity is 3.0 m/s, hence the
predicted systolic pulmonary artery pressure is 36 mm Hg. Bottom. Continuous mode
recording of pulmonary insufficiency in the same patient. The peak regurgitant flow velocity in
early diastole is 2.75 m/s and 1.75 m/s in end-diastole, indicating that the diastolic pulmonary
artery pressure is elevated as well.

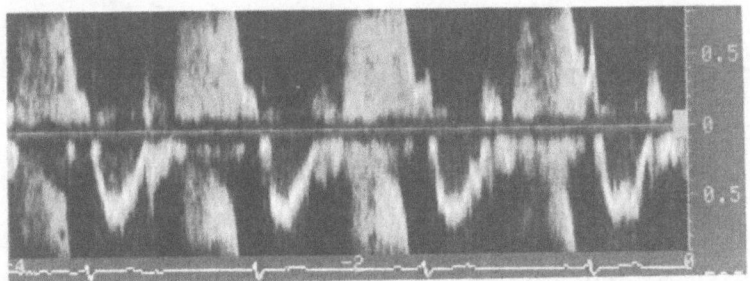

Fig. 5-101. Moderately severe pulmonary insufficiency with normal diastolic pressure in the pulmonary artery. The intensity of the regurgitant signal is stronger than that seen in cases of physiological pulmonary insufficiency.

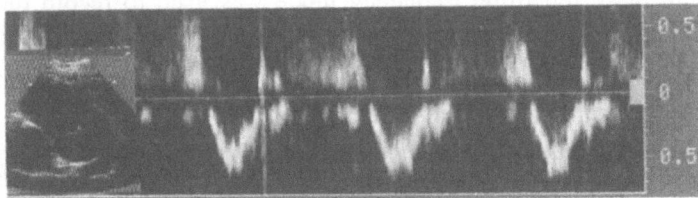

Fig.5-102. Pulsed mode recording in a mild pulmonary insufficiency. The position of the sample volume in the right ventricular outflow tract has shifted when the two dimensional image was frozen, and this signal was actually recorded at a distance of approximately 1.5 cm behind the pulmonary annulus.

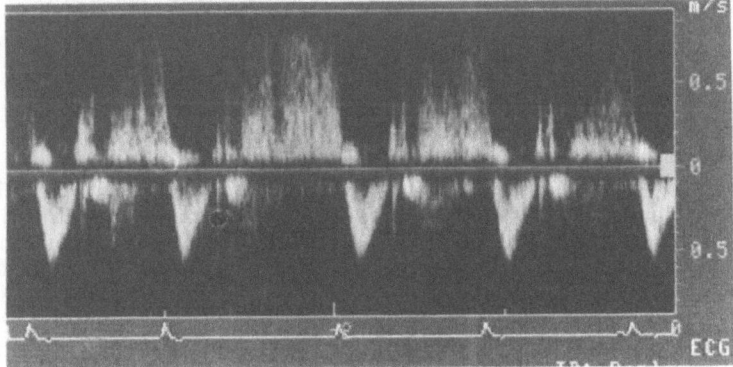

Fig.5-103. Continuous mode recording of a small pulmonary insufficiency in the normal patient.. Drop out of the regurgitant flow signal in early diastole may be seen in continusous mode recordings as well as in pulsed mode recordings.

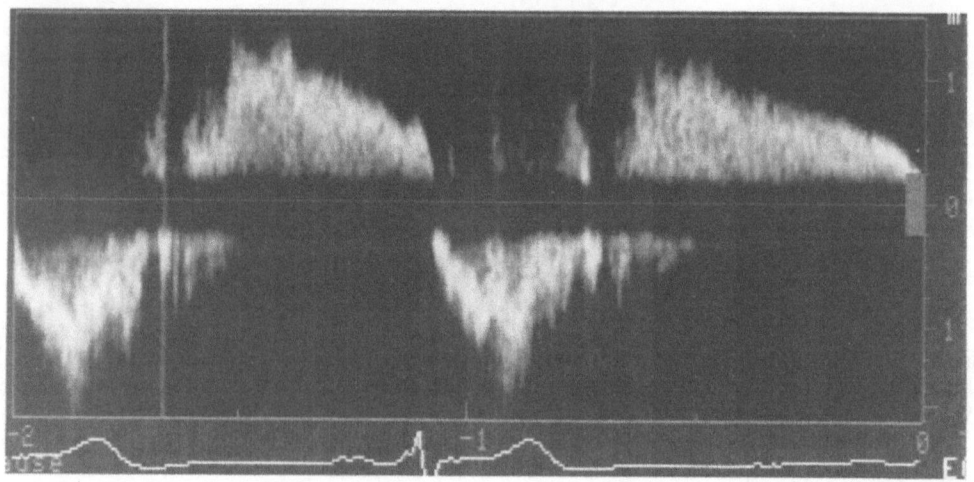

Fig. 5-104 . High pulse repetition frequency mode was used to record the pulmonary insufficiency in a patient with idiopathic dilatation of the pulmonary artery. The regurgitant flow was estimated to be moderately severe with color flow analysis. The pulmonary artery pressure was normal, hence the regurgitant flow velocity was not high. High pulsed repetititon frequency mode was therefore used to record the regurgitation.

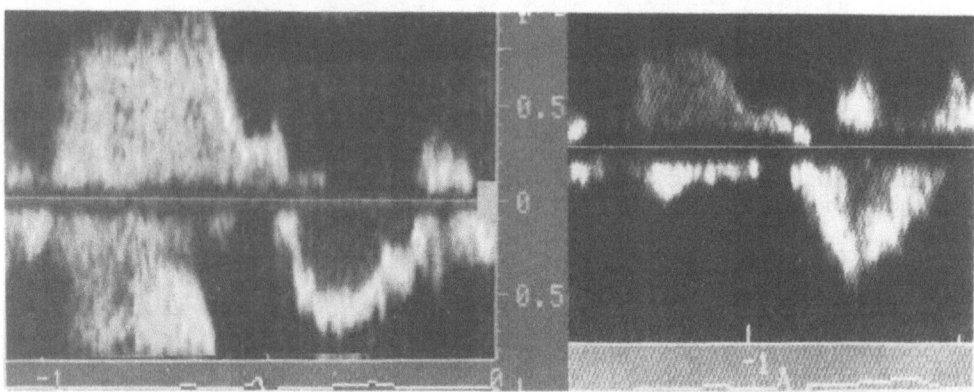

Fig. 5-105 . Pulsed Doppler mode was used to record the pulmonary insufficiency in 2 patients with a moderate and mild pulmonary regurgitation. The pulmonary artery pressure was normal, hence the regurgitant flow velocity was not high. The diastolic signal in figure A is stronger than in figure B because a larger volume of blood is back scattering ultrasonic energy.

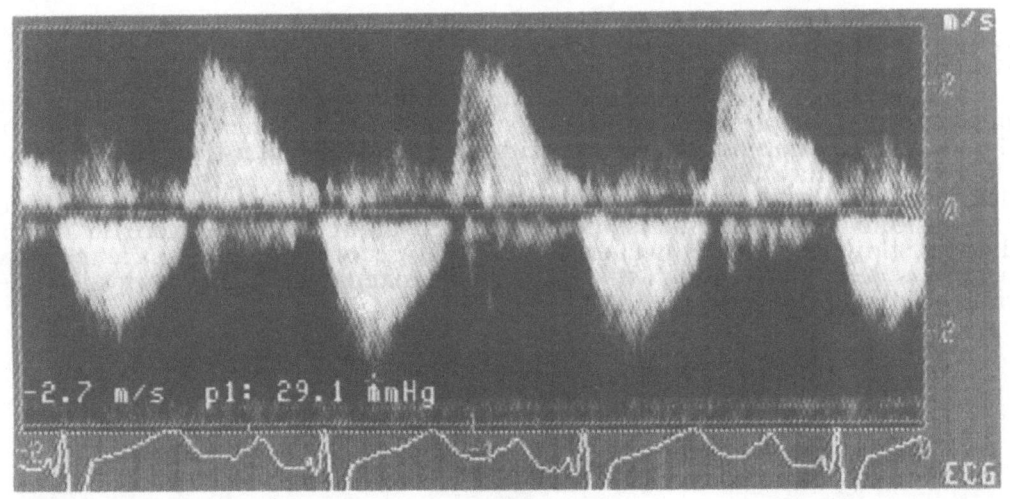

Fig. 5-106 . Continuous mode recording of moderate pulmonary insuffficiency following pulmonary valvotomy. The peak forward flow velocity is slightly increased (2.7 m/s), but there is no singificant residual obstruction.

Tricuspid Insufficiency

The pulsed mode flow mapping technique is the most frequently applied method of assessing tricuspid insufficiency. Either a parasternal or apical imaging window can be used to record the extension of the regurgitant flow signal into the right atrium. The sample volume is initially placed in the right atrium proximal to the tricuspid valve and methodically moved until an aliased holosystolic flow signal is recorded. Continuous mode may be used at the beginning of the examination to determine the jet orientation. Once the flow signal has been detected, the regurgitation can be tracked into the right atrium by switching to pulsed mode. The flow extension can then be used to estimate the degree of incompetence.

The regurgitant flow extension is affected by the cardiac output, right atrial dimensions, atrial compliance, regurgitant jet orientation, and right atrial pressure. The limited spatial orientation of pulsed mode can also introduce difficulties in interpreting the flow mapping results. In order to supplement the flow mapping information, the peak tricuspid flow velocity should be measured and the intensity of the forward flow signal compared to the regurgitant flow signal. The value of the peak tricuspid velocity should also be compared to the peak mitral velocity if the mitral valve is normal. The presence of increased cardiac output will be reflected by a concommitant increase in the peak flow velocities recorded across the other valves.

A small degree of tricuspid insufficiency can often be detected in normal subjects. The regurgitant flow signal is weak and localized to an area of the right atrium immediately behind the tricuspid annulus.

Flow patterns in the vena cavae and the hepatic veins will be affected by the presence of moderate to severe tricuspid insufficiency. When sampling flow in the hepatic veins or the superior vena cava, several characteristic changes in the flow pattern may be detected. The anterograde systolic peak velocity is decreased, while the anterograde diastolic flow velocity is augmented. Mid to end-systolic flow reversal is often recorded along with an increase in the diastolic flow velocity. However, the ability to record such changes in the flow pattern is dependent upon such factors as the size of the hepatic veins and the right atrial compliance.

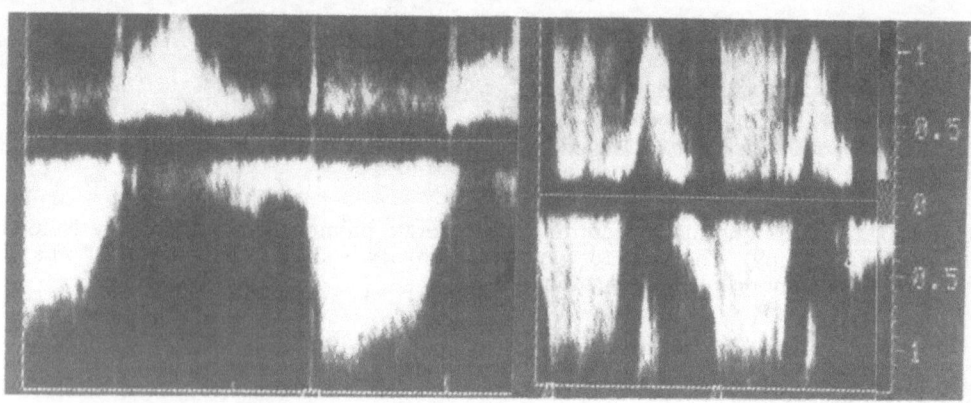

Fig. 5-107 . Moderately severe tricuspid insufficiency. A. The continuous mode recording form a parasternal window indicates that the right ventricular systolic pressure is not elevated. The peak regurgitant velocity is approxiamtely 2.5 m/s. B. Pulsed mode recording made with the sample volume 2.0 cm behind the tricuspid annulus.

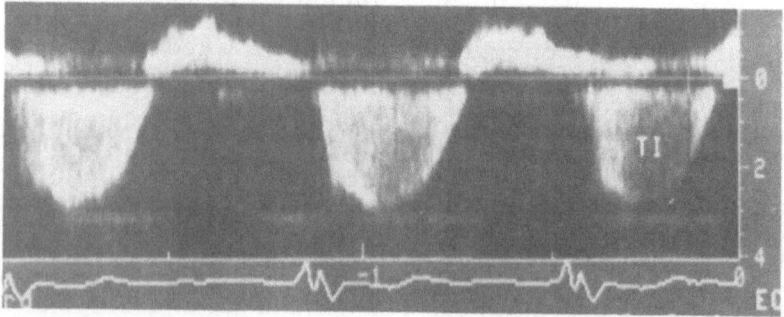

Fig.5-108. Tricuspid insufficiency with elevated systolic pulmonary artery pressure. The continuous mode recording from the apical window indicates that the systolic right ventricular pressure is increased. The peak regurgitant flow velocity is 3.0 m/s, corresponding to a predicted gradient of 36 mm Hg.

The value of the peak regurgitant velocity as recorded with continuous mode is not an indication of severity. The peak velocity is related to the right ventricular-right atrial pressure gradient in systole, and can be used to estimate this gradient by application of the modified Bernoulli equation. If there is no obstruction to right ventricular outflow, the systolic pressure difference between the right ventricle and the right atrium is approximately the same as the pressure difference between the pulmonary artery and the right atrium. By adding the estimated right atrial pressure to the calculated gradient, the systolic right ventricular pressure can be estimated noninvasively. When the right ventricular and right atrial pressures are within normal limits, the maximal regurgitant velocity ranges from 2.0 to 2.6 m/s. The right atrial pressure can be estimated from a clinical assessment of the neck veins, by an indwelling central venous pressure line, or it may be considered negligeable. Our findings in the experimental canine model indicate that the correlation between the Doppler and catheterization values of the right ventricular systolic pressure is dependent to some degree on the right atrial pressure. When the right atrial pressure is less than 10 mm Hg, the effect of neglecting the right atrial pressure is statistically insignificant. In the clinical situation then, it is acceptable to neglect the right atrial pressure when the right atrial pressure is normal or slightly increased. When the right atrial pressure is significantly increased as in right ventricular failure or on severe tricupsid regurgitation, the right atrial pressure must be added to the gradient when estimating the right ventricular systolic pressure. Failure to add the right atrial pressure in these cases will result in an underestimation of the right ventricular pressure.

The most frequently encountered source of error lies in the estimation of the peak regurgitant velocity. If the true peak velocity is not recorded, the calculated gradient will be errroneously low. The value of the velcotiy is squared in the modified Bernoulli equation, so any error made in the estimation of the velocity will be squared. The audio signal should be used to align the continuous wave beam with the regurgitant jet in order to ensure optimal beam-to-flow alignment.

Fig. 5-109. Overleaf. Multimodality assessment of tricuspid insufficiency. A. The color flow display of the right ventricular inflow using the rainbow color assignment. B. The regurgitant flow is seen as a predominantly blue flow bolus containing regions of color aliasing. C. When an optimal flow display of the regurgitant jet has been obtained, the continuous mode cursor is utilized to record the regurgitant flow velcoity curve. The peak regurgitant velocity is 4.3 m/s, hence the predicted gradient is 74 mm Hg. D. Pulsed mode recording of hepatic vein flow from the subcostal window. The diastolic flow component is accentuated. E. A small amount of pulmonary insufficiency was detected upon examination of the right ventricular outflow tract. F. Continous mode recording of the pulmonary insufficiency from the same position. The peak regurgitant velocities indicate that the diastolic pulmonary artery pressure is also elevated.

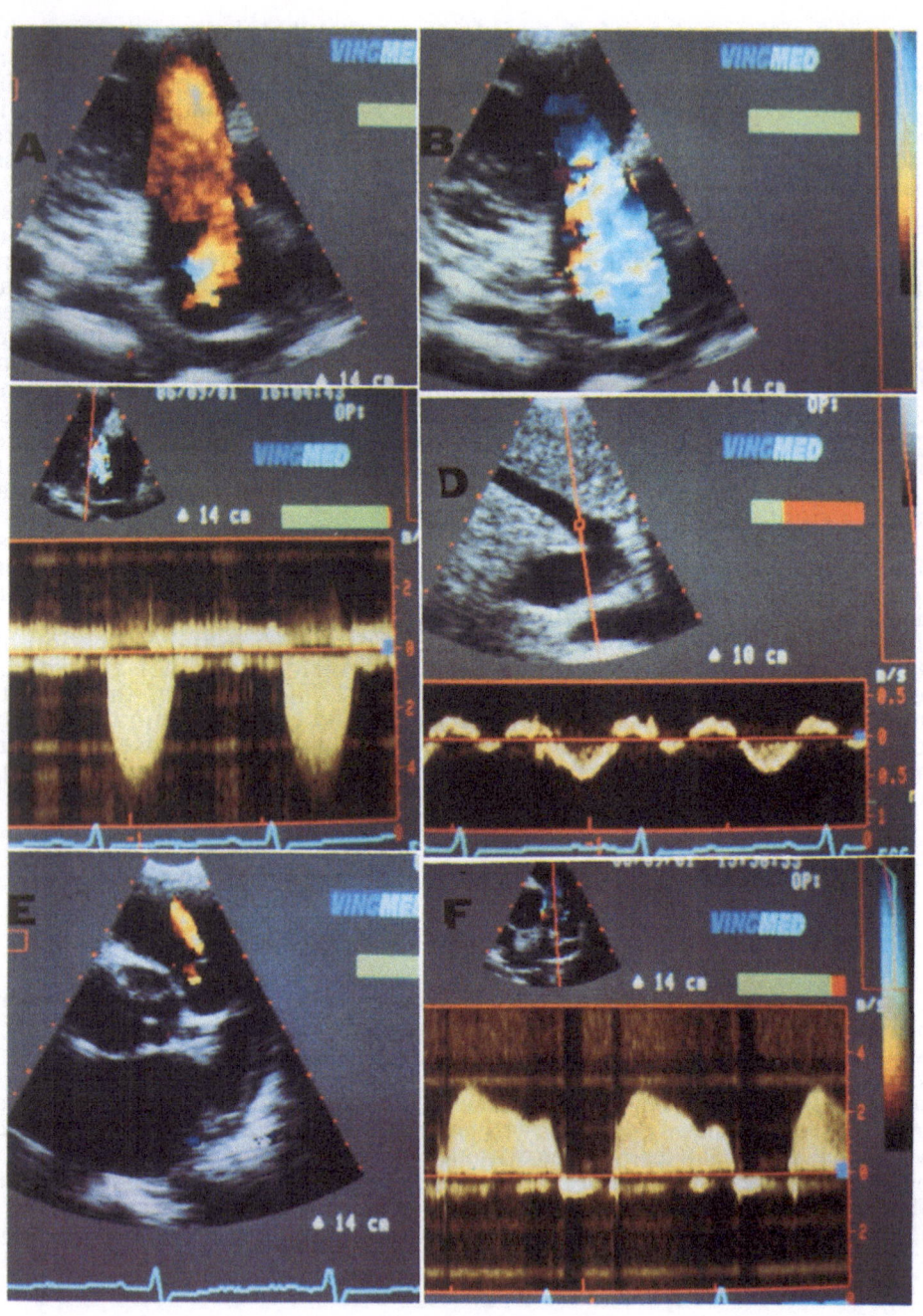

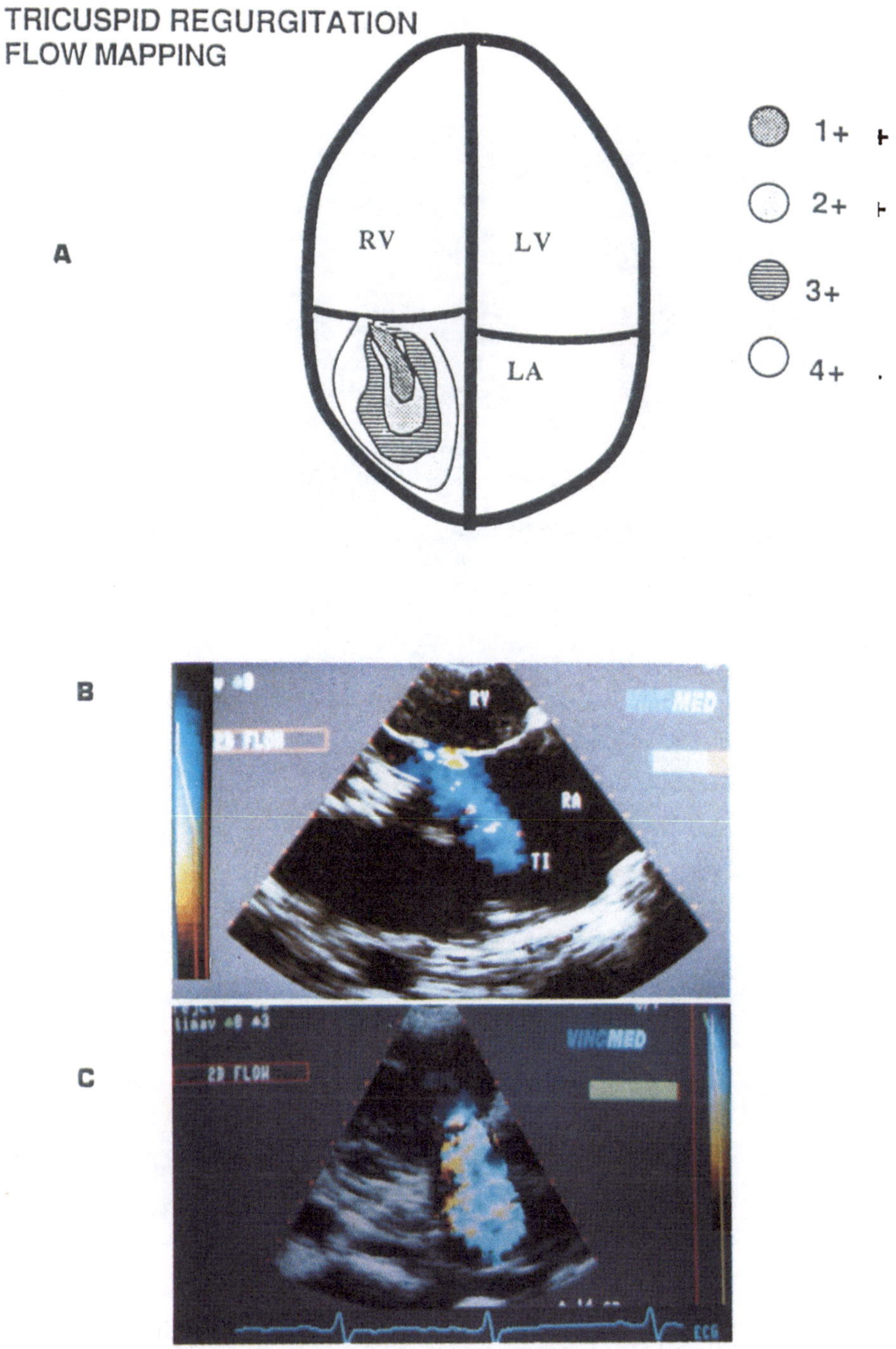

TRICUSPID REGURGITATION FLOW MAPPING

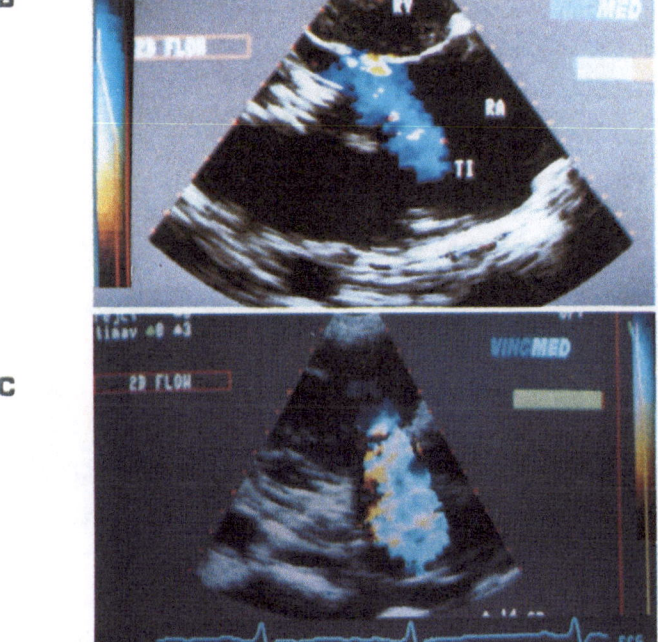

Fig.5-110. Color Flow mapping in tricuspid regurgitation. A. The axial and lateral extension of the regurgitant flow may be used to estimate the severity of the insufficiency. Flow extension is influenced by several factors such as the right ventricular function, the size of the right atrium, and the right atrial compliance. B. Moderate tricuspid insufficiency imaged from a parasternal position. C. Severe tricuspid insufficiency imaged from a similar position. The flow extension in the axial and lateral directions is far greater than that seen in B.

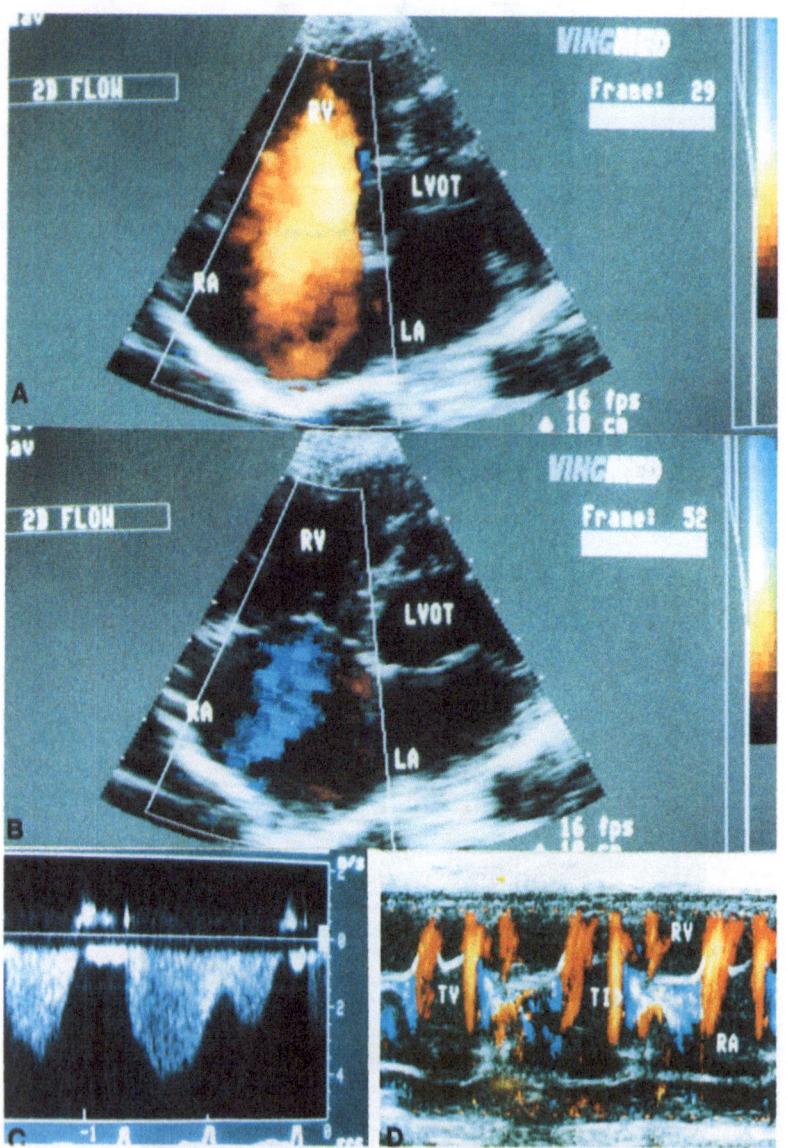

Fig. 5-111 A. Two dimensional display of right ventricular inflow from the apical window. B. In systole, a small flow bolus is seen to emanate from the tricuspid annulus. C. The continuous mode recording from the same position. Note diastolic flow across the tricuspid valve is recorded following a premature contraction, and the regurgitant velocity is much less than that recorded in the other beats. D. The color TM mode yields god temporal resolution .

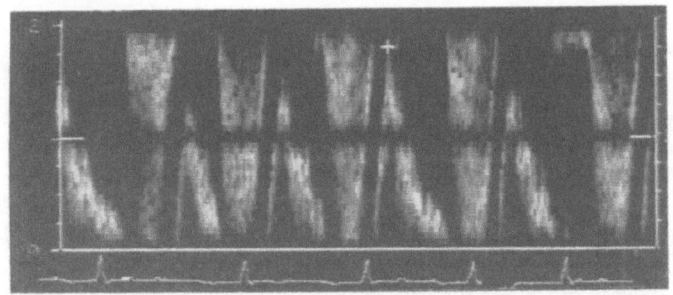

Fig.5-112 . Severe tricuspid insufficiency recorded with pulsed mode at the level of the tricuspid valve. Spectral unwrapping has been used in an attempt to resolve the peak forward and reverse flow velocities. The peak tricuspid velocity is 1.8 m/s, but the peak regurgitant velocity can not be measured because the peak of the flow velocity curve is still unresolved. The relatively narrow bandwidth of the regurgitant flow signal indicates that the regurgitation is significant.

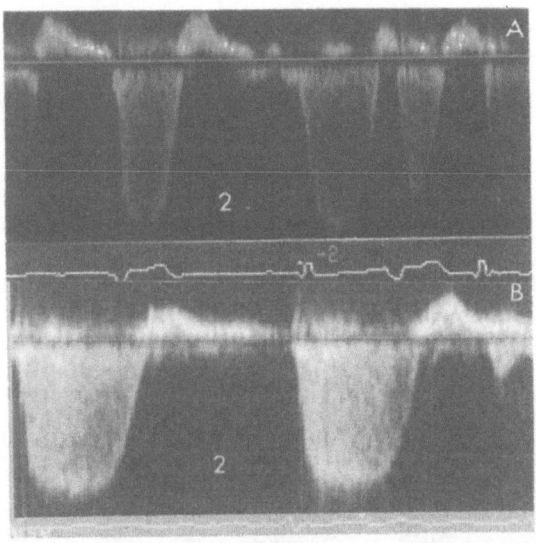

Fig.5-113 . Mild (A) and severe (B) tricuspid regurgitation in the presence of normal pulmonary artery pressure. The peak velocities of the two traces are approximately the same although the peak velocity in A is less clearly recorded owing to the small volume of regurgitant flow. The relative intensity of the regurgitant flow signal is a good indicator of severity when used in conjunction with flow mapping techniques.

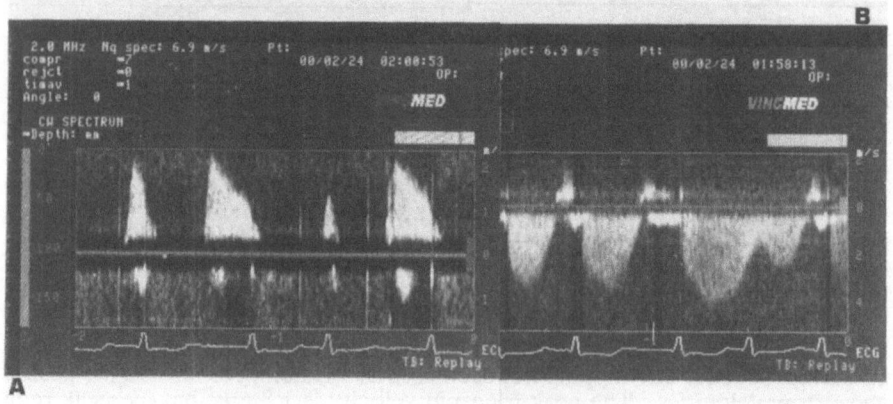

Fig.5-114. The continuous mode recording from the same patient as in figure 1-111. Note that the diastolic flow across the tricuspid valve is recorded following a premature contraction, and the regurgitant velocity is much less than that recorded in the other beats. It can be seen in the top panel that the mitral valve also fails to open following an extra systole

SYSTOLIC RIGHT VENTRICULAR PRESSURE

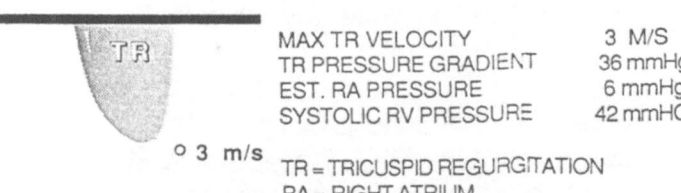

MAX TR VELOCITY	3 M/S
TR PRESSURE GRADIENT	36 mmHg
EST. RA PRESSURE	6 mmHg
SYSTOLIC RV PRESSURE	42 mmHG

○ 3 m/s

TR = TRICUSPID REGURGITATION
RA = RIGHT ATRIUM
RV = RIGHT VENTRICAL

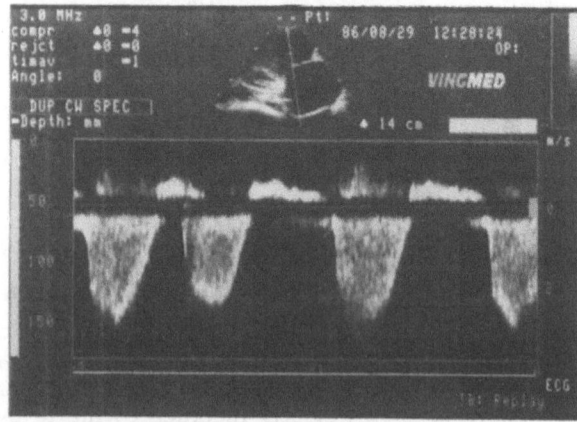

Fig.5-115 . Estimation of the systolic right ventricular pressure when the right atrial pressure is elevated. The value of the right atrial pressure must be added to the calculated gradient when the right atrial pressure is increased to avoid underestimation of the systolic right ventricular pressure.

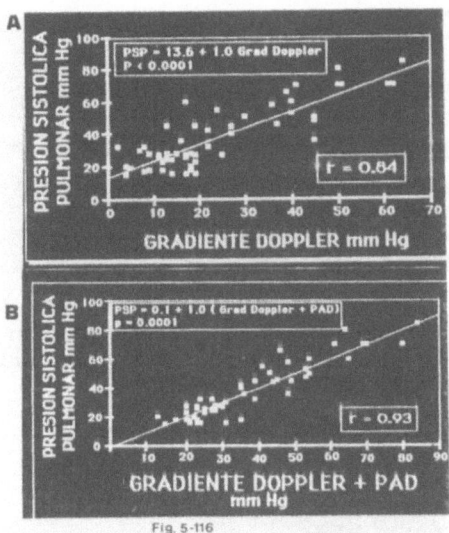

Fig. 5-116

Fig. Fifty-five simultaneous measurements of the pulmonary artery systolic pressure (PSP) and the Doppler estimated right ventricular-right atrial gradient (Gradiente Doppler) were performed in a series of open-chested dogs. The right ventricular pressure was altered by pulmoanry artery banding and volume loading. In some cases, the invasively measured right atrial pressure exceeded 10 mm Hg. Top. Correlation between Doppler gradient and the systolic pulmonary artery pressure (r = 0.84). Bottom. The correlation between the Doppler estimated systolic pulmonary artery pressure and the right ventricular pressure when the invasively measured right atrial pressure was added to the Doppler gradient. A better correlation is noted (r = 0.93).

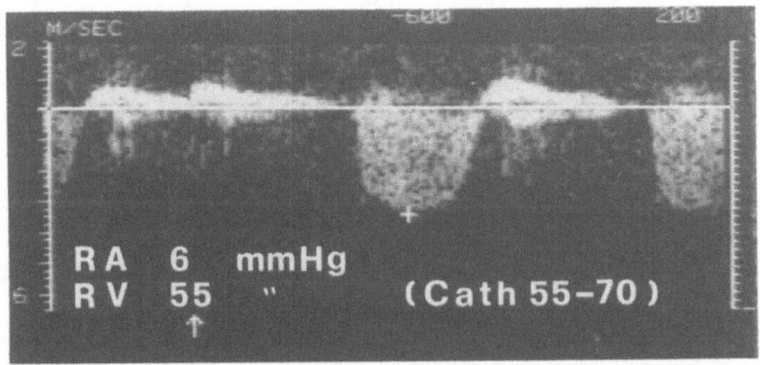

Fig.5-117 . Continuous mode recording of tricuspid insufficiency from the parasternal window. The peak regurgitant velocity was 3.5 m/s, corresponding to a predicted gradient of 49 mm Hg. The clinical estimate of the right atrial pressure (6 mm Hg) was added to the gradient to obtain the predicted systolic right ventricular pressure (55 mm Hg). The invasively measured value (Cath) was 55 to 70 mm Hg.

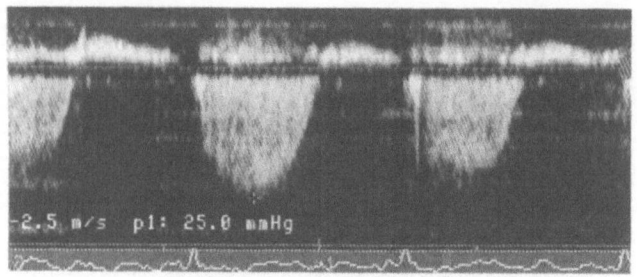

Fig.5-118 Continous mode recording of tricuspid insufficiency in a patient with normal pulmonary artery pressure. The peak regurgitant velocity is 2.5 m/s, corresponding to a predicted systolic pulmonary artery pressure of 25 mm Hg.

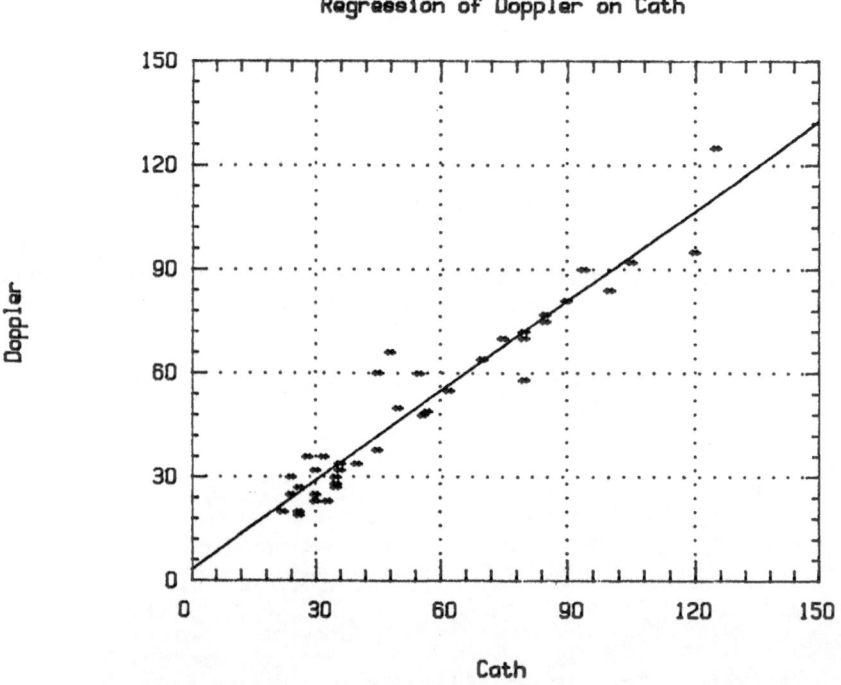

Fig.5-119. In this series of 35 patients with tricuspid insufficiency, simultaneous right ventricular and right atrial pressures were obtained invasively. The peak regurgitant flow velocity was used to predict the right ventricular pressure with continuous mode by adding the invasively measured right atrial pressure was added to the Doppler-derived gradient. This study by Skjaerpe and coworkers demonstrates that Doppler estimate of right ventricular pressure correlates very closely with the invasive estimate when the absolute value of the right atrial pressure is added to the Doppler gradient.

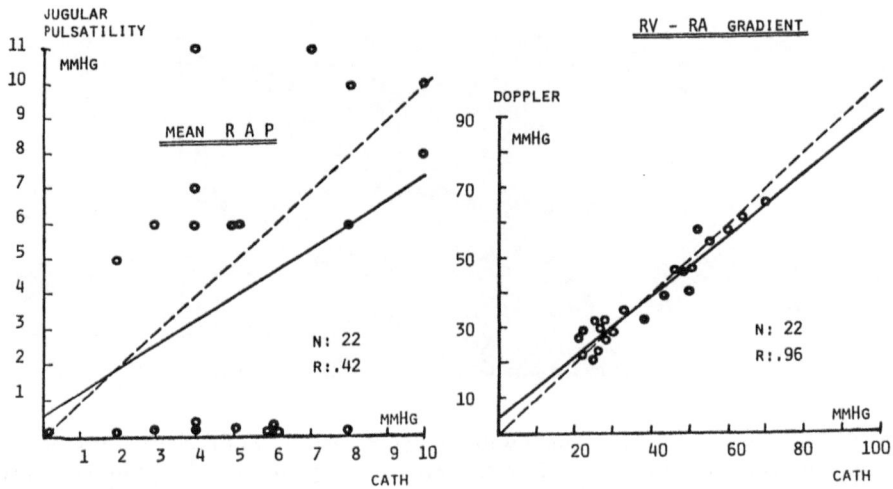

Fig. 5-120 . Right . This study by Sgalambro et al in a series of 22 patients with tricuspid regurgitation demonstrates the close correlation between the Doppler estimate of right ventricular pressure and the invasive value. The clinical estimate of the right atrial pressure was not added to the Doppler derived gradient in this study. Left. The clinical estimate of the mean right atrial pressure (by examination of the jugular pulsatility) was compared to the invasively measured right atrial pressure. A very poor correlation is noted (r = .42). This results of this study therefore suggest that it is generally not necessary to include an estimate of the right atrial pressure.

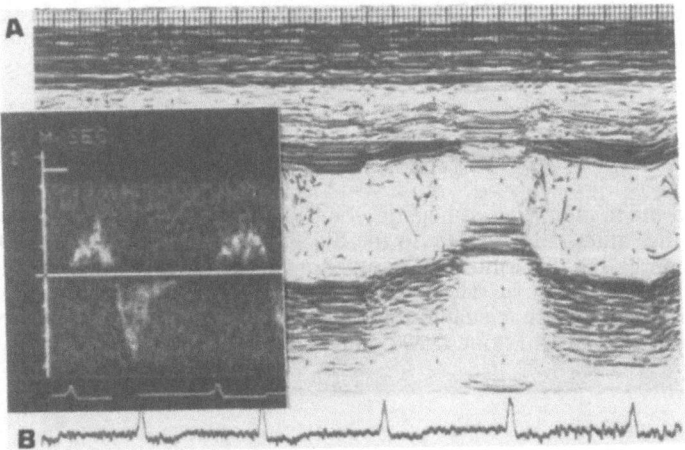

Fig 5-121 A. Contrast study of the inferior vena cava in a patient with tricuspid insufficiency. The systolic appearance of contrast in the inferior vena cava coincided with the onset of regurgitant flow in the pulsed mode recording of hepatic vein flow seen in B.

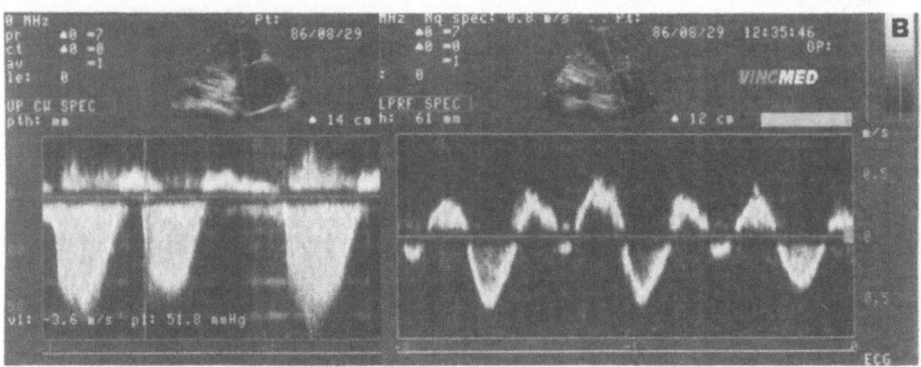

Fig.5-122. Severe tricuspid insufficiency with elevated systolic pulmonary artery pressure. A. The peak regurgitant velocity is 3.6 m/s, corresponding to a sytolic pulmonary artery pressure of 52 mm Hg. B. Pulsed mode recording of hepatic vein flow. Systolic flow reversal is seen and the distolic flow component is accentuated.

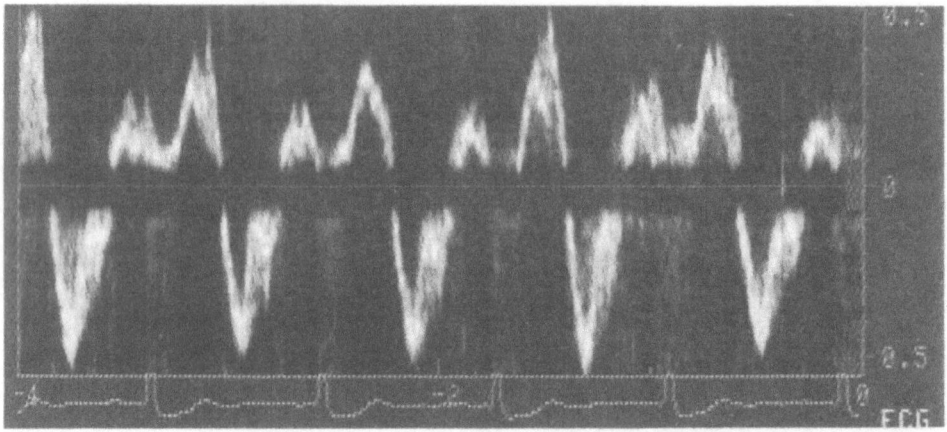

Fig.5-123 Pulsed mode recording of hepatic vein flow in severe tricuspid insufficiency. The average ratio of the antegrade systolic to the diastolic flow component (S/D ratio) may be calculated. In general, the diastolic flow component is accentuated in tricuspid regurgitation and the S/D ratio is less than 1.0. Holosystolic flow reversal is seen in this example and is a finding characteristic of severe tricuspid regurgitation. Note the beat to beat variation in the amplitude of the systolic and diastolic flow components.

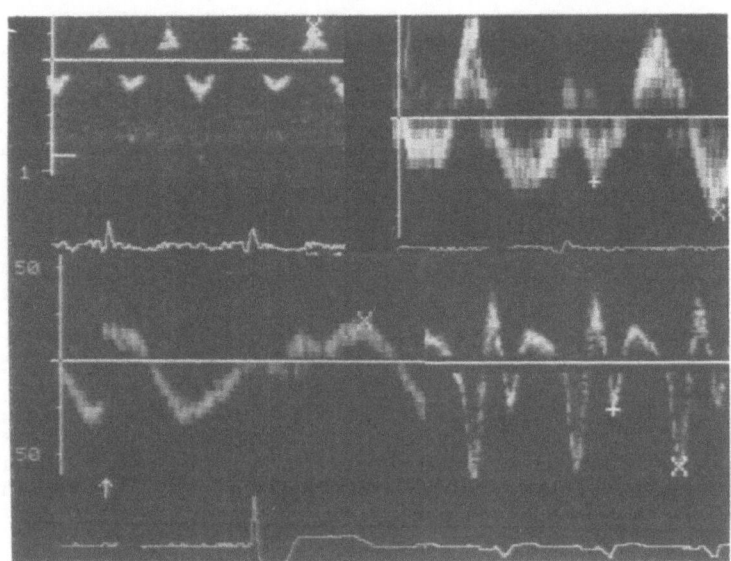

Fig.5-124. This series of case examples was obtained by recording the hepatic veinous flow in patients with (A) a 1+ tricuspid insufficiency, (B) a 2+ tricuspid insufficiency , (C) a 3+ tricuspid insufficiency, and a 4+ tricuspid insufficiency (D). The hepatic vein flow is generally easy to record in most patients , and can be an acceptable means of evaluating the severity of tricuspid regurgitation when other exam windows for flow mapping are suboptimal.

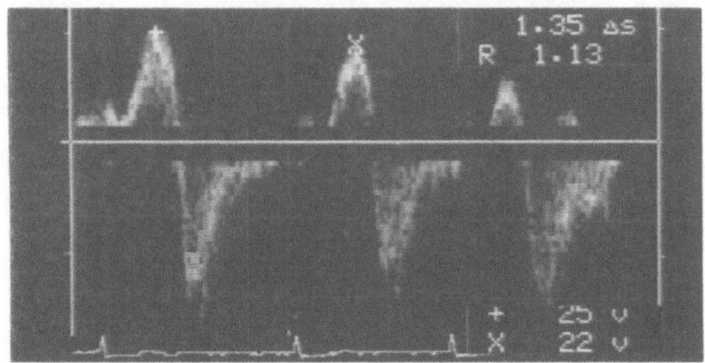

Fig. 5-125 . Hepatic vein flow in severe tricuspid regurgitation. When measuring flow velocities in the hepatic veins it is necessary to decrease the level of high pass filtering being used so that the desired information is not removed from the recording. The blacked out area around the spectral baseline indicates the frequency range which has been filtered.

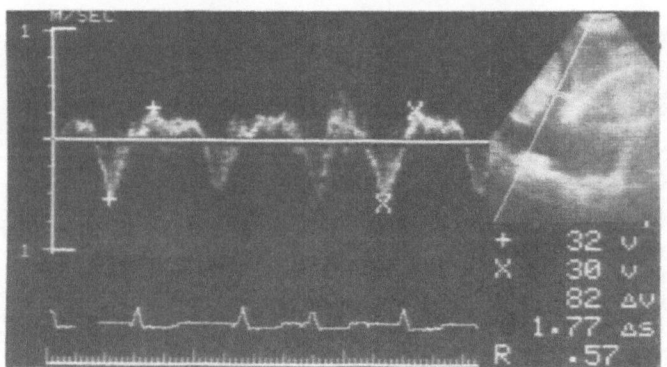

Fig.5-127. Pulsed Doppler is used to interogate the hepatic vein flow in this patient with a tricuspid regurgitation graded 3+ by pulsed Doppler techniques. It may be helpful to increase the sample volume size while searching for the hepatic veins , and then the sample volume length may be decreased to improve radial resolution.

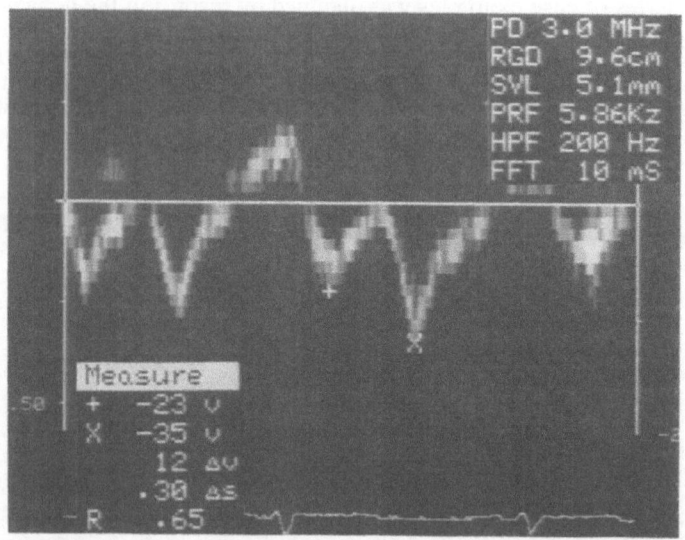

Fig.5-128 . Flow in the superior vena cava recorded from the right supraclavicular window in a patient with elevated right ventricular end-diastolic pressure. The typical diastolic "dip and plateau" pattern is recorded in the superior vena cava. The ratio of the diastolic flow component to the systolic flow component is .65

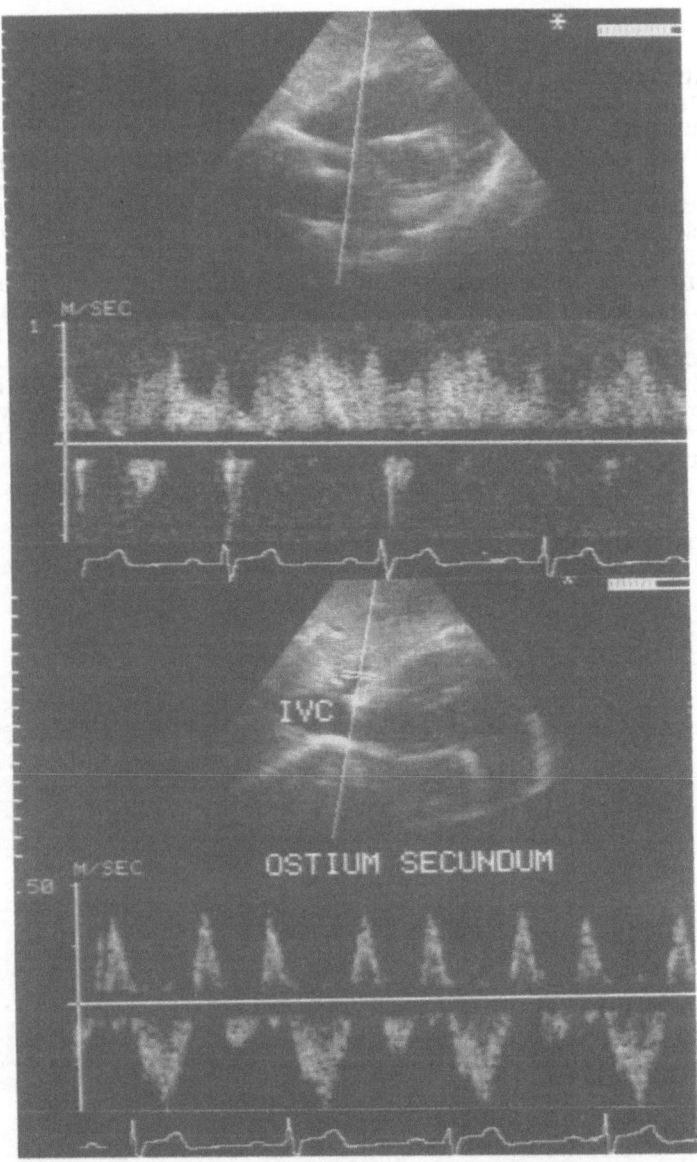

Fig. 5-129 . Top. Flow through an atrial septal defect recorded with continuous mode in an elderly patient from the subcostal window. The interrogation depth was too large for an optimal recording with pulsed mode, and the parasternal approach to recording the flow was not successful. Bottom. Pulsed mode recording of hepatic vein flow in the same patient.

Prosthetic Valves

Doppler ultrasound has been shown to be a useful diagnostic tool in the evaluation of prosthetic valve function . The prosthetic valve is initially examined in the same manner as the native valve; forward flow is carefully recorded in order to determine whether or not obstruction is present. The presence of regurgitation is detected by applying the flow mapping technique as in native valves. The peak and mean pressure gradients existing across the prosthesis can be estimated using the modified Bernoulli equation. When Doppler techniques are combined with echocardiographic technique, information on transvalvular flow as well as structural information can be obtained.With echocardiography alone, it may be difficult to ascertain whether or not a prosthesis is functioning normally. Doppler ultrasound allows one to examine the prosthetic flow pattern, and compare the results with the established values of peak velocity, peak gradient, and mean gradient for that type of prosthesis. The cardiac output of the patient at the time of the examination must be taken into consideration, since variations in cardiac output will change the values of the prosthetic valve flow velocity and the derived gradients.

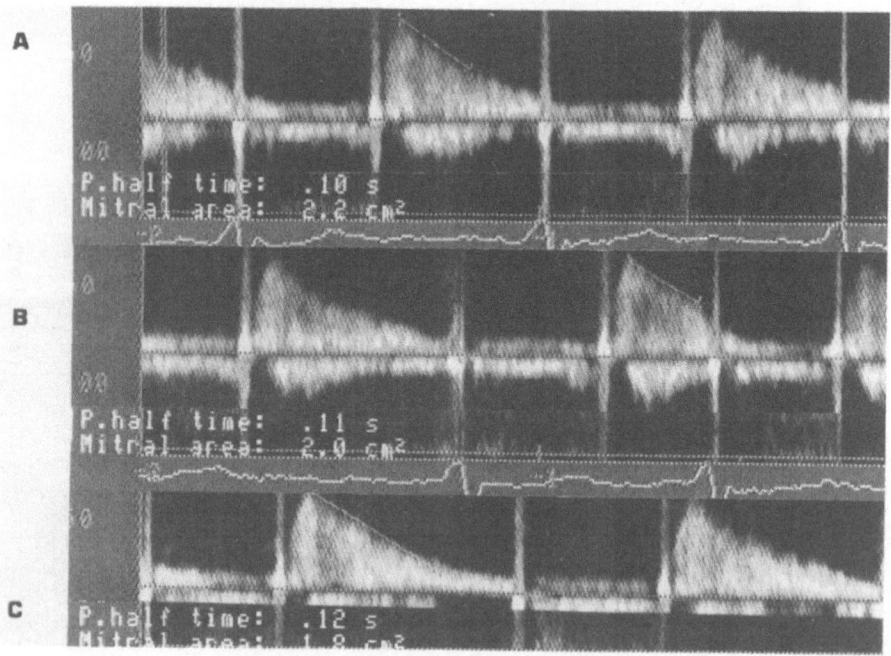

Fig.5-130. Variations in the value of the pressure half time due to atrial fibrillation. Continuous mode recordings of mitral flow in a patient with a Bjork-Shiley mitral prosthesis. In trace A, the pressure half time measured from the two flow curves is 100 ms. In trace B, the pressure half time measured for the beat shown is 110 ms. In trace C, the pressure halftime is 120 ms. This represents a 20 % increase in the value of the pressure half time measured in trace A.

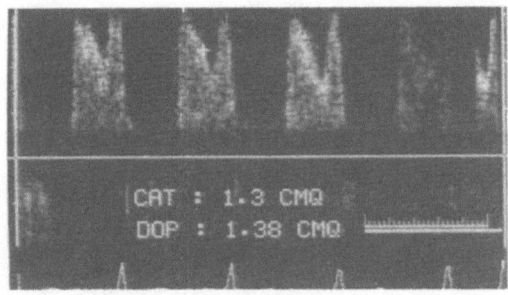

Fig. 5-131 . Continuous wave Doppler recording of flow through a Lieve mitral valve prosthesis. The average pressure half time was 158 ms, corresponding to an estimated valve cross sectional area of 1.38 sq cm. A valve area of 1.3 sq cm was estimated at catheterization.

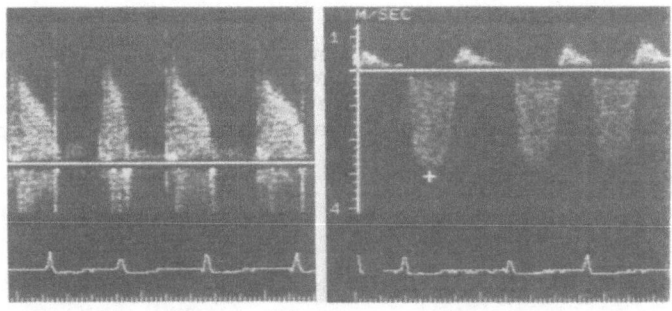

Fig.5-132 . A patient with a Hancock prosthesis in the mitral position was thought to have prosthetic incompetence by auscultation. Left. The continuous mode recording of the prosthetic flow showed a normally functioning prosthesis with no regurgitation. Right. The continuous mode recording of tricuspid flow in the same patient indicated that tricuspid regurgitation was present. The tricuspid regurgitation was graded as mild (2+) by pulsed Doppler techniques.

Ideally, a Doppler echocardiographic examination should be performed immediately after valve replacement in order to establish the baseline study for that particular patient. The baseline peak flow velocity, mean gradient and peak gradient can then be used as a reference when subsequent Doppler examinations are performed. A significant deviation in the Doppler-derived parameters without a change in cardiac ouput should be interpreted as a change in prosthetic valve function. If a weak regurgitant flow signal is heard or recorded after surgery, the presence of this flow signal should be noted in the patient's file.

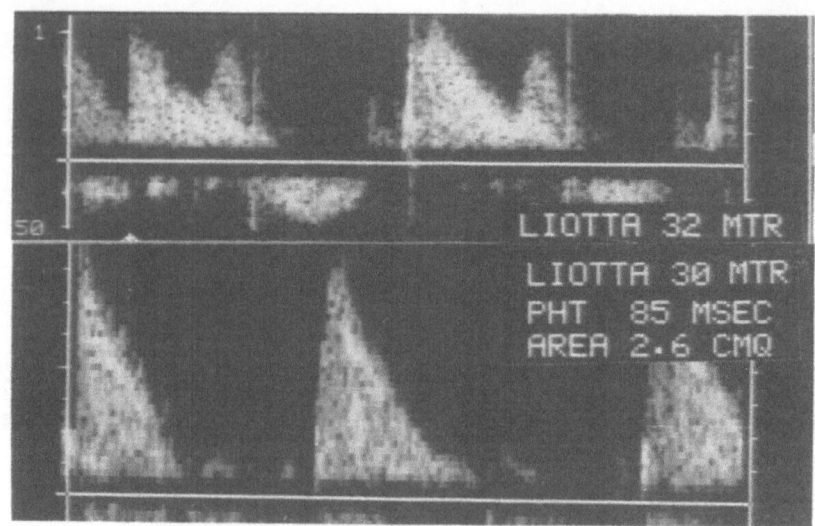

Fig.5-133 . Continuous mode recording of flow across two normally functioning Liotta mitral prosthesis. The patient in the top panel is in sinus rhythm, and a biphasic flow velocity curve is obtained. The spikes for valve opening and closure are clearly recorded. The patient in the bottom panel is in atrial fibrillation so a monophasic flow pattern occurs.

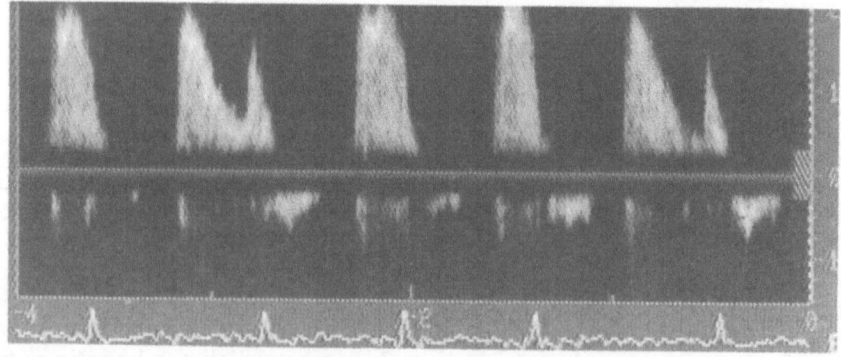

Fig. 134 . Continuous mode recording of flow across a normally functioning Sorin 25 mitral prosthesis. The patient is in atrial fibrillation , and a monophasic flow velocity curve is obtained. The spikes for valve opening and closure are clearly recorded. The obtained half time measurement is 90 ms, corresponding to a valve area of 2.44 sq cm.

The jet through an obstructed valve prosthesis is frequently eccentric although a parallel alignment between the continuous mode beam and the prosthetic flow may be acheived with the guidance of the audio signal.

Pulsed mode is then utilized in order to rule out the presence of prosthetic valve regurgitation. The sample volume is positioned in the left atrium immediately behind the prosthesis, and swept laterally in the search for the regurgitant flow signal. Once the flow signal has been localized, the sample volume should be moved further into the retrograde chamber to determine the flow extension. The sample volume should alos be swept laterally to determine the regurgitant signal distribution in the lateral direction. It should be noted however, that the valve hardware may absorb a considerable amount of ultrasound so that little ultrasound actually reaches the left atrium from the apical position. The ultrasonic beam is heavily attenuated by the valve apparatus, and it may be difficult to detect the regurgitant flow signal. The regurgitation may be missed entirely from the apical position if the regurgitation is mild.

In order to minimize the effects of attenuation, an intermediate transducer position between the apex and the sternum can be employed. The interrogation depth is then reduced, and so is the attenuation effect By using an off-axis position, one can position the sample volume so that the beam bypasses most of the valve hardware. The off-axis position may also be advantageous since the regurgitant flow is frequently eccentric, and a more parallel beam-to- flow alignment can be acheived from this position as opposed to a more conventional apical four-chamber position.

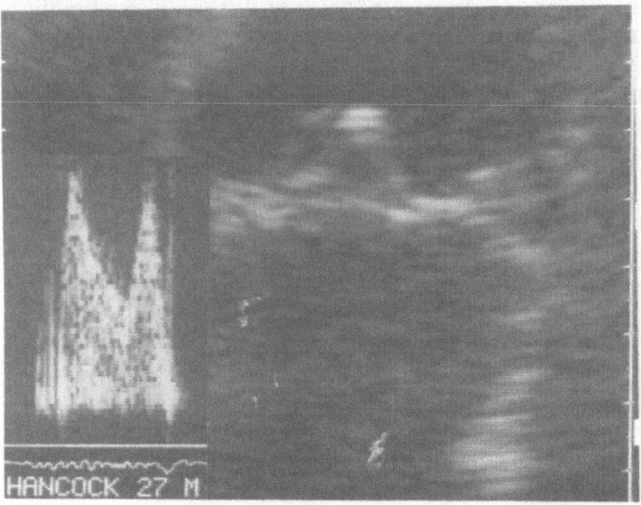

Fig.5-135. Continuous mode recording of normal flow through a Hancock 27 mitral prosthesis. The average pressure halftime is 95 ms which is slightly elevated for values in the native valve , but is common in prosthetic valves. While the two dimensional image of the prosthesis clearly demonstrated a normal valve motion, the Doppler study allowed direct observation of the valve function and the tranvalvular flow.

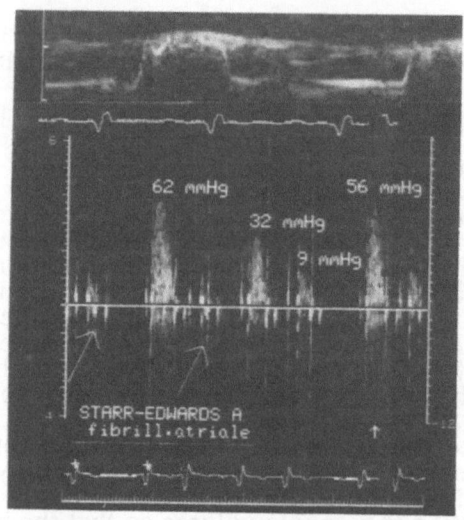

Fig. 5-136 . Continuous mode recording of flow through a Starr-Edwards aortic valve prosthesis from the apical window. The patient is in atrial fibrillation, and a marked beat to beat variation in the peak pressure gradient is noted. The peak gradient (mm Hg) is indicated above each of the flow velocity curves. Very little forward flow is recorded across the prosthesis in the first and third beats (arrows). The M-mode recording of the prosthetic valve demonstrates the failure of the prosthesis to open following the second R wave.

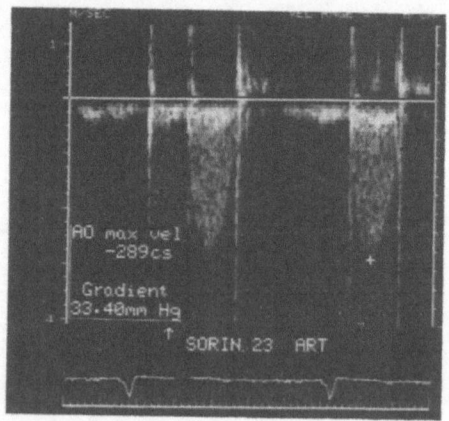

Fig. 5-137 . Continuous mode recordings of flow across a normally functioning Sorin aortic valve prosthesis from the apical (left) and subcostal (right) windows. The spectral envelope is better delineated and the peak velocity is slightly higher in the subcostal tracing. The estimated peak gradient is 24 mm Hg, and a small amount of regurgitation is present.

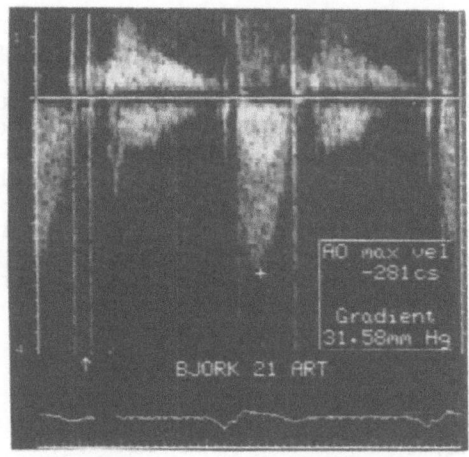

Fig. 5-138 Continuous wave Doppler recording of flow through a normal Starr-Edwards aortic prosthesis. Due to the presence of atrial fibrillation, there is a marked variation in peak flow velocity and peak pressure gradient. The peak pressure gradient (mm Hg) is indicated next to the three labeled flow curves. The average value of the peak gradient should be used when asessing prosthetic valve performance.

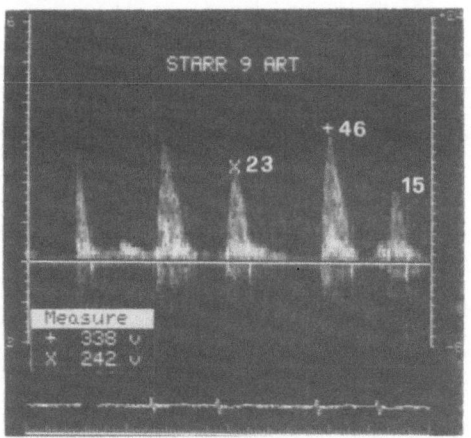

Fig. 5-139 . Continuous mode recording from the apex of flow through a normally functioning Bjork prosthesis. The maximal velocity is 2.8 m/s, and the maximal systolic gradient is approximately 32 mm Hg. The superimposed sytolic flow with a peak velocity of 0.8 m/s represents the left ventricular outflow.

Pulsed mode can also be used to ensure that there is no leakage through the sewing ring. The sample volume is placed behind the sewing ring and moved around the periphery of the ring to detect the retrograde flow. However, it is not possible to distinguish between valvular and paravalvular leakage with Doppler technique alone. The use of simultaneous pulsed mode and imaging or color flow mapping helps in establishing the diagnosis of paravalvular leakage.

Color flow analysis is helpful in the assessment of prosthetic mitral valve function because the left ventricular filling pattern may be examined. The different types of valves produce different filling patterns, and the orientation of the central jet also varies. In the case of ball-and-cage valves, there is no central jet since the blood flows around the ball and into the left ventricle. A central jet directed towards the interventricular septum is visualized when examining single disc or bioprosthetic valves.

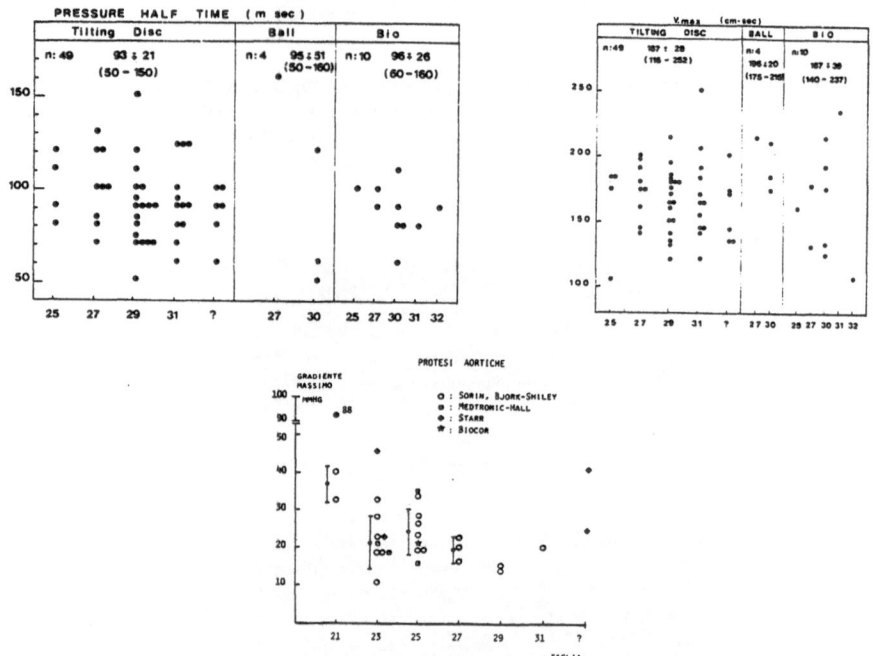

Fig. 5-140 . (A) The pressure halftimes calculated for normally functioning mitral valve prostheses. The average pressure halftime and the normal range of values are listed for each type of mitral prosthesis. (B) The maximum flow velocities recorded in normally functioning mitral prostheses.(C) The prosthesis valve size was compared to the peak gradient in a series of 30 normally functioning aortic valve prostheses. A wide range of peak gradients can be found for a given valve size. In order to correctly interpret the Doppler recording of prosthetic valve flow, a baseline study after surgery is essential. (Taglia = Valve Size, Gradiente Massimo = Peak Gradient).

Aortic Valve Prostheses

Flow through an aortic valve prosthesis can most often be succesfully examined from the apical or right parasternal window. The suprasternal window is less successful in recording flow across prosthetic aortic valves compared to native valves, probably due to the variability of the jet direction in valve prostheses. Continuous mode should initially be employed so that a parallel or nearly parallel beam-to-flow alignment is acheived. The peak velocity of prosthetic valve flow is higher than that of a normal native valve because the prosthesis restricts left ventricular ejection to some degree. If the peak flow velocity is only moderately increased, one may switch to high pulse repetition frequency mode to record the antegrade flow across the prosthesis.

Once an adequate spectral flow pattern has been recorded, the peak and mean pressure gradient should be estimated and compared with the established ranges for the given type and size of the prosthesis. The left ventricular function should be taken into account when evaluating prosthetic valve performance. The reported normal ranges for a certain type and size prosthesis may differ (at times, considerably) due to the variability of the measurement process. The value of the mean and peak gradient will change from beat to beat, and at least three measurements should be made when estimating the average value of the Doppler-derived gradients. Because of the variability in the currently established normal ranges, mild prosthetic valve obstruction may not be detected.

When the calculated peak gradient is considerably larger than the upper limits of the normal range for the valve type, valvular obstruction should be suspected. Wilkes et al have reported a case of Doppler-detected subvalvular membrane in a patient with a Hancock aortic prosthesis; the M-mode and two-dimensional recordings did not reveal any abnormalities. The estimated peak gradient created by the obstruction was confirmed at catheterization .

The values of the peak and mean gradients are dependent upon the flow through the aortic prosthesis. When the left ventricular function is reduced, the Doppler-derived gradients may be lower than predicted. The presence of moderate prosthetic valve regurgitation will result in augmented flow through the prosthesis, thereby increasing the estimated peak and mean pressure gradient. Generally, in the presence of normal left ventricular function, the peak Doppler-derived gradient should be less than 50 mm Hg in aortic valve prostheses.

Prosthetic valve regurgitation may be detected by applying the flow mapping technique of conventional pulsed mode. It is usually more difficult to record regurgitant flow in cases of mechanical prostheses, because the valve hardware absorbs a considerable amount of ultrasonic energy. The use of an intermediate transducer position between the apex and the sternum can minimize the effects of ultrasonic attenuation by the prosthesis. A small amount of regurgitant flow can frequently be recorded in normally functioning prosthetic valves, although it may be missed with real-time flow imaging.

Marras and coworkers detected the presence of insignificant regurgitation in 80% of patients with normal Sorin and Bjork-Shiley aortic prostheses; the regurgitant flow signal was successfully recorded with both pulsed and continuous modes. Olson et al reported the presence of minimal regurgitation as a common normal finding in their study of patients with Lillehei-Kaster aortic prostheses.

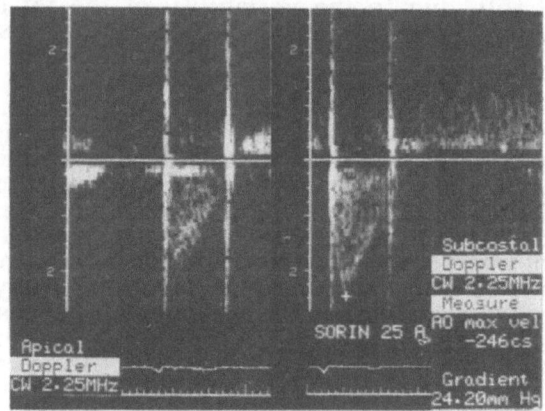

Fig. 5-141. Continuous mode recordings of flow through a normal Sorin aortic valve prosthesis from the apical window (left) and subcostal window (right). The flow velocity curve is more clearly recorded from the subcostal window, and the peak velocity is higher than that obtained from the apical approach.

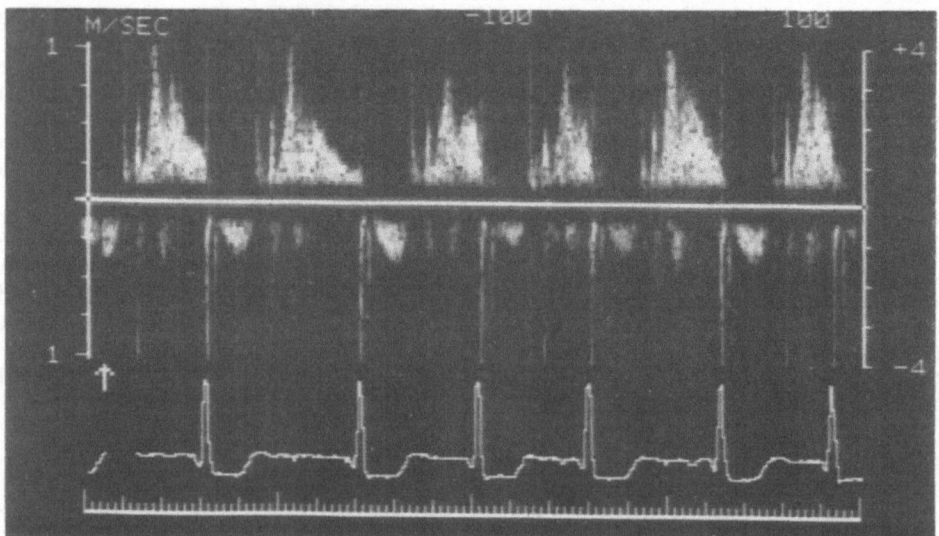

Fig.5-142. Timing of prosthetic valve opening and closure in a patient with a mitral prosthesis and an aortic valve prosthesis. The first spike occurring at the same time as the R wave on the electrocardiogram corresponds to the prosthetic mitral valve closure. The following spike is aortic valve opening , the following is aortic valve closure, and the forth spike is from the opening of the prosthetic mitral valve.

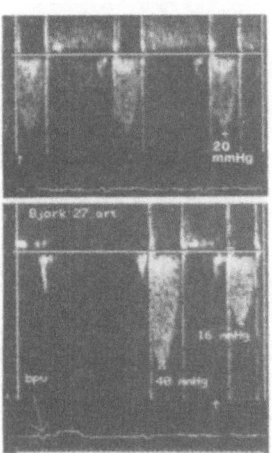

Fig.5-143 . Continuous mode recording of flow through a normal Bjork 27 aortic valve prosthesis from the apical window. Top. The peak pressure gradient is approximately 20 mm Hg. Bottom. Following a premature ventricular contraction (bpv), no blood is ejected from the left ventricle. In the beat following the premature contraction, a larger volume of blood is ejected, resulting in a higher than normal flow velocity (3.16 m/s). A lower peak velocity (2.0 m/s) is recorded in the second beat after the premature contraction. The peak gradients are indicated for these beats.

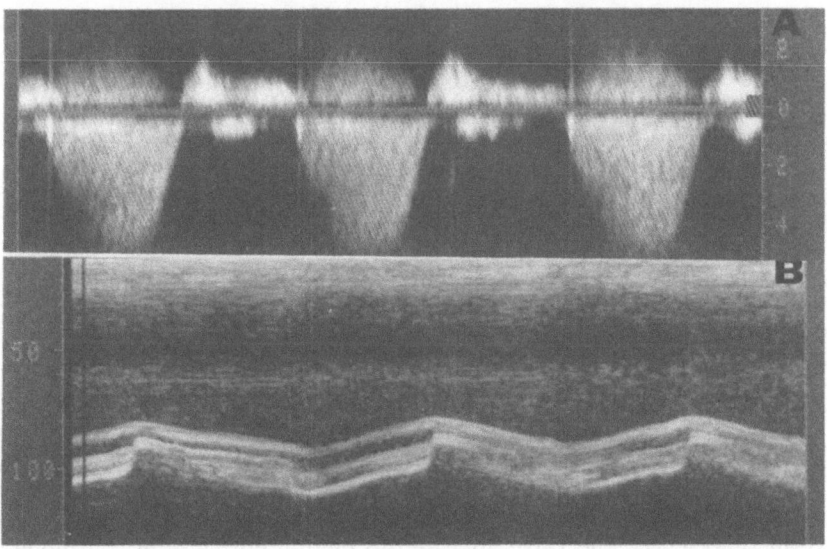

Fig.5-144 Endocarditis in a patient with a Hancock bioprosthesis. The prosthetic valve M-mode demonstrated a shaggy appearing echo on the valve. The insufficiency was detected by continuous wave Doppler first, then pulsed Doppler was used to map the regurgitant flow extension.

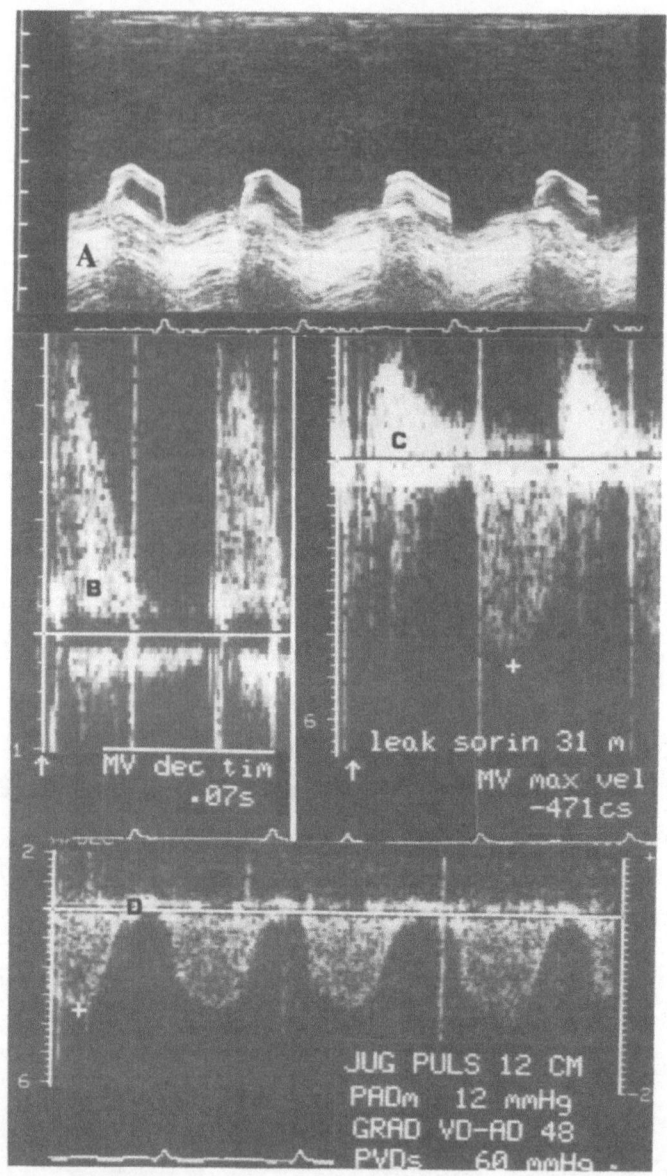

Fig.5-145 This study was obtained from a patient with a moderately severe degree of prosthetic mitral valve incompetence. The valve appeared to fuction normally by M-mode (A). The pressure gradient is increased due to the increased forward flow velocity, but the half time is only slightly prolonged(B). The insufficiency is demonstrated in figure C was sampled by continuous wave. A high velocity tricuspid regurgitant jet was detected and used to estimate the systolic right ventricular pressure. This measurement indicates that pulmonary hypertension is present.

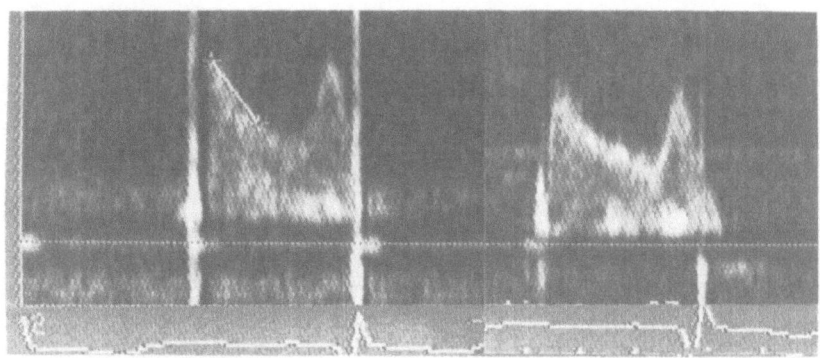

Fig.5-146. Normal flow through a Sorin mitral prosthesis with a pressure half time of 140 ms.

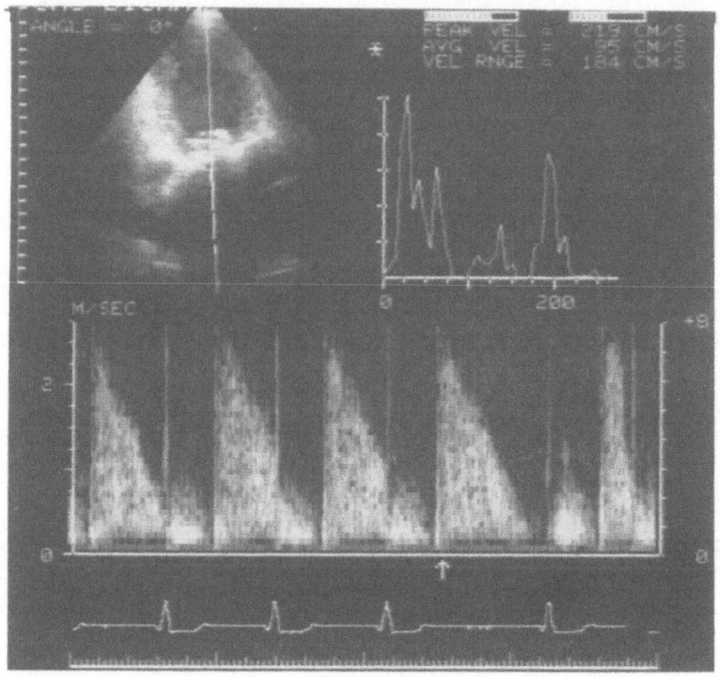

Fig.5-147. Continuous mode recording of flow through a Hancock porcine heterograft in the mitral position. The maximal velocity is 2.5 m/s, and the peak diastolic gradient is 25 mm Hg. The average pressure halftime of 196 ms indicates that moderate obstruction is present. Porcine valves generally have a longer pressure half time than disc or ball valves, but a pressure halftime of nearly 200 ms is clearly abnormal. In this case, the prolonged pressure half time was due to leaflet calcification.

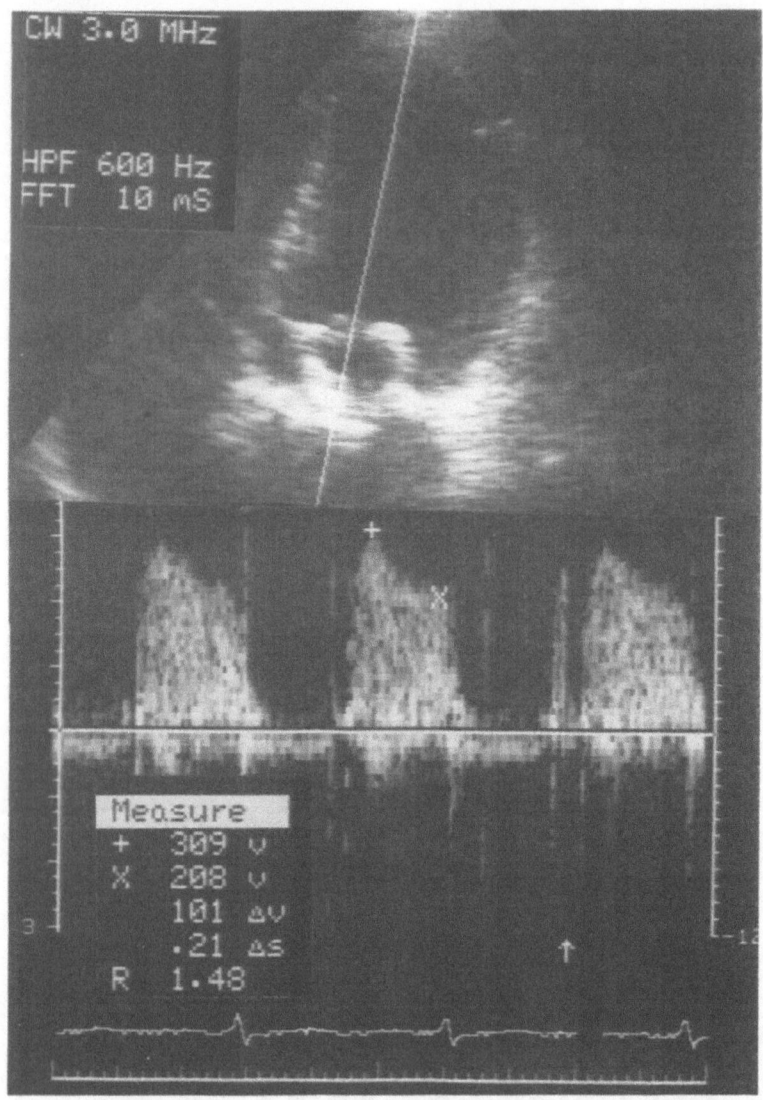

Fig. 5-148. Continuous mode recording of flow through an Angell-Shiley mitral prosthesis. The prosthesis was clearly visualized by two dimensional echocardiography, and a thickened appearence of the prosthetic valve leaflets was noted. Continuous wave Doppler was used to measure the peak mitral flow velocity so that the gradient and pressure half time could be calculated. The prolonged pressure half time of 180 ms and elevated pressure gradient was caused by prosthetic leaflet calcification.

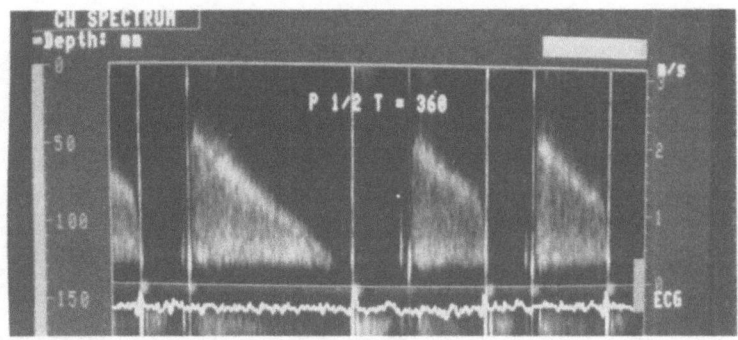

Fig. 5-149 This study was obtained in a patient with a mechanical prosthesis in the mitral position. The severe obstruction is due to the presence of a thrombosis. A peak velocity of 2.30 m/s yields a pressure gradient of 21. mm Hg. The pressure half time is signifigantly prolonged (360 ms) and indicates a severe obstruction is present.

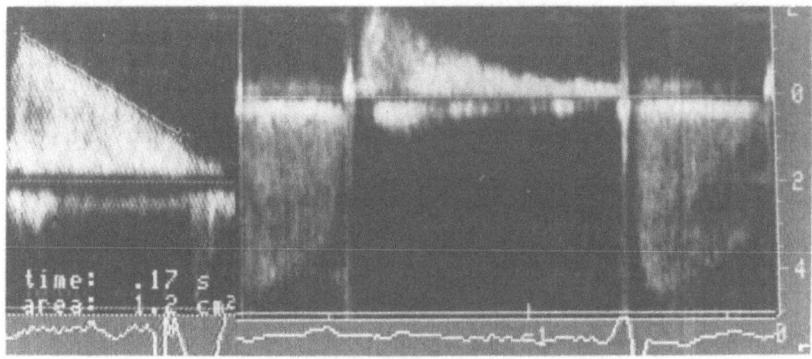

Fig. 5-150 . Continuous mode recording from the apex of flow through a normally functioning Bjork prosthesis in the mitral position. The maximal velocity is 1.5 m/s, and the maximal systolic gradient is approximately 9 mm Hg.   A small leak across the valve is detected by continuous wave Doppler. The presence of a small prosthetic valve leakage is frequently detected in normally functioning valves.

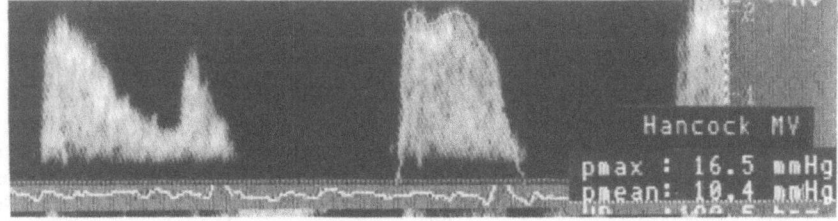

Fig. 5-151. Normal Hancock mitral valve prosthesis . Note the beat to beat difference in pressure halftimes. In irregular rhythms the halftime should be measured over several complex's.

183

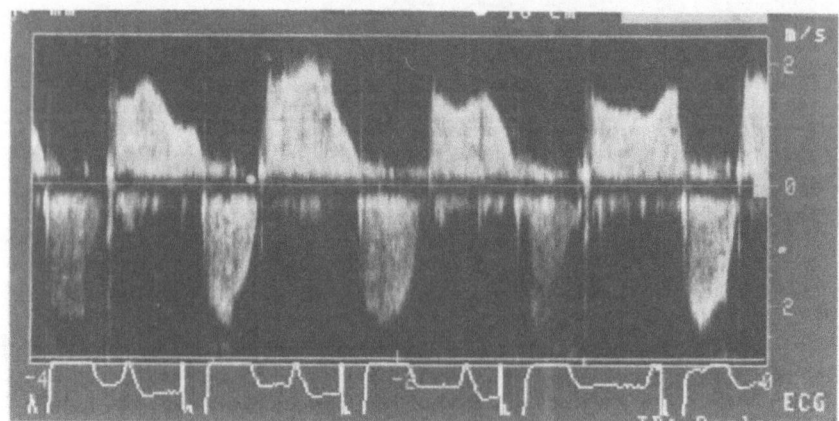

Fig.5-152 Severe prosthetic valve dysfunction. Continuous mode recording of flow through a Hancock tricuspid valve prosthesis from the parasternal position. Note the abnormal configuration of the flow velocity curve and the marked change in the flow pattern from beat to beat. Significant regurgitation was also present but an optimal flow pattern of the forward and retrograde flow could not be obtained at the same time due to the different orientation of the two jets. The regurgitant flow signal can be seen here although it is not optimally recorded. The regurgitant peak velocity indicates that normal systolic pulmonary artery pressure is present.

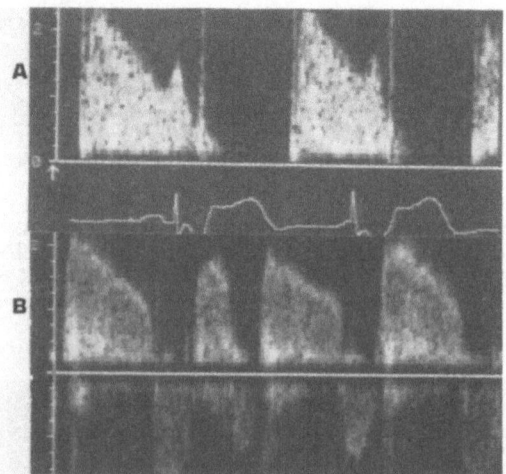

Fig. 5-153. Continuous mode recordings of prosthetic valve flow in two patients with tricuspid prostheses. The top trace is of a normally functioning prosthesis; the pressure half time is approximately 110 ms and no regurgitation is detected. The bottom trace is an example of a seriously malfunctioning prosthesis. The mean pressure half time is 310 ms. Switching to pulsed mode, the regurgitant flow signal was detected in more than two-thirds of the right atrium.

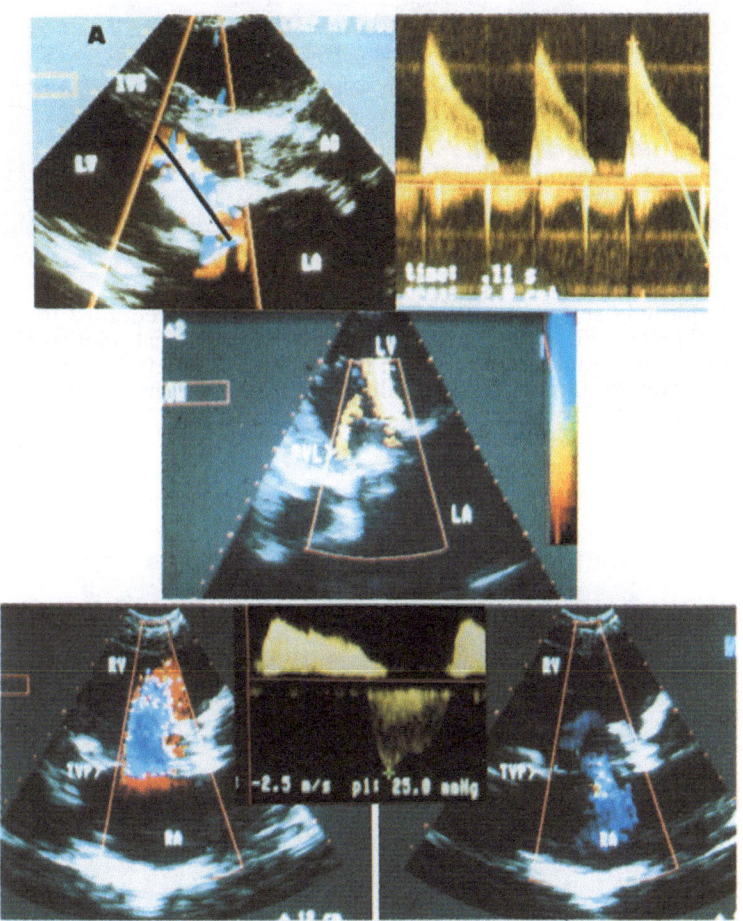

Fig. 5-154. A. Left. Color flow display of the flow across a normal Carpentier-Edwards mitral prosthesis from the parasternal window. A mosaic pattern is visualized, indicating that the flow velocity is higher than that of normal left ventricular inflow. The jet is oriented towrds the interventricular septum. Right. Continuous mode recording of prosthetic flow from the apical window. The pressure halftime is 110 ms, and the estimated orifice area is 2.0 sq cm. B. Color flow display of a prosthetic valve leak (PVL) in a patient with a mitral valve bioprosthesis. The left ventricular inflow is visualized in shades of yellow orange. The prosthetic valve leak can be seen as a small orange flame originating from the sewing ring of the prosthesis. C. Left. Color flow display of right ventricular inflow in a patient with a tricuspid valve bioprosthesis. The core region of inflow is moving at a velocity higher than the Nyquist value, and color aliasing is noted. Right. In systole, a small amount of regurgitation can be seen as a predominantly blue flowwith some regions of color aliasing. Insert. The continuous mode recording of the regurgitation confirms that the regurgitation is weak. The estimated systolic pulmonary artery pressure is normal.

185

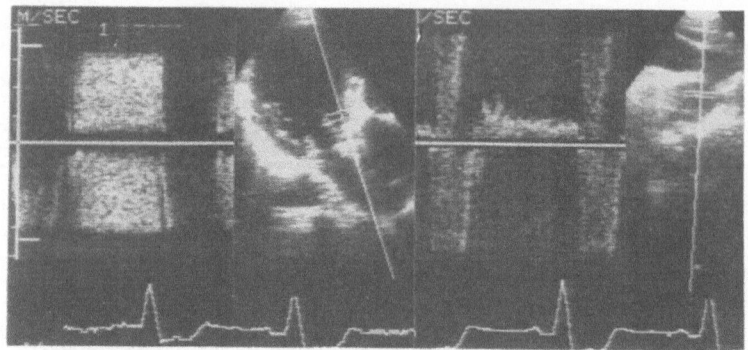

Fig.5-155. Moderately severe prosthetic valve incompetence recorded in a patient with a mechanical prosthesis. Left. Pulsed mode recording from the apical position of the regurgitant flow signal. The flow signal was detected in two-thirds of the left ventricular cavity. Right. Pulsed mode recording of flow in the descending aorta from the suprasternl window. Reverse flow is recorded throughout diastole.

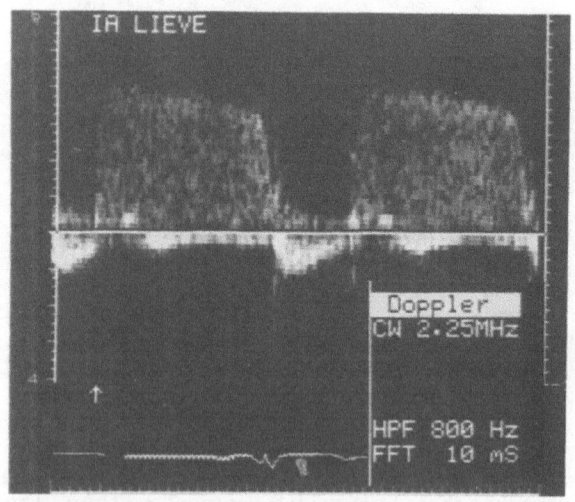

Fig.5-156 . Continuous mode recording from the apex of flow through a normally functioning Lieve aortic valve prosthesis. The maximal velocity was between 1.8 and 2.2 m/s, and the maximal systolic gradient approximately 15 mm Hg. A very weak aortic regurgitation signal is detected by continuous wave Doppler. This is a frequently observed finding in the normally functioning aortic valve prosthesis.

186

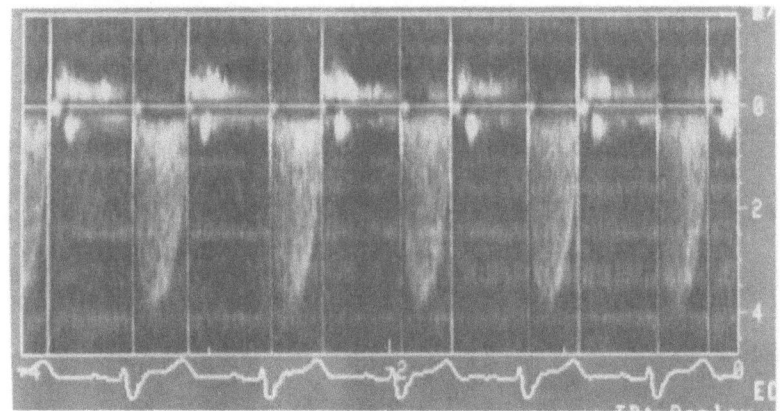

Fig .5-157 . Continuous mode recording from the apex of flow through an obstructed Bjork aortic valve prosthesis . The maximal velocity is 4.0 m/s, and the maximal systolic gradient is approximately 64 mm Hg. The opening and closing movements of the valve are clearly seen in this figure.

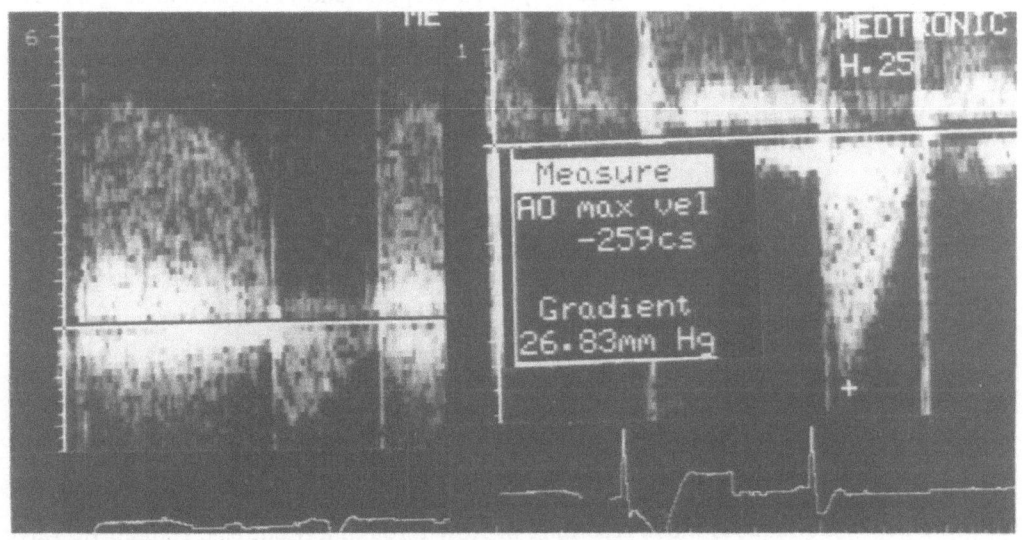

Fig.5-158. Right. Continuous mode recording of flow through a Medtronic Hall 25 aortic valve prosthesis from the apical window. The peak velocity is approximately 2.6 m/s, and the peak gradient is 27 mm Hg. Left . With a slight change in angulation, the forward flow is less optimally recorded but the aortic insufficiency is clearly detected.

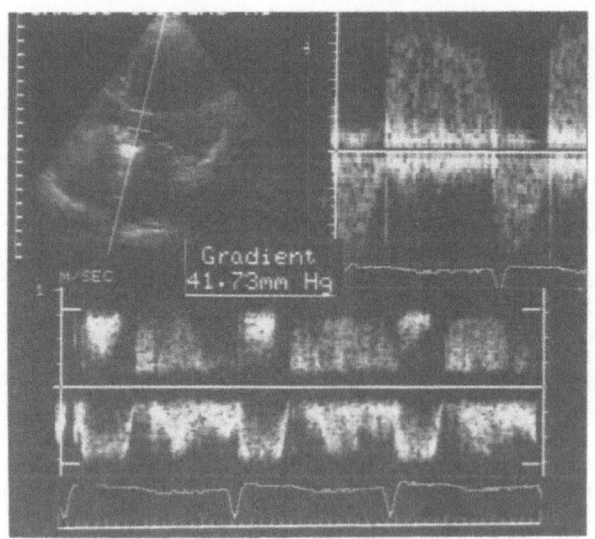

Fig.5-159. Aortic valve prosthesis. Bottom panel. Pulsed mode recording of the regurgitant flow signal with the sample volume placed immediately behind the prosthesis. The localization of this paravalvular leak was performed by pulsed Doppler and confirmed at surgery. The incompetence was graded as moderate by flow mapping techniques. The continuous wave Doppler was then used to measure the peak flow vlocity across the prosthesis.

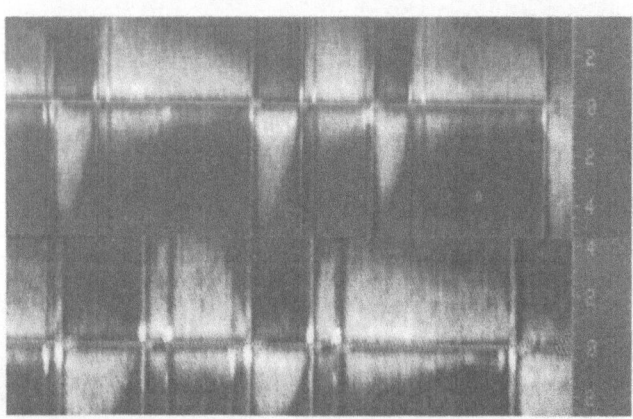

Fig. 160 . Top.   Continuous mode recording of flow through a Medtronic Hall aortic valve prosthesis from the apical window. The peak velocity is approximately 5.0 m/s, and the peak gradient is 100 mm Hg . Bottom . When the sweep speed is increased, one may appreciate the temporal relationship between aortic and mitral prosthetic valve opening and closing. The high amplitude signal from valve motion is filtered by the automatic gain control (AGC) , which accounts for the valve spike drop out on the spectral recording.

188

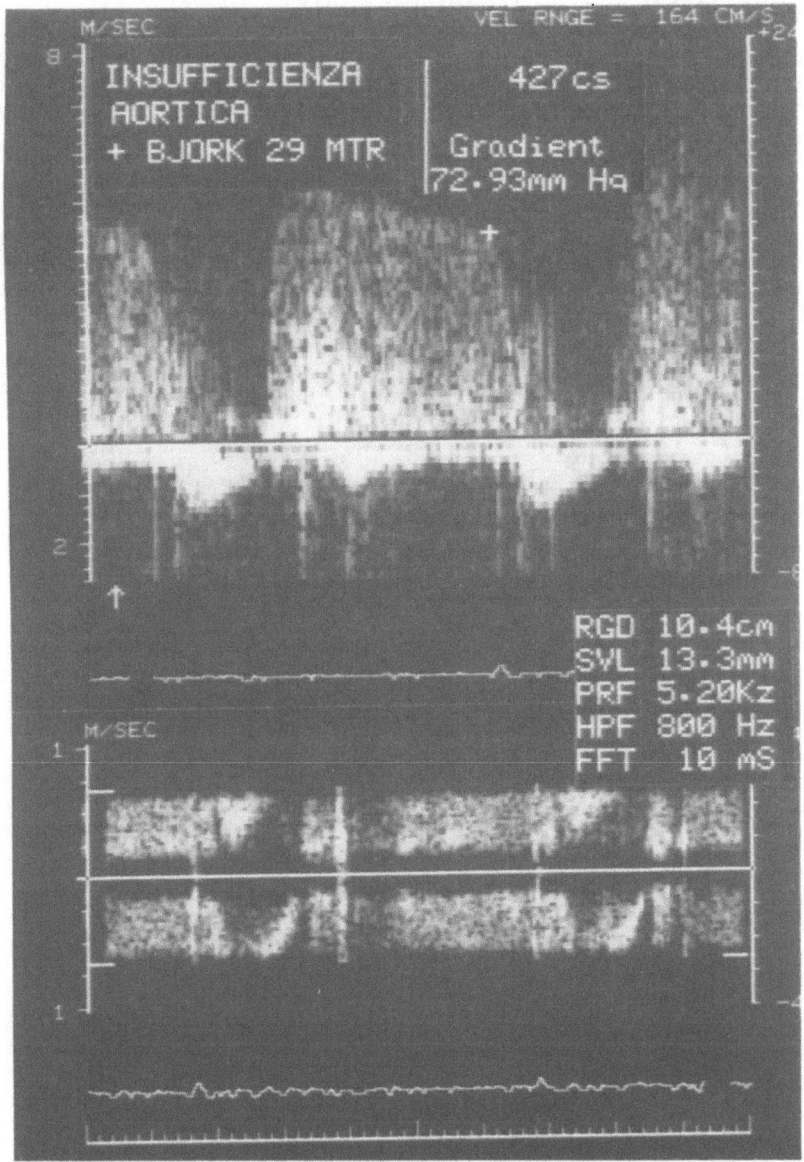

Fig. 5-161. Moderate aortic insufficiency in a patient with a Bjork Shiley aortic prosthesis. Top. Continuous mode recording of the regurgitation from the apical window. The end diastolic peak velocity is 4.27 m/s, hence the estimated end-diastolic gradient between the aorta and the left ventricle is 73 mm Hg. Bottom. Pulsed mode recording of the insufficiency from the same position.

Hypertrophic Obstructive Cardiomyopathy

Conventional Doppler techniques allow one to assess the severity of the intraventricular obstruction present in patients with hypertrophic cardiocmyopathy. From the apical window, the left ventricular outflow can be examined with pulsed mode. By moving the sample volume further into the outflow tract, the level at which the increased velocity originates can be determined. The pulsed mode recording of left ventricular outflow will be heavily aliased at the level of the narrowest flow trajectory. Continuous mode should then be utilized to measure the peak flow velocity through the narrowed outflow tract. It may be difficult to record the low intensity but high velocity signals from the blood passing through this obstruction. An independent Doppler transducer is usually required to adequately record the peak velocities in the outflow tract.

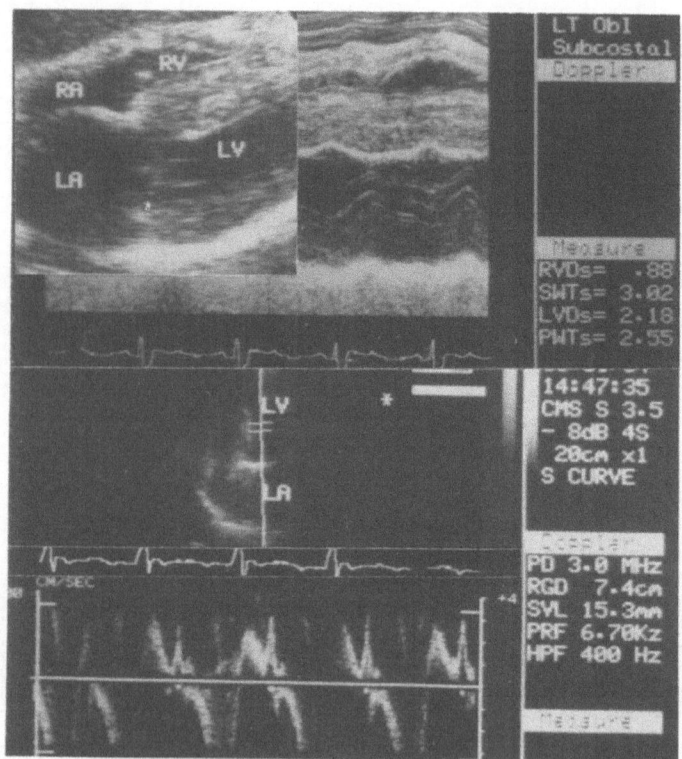

Fig. 5-162 . Subvalvular aortic obstruction. The M-mode recording of the left ventrical demonstrates the presence of marked left and right ventricular hypertrophy.The pulsed Doppler was used to localize the position of the obstruction in the left ventricular outflow tract .

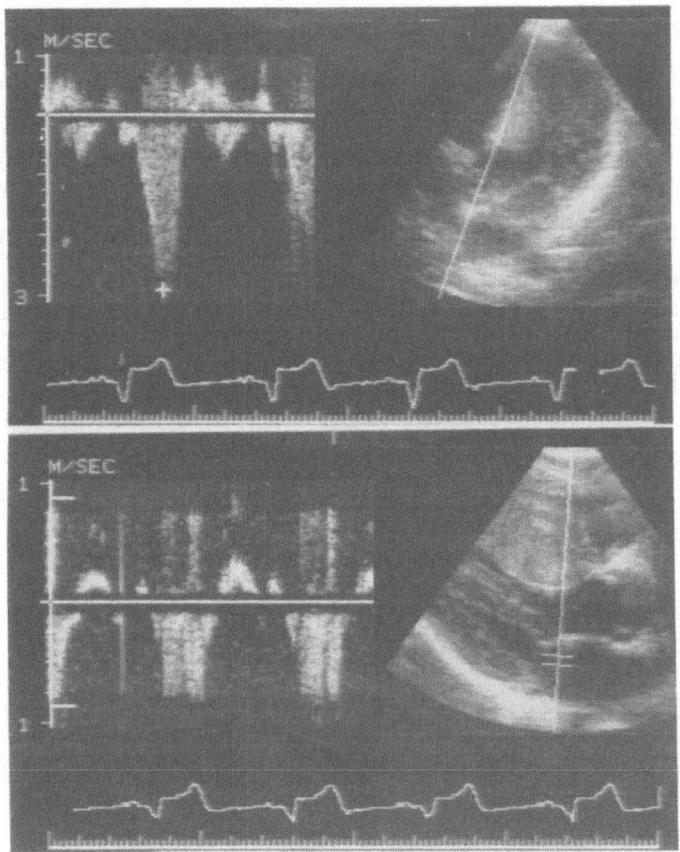

Fig.5-164 . Left ventricular outflow obstruction in a patient with hypertrophic cardiomyopathy. Top. Continuous mode recording from the apical window of the left ventricular ouflow. The peak outflow velocity was 2.9 m/s, corresponding to a peak intraventricular gradient of 34 mm Hg. Bottom. Pulsed mode recording from the parasternal window of the mild mitral regurgitation which was present.

The continuous mode recording of left ventricular outflow has a late systolic peak which is characteristic of a dynamic obstruction to flow. The systolic anterior motion of the mitral leaflets serves to further narrow the outflow tract, causing the development of high flow velocities in late systole. The faded appearance of the spectral flow pattern in late systole is caused by the reduced volume of blood which has passed through the obstructed outflow tract. A high pass filter setting greater than 800 Hz should be selected when attempting to record the low intensity but high velocity outflow signal. Once the peak velocity has been optimally recorded, the peak intraventricular pressure gradient can be estimated by application of the modified Bernoulli equation.

Mitral regurgitation can frequently be detected in patients with hypertrophic cardiomyopathy. The outflow jet is more superiorly directed than the regurgitant jet, and the two flows can easily be differentiated. In addition, the configurations of the spectral flow patterns are different. The regurgitant flow pattern peaks in mid-systole, whereas the outflow pattern peaks in late systole. The regurgitant flow signal can usually be detected throughout systole, spporting the conclusion that the regurgitation is not initated by the systolic anterior movement of the mitral valve leaflets.

The peak velocities recorded in the aorta from the apical window may be within normal limits, indicating that the outflow jet has dissipated by the time the left ventricular outflow reaches the aortic annulus. When recording flow in the ascending aorta from the suprasternal window, a high degree of variability may be noted in the spectral flow pattern. Yock and coworkers have suggested that this finding is consistent with the formation of late systolic eddy currents with differing directions in the ascending aorta.

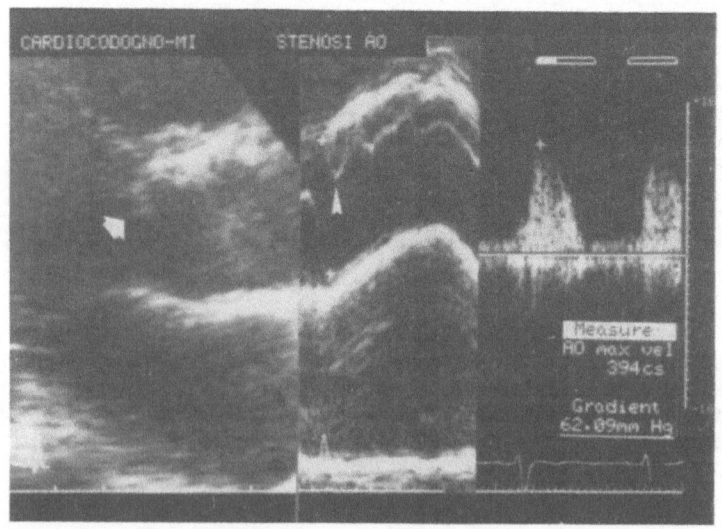

Fig. 5- 165 . Subvalvular aortic obstruction. Left. the white arrow points to the obstruction as seen in the parasternal long axis view of the left ventricle. Center. The M-mode recording of the aorta demonstrates the presence of mid-systolic notching (arrow) of the aortic valve. Right. Continuous mode interrogation of the outflow tract. The peak velocity is 3.94 m/s, corresponding to a peak intraventricular gradient of 62 mm Hg.

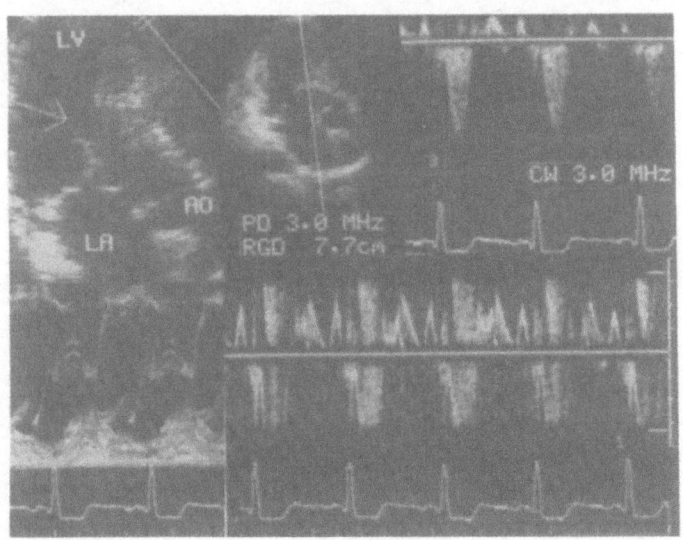

Fig.5-166. Mild intraventricular obstruction. Right. The systolic anterior motion of the mitral valve is seen in the two-dimensional image and in the M-mode recording. Center. Pulsed mode recording of the left ventricular outflow at the level of the obstruction. Right. Continuous mode recording of the left ventricular ouflow, with a peak outflow velocity of 2.0 m/s. This indicates the presence of mild intraventricular obstruction; the peak resting gradient is 16 mm Hg.

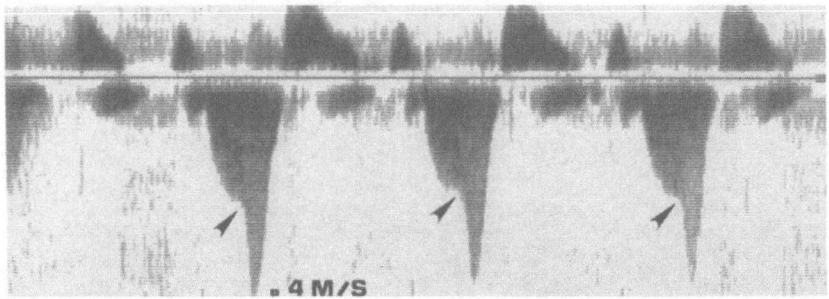

Fig.5-167.   Obstructive cardiomyopathy. Continuous mode recording of left ventricular outflow obtained from the apical window. The positive biphasic diastolic flow represents the mitral flow. The onset of flow in the f=left ventricular outflow tract is normal, but the presence of a dynamic obstruction causes a rapid mid-systolic increase in the peak flow velocity (arrow) from 2.0 to 4.0 m/s. The peak intraventricular gradient is 64 mm Hg, whereas the gradient estimated by inclusion of the initial outflow velocity is 48 mm Hg. Note the time delay between the cessation of mitral flow and the onset of left ventricular outflow. Such a delay helps to differentiate the outflow signal from that of mitral regurgitation.

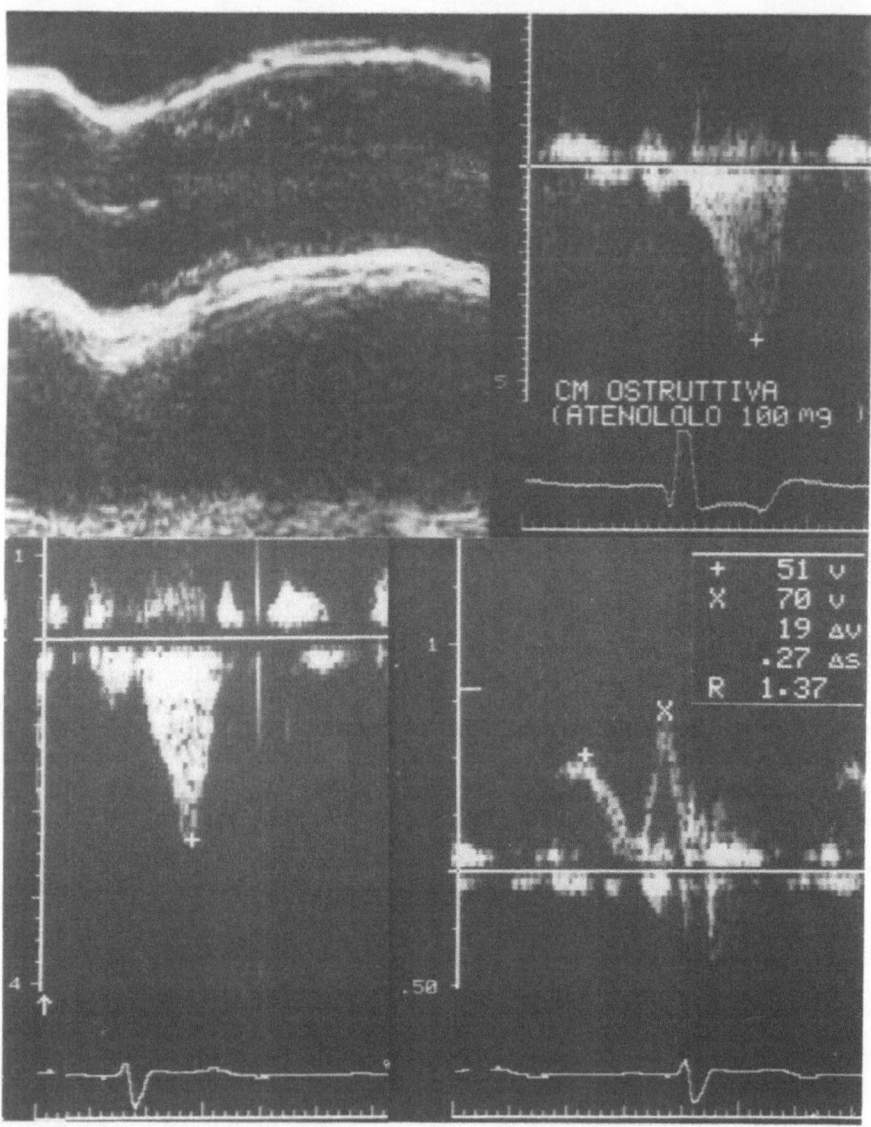

Fig.5-168 . Obstructive cardiomyopathy. A. The M-mode recording of the aorta demonstrates partial closure of the aortic valve. B. Continuous mode recording of left ventricular outflow from the apical window. The peak outflow velocity is 2.4 m/s, corresponding to a peak intraventricular gradient of 23 mm Hg at rest. C. Following the administration of 100 mg of atenolol, the peak intraventricular gradient increases to 64 mm Hg. D. Pulsed mode recording of mitral flow from the apical window. The amplitude of the atrial flow component is greater than the rapid filling component.

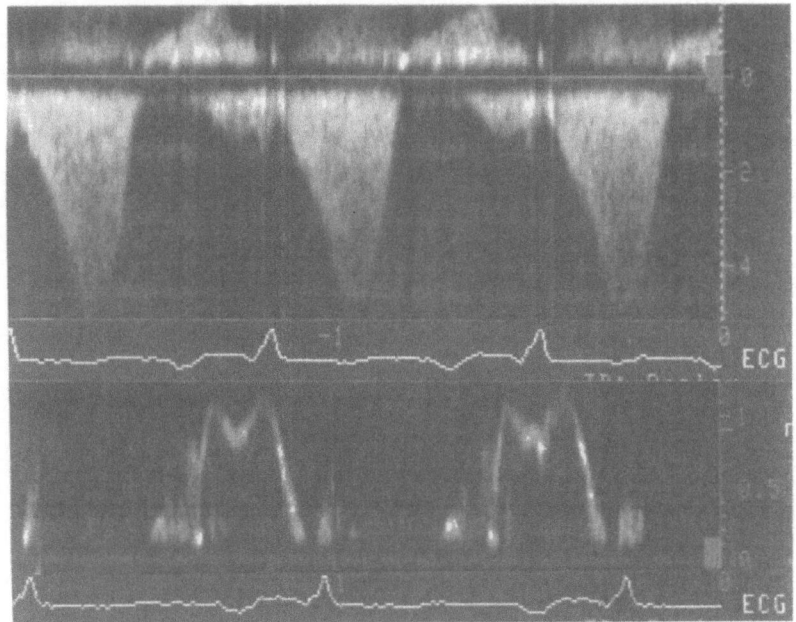

Fig.5-169. Top. Continuous mode recording of left ventricular outflow in cardiomyopathy. The peaking of the flow velocity curve in late systole is characteristic of a dynamic outflow obstruction. The maximal flow velocity of 5.0 m/s indicates the existence of a peak intraventricular pressure gradient of 100 mm Hg . Bottom. Pulsed mode recording of mitral flow in the same patient. The average pressure half time is 80 ms, and is slightly more prolonged than a normal mitral valve. The amplitude of the atrial flow component is slightly greater than that of the rapid filling component.

Dilated cardiomyopathy

The pulsed mode recordings of the left ventricular filling pattern in patients with dilated cardiomyopathy reflect the depressed left ventricular performance found in such patients. The mitral flow velocity curve has an accentuated atrial flow component while the rapid filling component has a reduced peak flow velocity. In the presence of moderate mitral regurgitation, this pattern may no longer be recorded. The magnitude of the rapid filling component may equal or exceed that of the atrial flow component as a result of the augmented flow across the mitral valve and the increased left atrial pressure in early diastole. This effectively masks the abnomal appearance of the left ventricular filling pattern.

The flow pattern in the ascending aorta is usually normal in appearance, but the peak velocity may be lower than 0.7 m/s. If the ascending aorta is clearly visualized and a technically adequate aortic flow pattern is recorded, an estimation of the cardiac output can be made. The Doppler-derived cardiac output may also be used to follow cardiomyopathy patients undergoing vasodilator therapy on a long term basis.

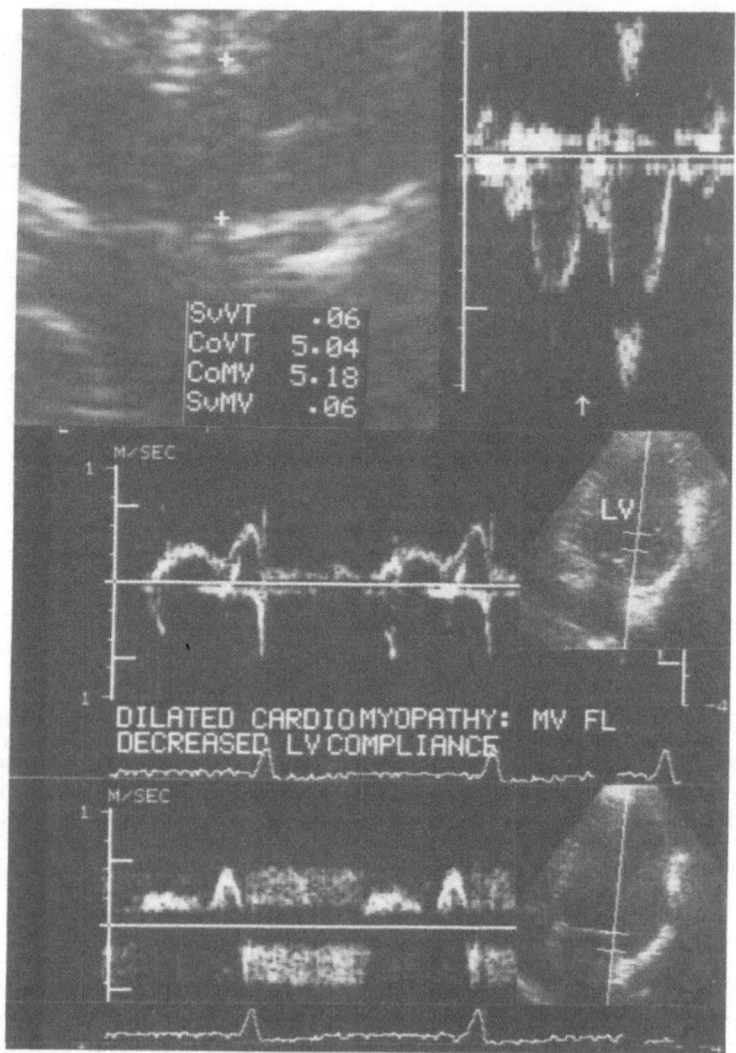

Fig 5-170. Dilated cardiomyopathy. Top. Calculation of the cardiac output at the level of the aortic valve. The diameter of the aortic annulus was measured from the parasternal long axis view, and the pulsed mode recording of aortic flow was obtained from the apical window. The estimated stroke volume calculated by the mean velocity method (SvMV) and the velocity time integral method (SvVT) was 60 ml. The cardic output calculated by both methods was nearly the same (approximately 5.0 l/min). Center. Pulsed mode recording of mitral flow from the apical window. The amplitude of the A component was greater than that of the E component, indicating the presence of decreased left ventricular compliance. Bottom. By shifting the sample volume ot the atrial side of the mitral orifice, a mild degree of mitral regurgitation was detected.

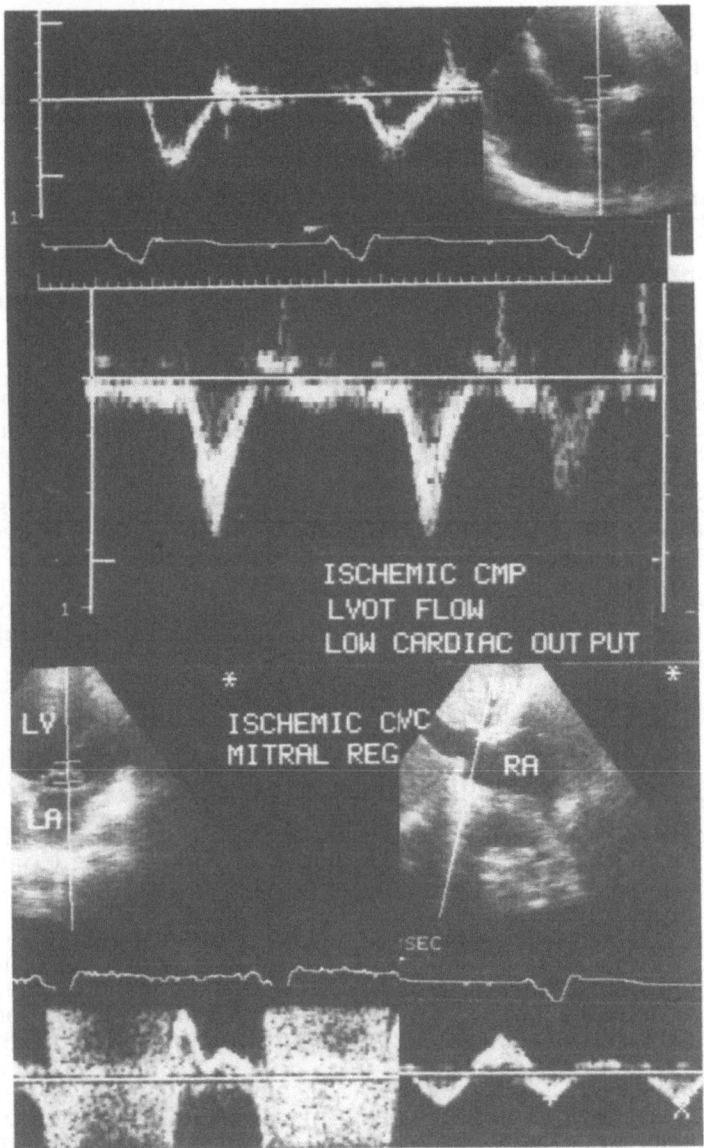

Fig.5-171 . Ischemic cardiomyopathy. Top. Pulsed mode recording of left ventricular outflow, with the sample volume positioned behind the aortic valve. The peak velocity is approximately 0.6 m/s. Center. Pulsed mode recording of left ventricular outflow with the independent Doppler transducer. Bottom left. Pulsed mode recording from the apical window of the moderate mitral regurgitation which was present. Bottom right. Pulsed mode recording of flow in the hepatic veins from the subcostal window.

References

1. Holen J, Simonsen S. Determination of the pressure gradient in mitral stenosis with Doppler echocardiography. Br Heart J 41;529-535, 1979.
2. Hatle L, Angelsen BA, Tromsdal A. Noninvasive assessment of aortic stenosis by Doppler ultrasound. Br Heart J 43;284-292, 1980.
3. Hatle L, Angelsen BA, Tromsdal A. Noninvasive assessment of atrioventricular pressure halftime by Doppler ultrasound. Circulation 60;1096-1104, 1979.
4. Stamm BR, Martin RP. Quantification of pressure gradients across stenotic valves by Doppler ultrasound. J Am Coll Cardiol 2;707-718, 1984.
5. Hatle L, Brubakk A, Tromsdal A, Angelsen BA. Noninvasive assessment of the pressure drop in mitral stenosis by Doppler ultrasound. Br Heart J 40;131-140,1978.
6. Bommer WJ, Mapes R, Miller, et al. Detection of aortic insufficiency by pulsed Doppler echocardiography (abstr). Am J Cardiol 47:412, 1981.
7. Ciobanu M, Abbasi AS, Allen M, et al. Pulsed Doppler echocardiography in the diagnosis and estimation of severity of aortic insufficiency. Am J Cardiol 49:339-343, 1982.
8. Valdes-Cruz LM, Horowitz S, Mesel E, et al: A pulsed Doppler echocardiographic method for calculation of pulmonary and systemic flow: Accuracy in a canine model with ventricular septal defect. Circulation 68:597-602, 1983.
9. Takeda P, Kwan OL, Water J, et al: Aetermination of peak aortic pressure gradient by continuous wave Doppler measurements of maximal blood flow velocity: Experimental validation (abstr). J Am Coll Cardiol 1:657, 1983.
10. Diebold B, Perronneau P, Blanchard D, et al. Noninvasive quantification of aortic regurgitation by Doppler echocardiography. Br Heart J 49:167-173, 1983.
11. Lesbre JP, Isorni C, Lespererance J, et al. Les dysfonctions de bioprostheses: Apport respectif de L'echocardiographie et du Doppler. Arch Mal Coeur 79;9:1278-1286, 1986.
12. Wallmeyer K, Wann LS, Sagar KB, et al. The influence of preload and heart rate on Doppler indexes of left ventricular performance: Comparison with invasive indexes in an experimental preparation. Circulation 74;1:181-186, 1986.
13. Simpson IA, Reece IJ, Houston AB, et al. Noninvasive assessment by Doppler ultrasound of the Wessex porcine, low profile Ionescu-Shiley, and Hancock pericardial prostheses. Br Heart J 56:83-8, 1986.
14. Zhang Y, Nitter-Hauge, Myhre E. Determination of the mean pressure gradient in mitral stenosis by Doppler echocardiography. Eur Heart J 6:858-64, 1985.
15. Vandenbossche JL, Kramer BL, Massie BM, et al. Two-dimensional echocardiographic evaluation of the size, function, and shape of the left ventricle in chronic aortic regurgitation: Comparison with radionuclide angiography. J Am Coll Cardiol 4:1195-1206, 1984.
16. Ihlen H, Amlie JP, Dale JP, et al. Determination of cardiac output by Doppler echocardiography. Br Heart j 51:54-60, 1984.

17. Wranne B, Ask P, Loyd D. Quantification of heart valve regurgitation: A critical analysis from a theoretical point of view. Clin Physiol 5:81-88, 1985.
18. Seitz WS, Hosenpud JD, Schutz. An orifice formula independendent of mitral pressure gradient for the evaluation of prosthetic mitral valve obstruction. Eur Heart J 5:932-940, 1984.
19. Krayenbuehl HP. Myocardial function. Eur Heart J 6; supplement C, 33-39, 1985.
20. Come PC, Buckley BH, Goodman ZD, et al. Hypercontractile cardiac states simulating hypertrophic cardiomyopathy, Circulation 55:90-8, 1977.
21. Barlow JB, Pocock WA. Mitral valve prolapse: The specific billowing mitral leaflet syndrome or an insignificant nonejection systolic click. Am Heart J 97:277-85, 1979.
22. Maron BJ, Epstein SE. Hypertrophic cardiomyopathy. Am J Card 45;141-54, 1980.
23. Ohlsson J, Wranne B. Noninvasive assessment of valve area in patients with aortic stenosis. J Am Coll Cardiol 7; 3:501-8, 1986.
24. Spirito P, Maron BJ, Bonow RO. Noninvasive assessment of left ventricular diastolic function: Comparative analysis of Doppler echocardiographic and radionuclide angiographic techniques. J Am Coll Cardiol 7;3:518-26, 1986.
25. Freedman RA, Yock PG, Echt DS, Popp RL. Effect of variation of PQ interval on patterns of atrioventricular valve motion and flow in patients with normal ventricular function. J Am Coll Cardiol 7;3:595-602, 1986.
26. Holen J, Nitter-Hauge S. Evaluation of obstructive characteristics of mitral disc valve implants with ultrasound Doppler techniques. Acta Med Scan 1977;201:429.
27. Holen J, Hoie J, Semb B. Obstructive characteristics of Bjork-Shiley, Hancock, and Lillehei-Kaster prosthetic mitral valves in the immediate postoperative period. Acta Med Scand 1978; 5:204.
28. Holen J, Simonsen S, Froysaker T. An ultrasound Doppler technique for the noninvasive determination of the pressure gradient in the Bjork-Shiley mitral valve. Circulation 1979;59:436.
29. Nitter-Hauge S. Doppler ultrasound used in the control of patients with mitral disc prostheses. Eur Heart J 1984;5 (suppl II):231.
30. Williams GA, Nelson J, Hrosek D, Kennedy HL. Evaluation of prosthetic mitral valves with two dimesional Doppler echocardiography. Eur Heart J 1985; 5(suppl I):11.
31. Labovitz AJ, Mrosek D, Nelson J, Kennedy HL, Williams GA. Doppler evaluation of prosthetic aortic valves. Eur Heart J 1984;5 (suppl I): 191.
32. Veyrat C, Cholot N, Abitbol G, Kalmanson D. Noninvasive diagnosis and assessment of aortic valve disease and evaluation of aortic prosthesis function using echo pulsed Doppler velocimetry. Br Heart J 1980; 43: 393.
33. Raisaro A, Recusani F, Sgalambro A, Tronconi L. Determination of regurgitant flows in prosthetic heart valve dysfunction (abstr). Eur Heart j 1984; 5 (suppl I):11.

34. Recusani F, Scheuble C, Sgalambro A, Cereze P, et al. PUlsed Doppler echocardiography in mechanical prosthetic heart valve malfunction (abstr). Eur Heart J 1984; 5 (suppl I) : 11.
35. Gross CM, Wann LS. Dop[p[ler echocardiographic diagnosis of porcine bioprosthetic cardiac valve malfunction. Am J Cardiol 1984; 53: 1203.
36. Nitter-Hauge S. Doppler echocardiograp[hy in the study of patients with mitral disc valve prostheses. Br Heart J 1984;51: 61.
37. Gardin JM, Burn CSm Childs WJ, Henry WL. Evaluation of blood flow velocity in the ascending aorta and the main pulmonary artery of normal subjects by Doppler echocardiography. Am Heart J 1984; 107: 310.
38. Smith MD, Handshoe R, Handshoe S, Kwan OL, De Maria AN. Comparative accuracy of two-dimensional echocardiography and Doppler pressure half time in assessing severity of mitral stenosis in patients with and without prior commissurotomy. Circulation 1986; 73: 100.
39. Libanoff AJ, Rodbard S. Atrioventricular pressure half time: Measurement of the mitral valve orifice area. Circulation 1968; 38: 144.
40. Robson DJ, Flaxman JC. Measurement of the end-diastolic pressure gradient and mitral valve area in mitral stenosis by Doppler ultrasound. Eur Heart J 1984; 5: 660.
41. Holen J, Simonsen s. Determination of the pressure gradient in mitral stenosis with Doppler echocardipgraphy. Br Heart j 1979; 41: 529.
42. Zhang Y, Nitter-Hauge S, Myhre E. Determination of the mean pressure gradient in mitral stenosis by Doppler echocardiography. Eur Heart J 1985; 6: 858.
43. Takenada K, Dabestani A, Gardin JM, et al. Pulsed Doppler echocardiographic study of left ventricular filling in dilated cardiomyopathy. Am J Cardiol 1986; 58: 143.
44. Nolan SD, Dixon SH, Fisher RD, Morron AG. The influence of atrial contraction and mitral valve mechanics on venricular filling. A study of instantaneous mitral valve flow in vivo. Am Heart J 1969; 77: 784-91.
45. Weinstein IR, Marbarger JP, Perez JE. Ultrasonic assessment of the St. Jude prosthetic valve: M-mode, two-dimensional, and Doppler echocardiography. Circulation 1983; 68: 897.
46. Marras A, Sgalambro A, Lombardi, et al. Valutazione con ecografia Doppler di protesi aortiche normofunzionanti (abstr). G. Ital Cardiol 1986; 16 (suppl I): 73.
47. Hansen DE, Cahill PD, DeCapli WM, et al. Valvular-ventricular interaction: Importance of the mitral apparatus in canine left ventricular systolic performance. Circulation 1986, 6; 1310-1320.
48. Force T, Kemper A, Perkins L, et al. Overestimation of infarct size by quantitative two dimensional echocardiography: The role of tethering and of analytic procedures. Circulation 1986; 73, 6: 1360-8.

49. Skjearpe T.   Noninvasive quantitation of effective valve area in aortic stenosis with Doppler ultrasound and echocardiography (abstr). Sixth Symp on Echocardiology, Rotterdam, 1985.
50. Dennig K, Rudolph W. Doppler echocardiographic assessment of normal and malfunctioning mitral valve prostheses (abstr). Sixth Symp on Echocardiology, Rotterdam, 1985; 80.
51.   Diebold B, Raffoul H, Chevalier B, Degroote, et al.   A Doppler echocardiographic evaluation of percutaneous transluminal aortic valvuloplasty (abstr). Second Int Cong Cardiac Doppler, 1986;144.
52. Dabestani A, Takenada K, Henry WL. Pulsed Doppler hepatic vein flow in tricuspid regurgitation and atrial septal defect (abstr). J Am Coll Cardiol 1986; 7,2:145A.
53. Linker D, Skjearpe T, Samstad, Rossvoll O, Chapman J ,et al. Color flow mapping with an annular array transducer: An approach integrated with continuous and pulsed Doppler in adult and pediatric patients (abstr). Second Int Cong Cardiac Doppler, 1986; 122.
54.Robinson J, Gunstensen J, Lobo F, et al. Doppler-pathologic correlations in acute prosthetic valve failure leading to surgical replacement (abstr). Second Int Cong Cardiac Doppler, 1986;148.
55.Yock PG, Hatle L, Popp RL.   Pattern and timing of Doppler-detected intracavitary and aortic flow in hypertrophic obstructive cardiomyopathy. J Am Coll Cardiol 1986; 8: 1047-58.
56.   Currie PJ, Seward JB, Chan KL, et al.   Continuous wave Doppler determinaion of right ventricular pressure: A simultaneous Doppler Catheterization study in 127 patients. J Am Coll Cardiol 1985; 4: 750-6.
57. Sgalambro A, Recusani F, Raiaro, et al. Efficacia della ecocardiografia Doppler nella valutazione dei vizi mitralici (abstr). Eighth Nat Ital Ult Cong 1982: 279-282.
58. Sgalambro A, Recusani F, Raisaro A, et al. Profils de velocite' du flux mitral au Doppler pulse' dans le classement des retrecissements mitraux (abstr) In "Cardiovascular applications of Dopppler Echocardiography", Paris, 1982: 11-14.
59. Sgalambro A, Recusani, Raisaro A, et al. La diagnosi al Doppler pulsato di insufficienza aortica in presenza di stenosi mitralica (abstr). Bul Nat Soc Ital Card 1981, 26; 11: 1557-59.
60.   Pandian NG, Friedland L, McInerney K, Caldeira M.   Doppler echocardiographic study of superior vena cava blood flow: Definition of normal flow and detection of abnormal patterns in right heart disorders (abstr). J Am Coll Cardiol 1985, 5; 2: 500.
61. Sgalambro A, Lombardi F, Marras, et al. I Diffetti settali atriali negli adulti: Diagnosi e stima del Qp: Qs con eco bidimensionale e Doppler (abstr). J Ital Cardiol 1986, 16 (suppl I): 140.
62. Redel DA, Junck H. Description of blood flow velocity profiles inside the human main pulmonary artery with the use of color Doppler echocardiography (abstr).

63. Skjaerpe T, Hegrenaes L, Hatle L. Noninvasive estimation of valve area in patients with aortic stenosis by Doppler ultrasound and two-dimensional echocardiography. Circulation 1985, 72; 4: 810-17.

64. Peronneau PA. Flow velocity measurements in blood vessels by ultrasonic Doppler techniques. In Inserm Euromech 92, Cardiovascular and pulmonary dynamics 71; 105, 1977.

65. Schluter M, Langenstein BA, Hanrath P, et al. Mitral regurgitation detected by transesophageal pulsed Doppler echocardiography (abstr). Eur Heart J 1982, 2: 114.

66. Pierce GE, Morrow AG, Braunwald E. Idiopathic hypertrophic subaortic stenosis; Intraoperative studies of the mechanism of obstruction and the hemodynamic consequences. Circulation 1964, 30 (suppl IV):152-74.

67. Venco A, Recusani F, Sgalambro A. Diastolic movement of the mitral valve in hypertrophic cardiomyopathy: An echocardiographic study. Br Heart J 1980, 43: 159-63.

68. Henry Wl, Clark CE, Glancy Dl, Epstein SE. Echocardiographic measurement of the left ventricular outflow gradient in idiopathic hypertrophic subaortic stenosis. N Engl J Med 1973; 288: 989-993.

69. Sahn D, Valdes-Cruz LM, Scagnelli S, et al. Comparison of continuous wave and high pulse repetition frequency 2D echo Doppler for pressure gradient estimation in animal and human patients (abstr). Circulation 1983, 68 (suppl III)

70. Stevenson JG, Kawabori I, Brandestini MA. A twenty month experience comparing conventional pulsed Doppler echocardiography and color coded multigate Doppler for detection of atrioventricular valve regurgiation and its severity. In "Echocardiology", edited by H Rijsterbogh, Martinus Nijhoff, The Hague, 1981 (p399-407).

71. Currie PJ, Hagler DJ, Seward JB, et al. Instantanteous pressure gradients in stenotic cardiac lesions: Simultaneous continuous wave Doppler and dual catheter correlation (abstr). J Am Coll Cardiol 1985. 5; 2: 401.

72. Houston AB, Sheldon CD, Simpson IA. Assessment of the value of continuous wave Doppler echocardiography in 121 infants and children with congenital heart disease (abstr). Sixth Symp on Echocardiology, Rotterdam, June 1985.

73. Wilkes HS, Berger M, Gallerstein PE, et al. Left Ventricular outflow obstruction with continuous wave Doppler ultrasound. J Am Coll Cardiol 1983, 53: 550-553.

74. Hatle L, Angelsen BA, Tromsdal A. Noninvasive assessment of aortic stenosis by Doppler ultrasound. Br Heart J 1980, 43: 284-92.

CHAPTER 6

DOPPLER ULTRASOUND IN CONGENITAL HEART DISEASE

James V. Chapman
Aurelio Sgalambro M.D.
Sandra A. Yanushka

The Pulmonary-to-Systemic Flow Ratio

The pulmonary-to-systemic flow ratio or Qp/Qs ratio is an important parameter used to assess shunt severity. Until recently, cardiac catheterization was the sole means of obtaining the data needed to derive this ratio. The Doppler estimation of the flow ratio involves the systematic interrogation of flow across the semilunar valves until a good quality flow velocity curve is recorded. The flow velocity curve should have a narrow spectral bandwidth, and the value of the peak velocity should be consistent from beat to beat. Using pulsed mode, the sample volume is placed slightly distal to the semilunar valve in the center of the lumen. Slight alterations in the sampling site should be made with the guidance of the audio signal to obtain an optimal Doppler recording. The dimensions of the grest vessels at the valvular level must then be determined using the appropriate two-dimensional images or M-mode recordings. If a blunt velocity profile is assumed to exist at the valve level and slightly downstream from the valve, the flow volume or stroke volume may be calculated using the following equation:

$$ SV = \int_{1}^{2} (\mathbf{V} dt)(\mathbf{A}) $$

where SV is the stroke volume, V is the spatial mean velocity, and A is the vessel cross-sectional area. Stroke volume may be defined as the number of milliliters or cubic centimeters of blood passing through a given vessel cross-section in one heartbeat. A flat velocity profile is assumed to exist at the orifice level, and the peak velocity may therefore be substituted for the spatial mean velocity since the two values are nearly equivalent. To determine the stroke volume, the peak velocity is integrated over the duration of systole and the resulting value multiplied by the vessel cross-sectional area.

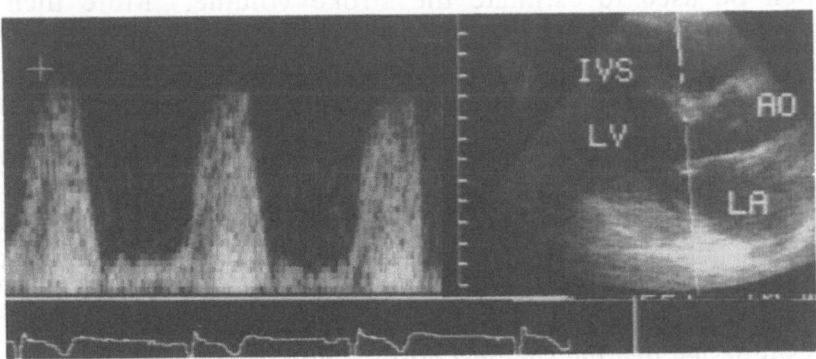

Fig. 6-1. Continuous mode recording of flow through a small muscular ventricular septal defect. Right. The continuous mode cursor is positioned through the muscular septum. Left. Continuous mode recording of shunt flow. The peak velocity is 4.2 m/s, and the calculated interventricular pressure drop is approximately 70 mm Hg. (AO = aorta, IVS = interventricular septum, LA = left atrium, LV = left ventricle.)

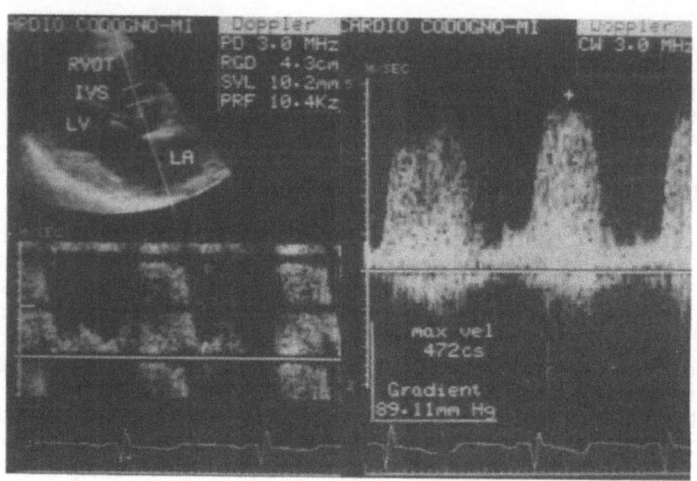

Fig. 6-2. Left. Pulsed mode recording of flow through a ventricular septal defect. Spectal unwrapping has been implemented so that positive velocities up to twice the Nyquist value can be measured. The peak velocity of shunt flow is still unresolved. Right. Continuous mode recording of the shunt flow. The peak flow velocity is 4.72 m/s, corresponding to an interventricular pressure drop of 89 mm Hg. Note the relatively high intensity of the low velocity signals. Low velocity diastolic flow through the defect is also recorded. (RVOT = right ventricular outflow tract, IVS = interventricular septum, LA = left atrium, LV = left ventricle.

The flow velocity integral may be calculated "on line" or may be determined by planimetry of the the area under the flow velocity curve. At least three attempts should be made to estimate the value of the flow velocity integral since there will be some beat-to-beat variation in its value. The average value should then be used to estimate the stroke volume. More then three measurements of the flow velocity integral should be made when the heartrate is irregular.

The vessel cross-sectional area is estimated by using the formula for the area of a circle ($\pi[(D/2)(D/2)]$) once the vessel diameter has been measured from the two-dimensional or M-mode recording. The aortic diameter can be measured from the long-axis view of the ascending aorta obtained from the second or third left intercostal space. The value of the aortic diameter at the level of the sinuses of Valsalva may be appreciably larger than that measured at the level of the annulus or at the sinotubular junction. Generally the internal diameter of the aorta measured at the annulus level is used in the calculation of the systemic output. Rein and coworkers obtained the closest correlation with thermodilution measurements of cardiac output when the annulus diameter was used to estimate the Doppler-derived cardiac output (42). Skjaerpe et al have also suggested that the smallest aortic diameter measured at the level of the annulus be used in determining the cardiac ouput (49).

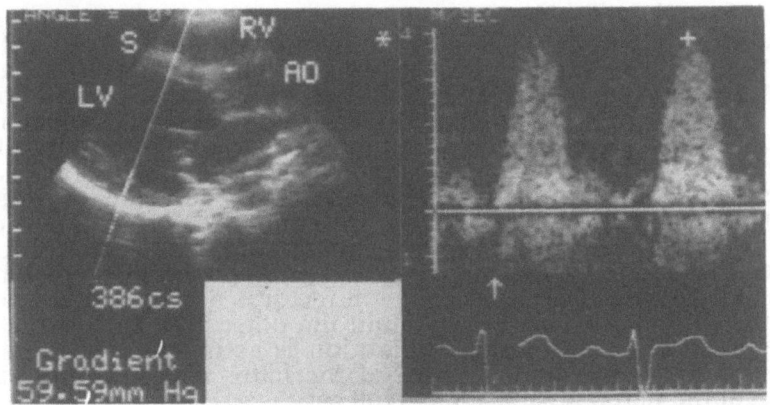

Fig. 6-3. Continuous mode recording of flow through a ventricular septal defect located in the muscular septum. The peak velocity is 3.86 m/s, and the estimated interventricular pressure drop is 60 mm Hg.

T he diameter of the pulmonary artery can best be estimated from the short-axis image obtained when the patient is rolled into an extreme left lateral position. If the patient is lying in the standard left lateral position, the pulmonary flow can easily be interrogated but it may be difficult to visualize the walls of the pulmonary artery.

There are several sources of error in the estimation of the stroke volume by Doppler technqiues. One of the most significant sources of error lies in the determination of the flow cross-sectional area. The flow cross-sectional area is assumed to be approximately the same value as the anatomic area, since it is the anatomic area which is estimated from the two-dimensional or M-mode recordings. The anatomic area is also assumed to be perfectly circular, and formula for the area of a circle is applied. The vessel diameter is squared in this formula, hence any error made when measuring the diameter will also be squared. The cross-sectional area varies with distance from the valve annulus and with the cardiac cycle. Finally, the vessel diameter should ideally be measured at the same level from which the pulsed mode recording was obtained, but this is difficult to verify. Changes in cardiac output will also affect the vessel dimensions. The assumption of a blunt velocity profile may also be a source of error (18).

The cardiac output is then calculated by multiplying the stroke volume by the measured heart rate. The output for both the pulmonary and systemic circulations should be calculated from the Doppler tracings of the pulmonary and aortic flow, respectively. Once these outputs have been determined, the pulmonary-to-systemic flow ratio is obtained by dividing the Doppler-derived pulmonary output by the systemic output. Good correlation between the Doppler-derived flow ratio and the invasively derived flow ratio have been reported by several investigators (51, 52). In general, a shunt is considered hemodynamically significant when the pulmonary-to-systemic flow ratio is greater than 2.0.

In cases of moderate to large ventricular septal defects and patent ductus arteriosus, there is turbulent flow in the pulmonary artery. The existence of turbulence gives rise to difficulty in the adequate recording of pulmonary flow, and a fair amount of variation in the pulmonary flow pattern may be observed. The presence of pulmonary stenosis would also preclude the use of the conventional method of estimating the pulmonary-to-systemic flow ratio. In such cases, the pulmonary output may be calculated by measuring the pulmonary venous return at the mitral orifice, as described by Fisher et al (16). The mitral orifice area changes throughout diastole, and a corrected mean orifice area is therefore used to estimate the flow cross-sectional area. The maximal orifice is measured from the appropriate two-dimensional short-axis still frame, while the correction factor is derived from the M-mode recording of the mitral valve. To obtain the correction factor, the maximal (Lmax) and mean (Lmn) leaflet separation is estimated from the M-mode mitral valve recording, and the ratio of the latter to the former calculated. The output at the mitral level is then given as:

$$CO = (\textstyle\int V_{mv}\, dt)(A_m)(Lmn/Lmax)$$

CO = cardiac output at the mitral orifice
V_{mv} = maximum mitral flow velocity
dt = the duration of diastole
A_m = the maximal mitral orifice area

The mitral flow velocity integral ($[\int Vmv\, dt]$) may be calculated on line or by planimetry of the area under the mitral flow velocity curve. The pulmonary venous return is then determined by muliplying the flow velocity integral by the corrected mitral orifice area. To obtain the pulmonary-to-systemic flow ratio, the output measured at the mitral orifice is divided by the output measured at the aortic orifice. Variations in heart rate will alter the value of the outputs measured at the mitral and aortic valve levels, and at least three attempts should be made to estimate the mitral and aortic outputs.

Ventricular Septal Defects

In the absence of cyanosis, the characteristic Doppler finding in ventricular septal defect is a disturbed systolic flow signal recorded in the right ventricle. The two-dimensional/Doppler examination is performed from the parasternal transducer position in most cases. Continuous mode is used to scan the right ventricular cavity for the presence of the abnormal flow signal. When the continuous wave beam intersects the jet of shunted blood, harsh tones may be heard in the audio signal. Mainly low velocity

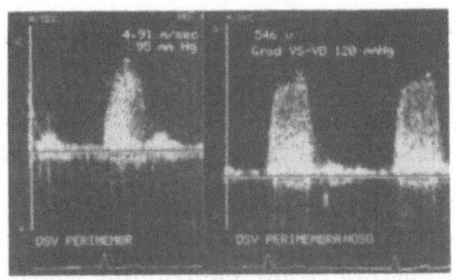

Fig. 6-4. Left. Continuous mode recordings of flow through a perimembraneous ventricular septal defect. The calculated pressure difference is 95 mm Hg. Right. A similar recording made in an older patient with a perimembraneous defect. The peak flow velocity is higher than in the first example, and the estimated interventricular gradient is 120 mm Hg. (DSV Perimembranous = perimembraneous ventricular septal defect).

components of high intensity will be recorded at a suboptimal beam-to-flow angle. The beam should be carefully re-aligned to acheive a parallel orientation to the jet by using the audio signal and the quality of the spectral trace for guidance. By selecting a high pass filter setting of at least 600 Hz, it is easier to record the high velocity components in the shunt flow signal. At a parallel position to flow, high frequencies will be heard in the audio signal and the envelope of the flow velocity curve will be clearly defined. A recording of shunt flow should then be made.

The relative flow signal intensity has been proposed as a qualitative indication of shunt severity. However, a parallel alignment with the shunt flow must be acheived before attempting such an assessment. If the beam-to-flow angle is large or the ultrasound beam is placed beside the core flow region, the signal intensity may be underestimated. The high frequency components in the shunt flow signal will not be adequately recorded. When the cardiac output is reduced or when the pulmonary resistance is increased, the flow signal intensity will be decreased. In cases of multiple septal defects, the Doppler beam may acheive a parallel position with respect to one of the jets. The flow signals arising from the nearby septal defects may result in a Doppler recording which is difficult to interpret. The most effective means of estimating shunt severity by Doppler technique is to calculate the pulmonary-to-systemic flow ratio as previously described.

After recording the peak flow velocity through the septal defect, the modified Bernoulli equation can be applied to estimate the interventricular pressure gradient (ΔP):

$$\Delta P = 4(Vm)^2$$

where Vm is the maximum shunt flow velocity. If the systolic blood pressure (SBP) is known, then the systolic right ventricular pressure (RVPS) can be calculated:

$$RVPS = SBP - \Delta P$$

Overestimation of the systolic right ventricular pressure can occur if the highest velocities in the jet are not recorded. The examiner should carefully evaluate the septal defect flow to ensure that the highest frequencies in the jet are being interrogated. In cases of apical septal defects, it can be difficult to orient the continuous wave beam so that the highest velocities are intercepted. The subcostal window usually provides the most parallel beam-to-flow orientation in such cases.

By switching to pulsed mode, the source of the systolic flow and the site of the ventricular septal defect can be localized. The same transducer angulation and position which resulted in an optimal continuous mode recording should be utilized in the pulsed mode examination. The sample volume is employed to track the systolic flow signal to its septal origin. When the sample volume is positioned within the defect itself, low frequency signals arising from wall motion will be recorded. Because the shunt flow velocities exceed the Nyquist limit, aliasing will occur in the systolic audio signal and in the flow velocity curve. The use of a lower frequency Doppler transducer and a spectral unwrapping algorithm may allow the peak flow velocity to be resolved in pulsed mode. Alternatively, high pulse repetition frequency mode can be utilized to record the high shunt flow velocities with a limited degree of range resolution. Usually, however, continuous mode is needed to accurately record the high velocities encountered in cases of acyanotic ventricular septal defect.

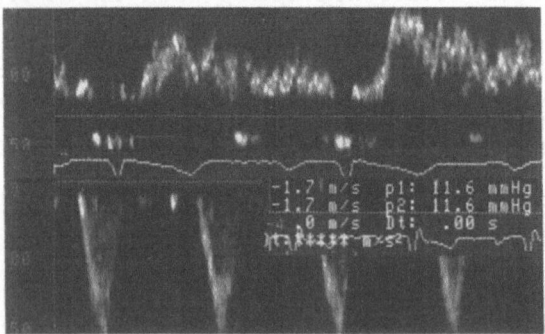

Fig. 6-5. Top and center. Pulsed mode recording of flow through an atrial septal defect, with a peak velocity of 1.0 m/s. The top trace contains 4 seconds of flow velocity information, while the center trace contains 2 seconds of flow velocity information. Bottom. High pulse repetition frequency mode recording of pulmonary flow in the same patient. The contour of the flow velocity curve resembles the contour of the flow velocity curve recorded in the normal descending aorta. The peak velocity is 1.7 m/s.

Low velocity diastolic flow through the septal defect can frequently be recorded with pulsed or continous mode. A biphasic diastolic flow pattern may be detected when the heart rate is low.

The pulsed mode finding of disturbed flow in the right ventricular cavity is sensitive but not specific for the diagnosis of ventricular septal defect. The presence of infundibular stenosis may result in the recording of increased flow velocity as well as flow disturbance in the right ventricular outflow tract. In cases of moderate to large atrial septal defect, flow disturbances may be recorded downstream in the right ventricular cavity owing to the series effect. The origin of the flow disturbance must be traced to the interventricular septum in order to establish the presence of a ventricular septal defect with pulsed mode.

Atrial Septal Defects

The characteristic pulsed Doppler finding in atrial septal defect is an early to mid-systolic flow signal recorded in the right atrium. There is rarely a significant pressure difference between the two atria hence the shunt flow velocity tends to be low. The maximal flow velocity is usually 1.0 m/s or less. In the absence of complicating lesions, the shunt direction is left-to-right because the right atrium has a higher capacitance than the left atrium. Two-dimensional echocardiography is quite successful in the visualization of large oval secundum defects, but only moderately successful when the defects are narrow or lie close to the fossa ovalis where much artifactual dropout occurs.

The pulsed Doppler/two-dimensional examination is most frequently performed from the subcostal window; a modified four-chamber view is obtained and the interatrial septum is visualized. The sample volume is placed on the right septal border and methodically moved along the septum until an abnormal systolic flow signal is heard. In the case of a moderate to large defect, the range gate may be positioned directly within the area of echo dropout and re-positioned slightly until the maximal signal intensity is heard in the audio signal. A systolic flow disturbance may also be recorded on the left side of the interatrial septum in large defects, although the magnitude of the disturbance will be less than that recorded in the right atrium.

The parasternal window may also be used to record flow through an atrial septal defect. The interatrial septum is usually not fully visualized from the parasternal position as it is from the subcostal window. However, a better angle to flow can sometimes be acheived from the parasternal approach and a more clearly defined systolic flow pattern can be recorded. The reduced interrogation depth of the parasternal window when compared to the subcostal window is an advantage when ruling out the presence of an atrial septal defect in an adult patient. The low intensity flow signal may not be well recorded from the subcostal window, whereas it may be quite clearly recorded from the parasternal window.

209

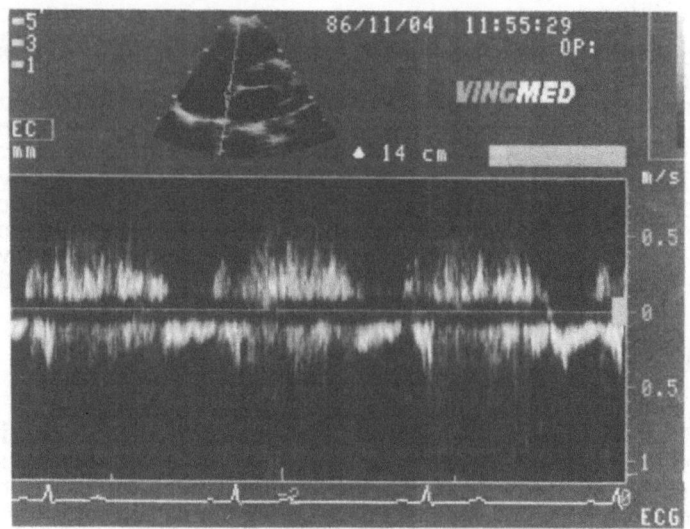

Fig. 6-6. Pulsed mode recording of atrial septal defect flow recorded from a low parasternal position. The sample volume is positioned near the right border of the interatrial septum, and a low velocity systolic flow is recorded moving into the right atrium.

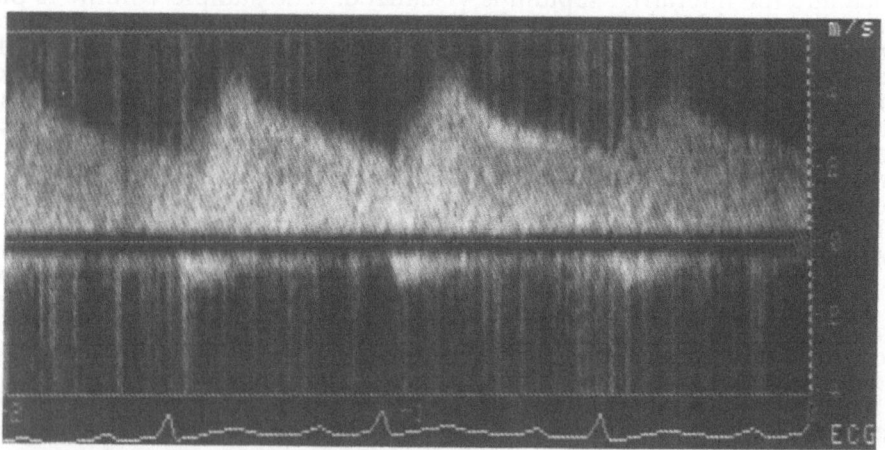

Fig. 6-7. Continuous mode recording of shunt flow in patent ductus arteriosus. The negative systolic flow represent pulmonary flow, while the continuous positive flow represents the ductal shunt flow. The peak shunt flow velocity is 4.5 m/s, indicating that the aortopulmonary pressure gradient is 81 mm Hg.

If the maximal systolic flow disturbance is located near the atrial entrance of the superior vena cava, a sinus venosus defect should be suspected. This type of atrial septal defect often coexists with some degree of anomalous pulmonary venous return. The existence of this abnomality can be established or ruled out in the course of the Doppler examination. When anomalous pulmonary venous return is present, bi-directional shunting may be recorded although the net direction of the atrial shunt will be right-to-left.

The increased flow volume in the right atrium will result in augmented flow across the tricuspid and pulmonary valves, and higher than normal peak flow velocities will be recorded. If the atrial shunt is large, the tricuspid flow pattern may resemble a normal mitral flow pattern. The pulmonary flow velocity may be twice the value of the peak aortic flow velocity, and disturbed flow in the right ventricular outflow tract can be recorded. The pulmonary-to-systemic flow ratio should be estimated by Doppler techniques in order to estimate the severity of the shunt.

In cases of primum defects, left ventricular outflow should be examined from the apical transducer position to exclude the presence of outflow obstruction. In response to the volume overload, the right ventricle may displace the septum into the left ventricular outflow tract. When this occurs, higher than normal outflow velocities will be recorded. The proximity of a primum defect to the atrioventricular valves may result in a loss of leaflet coaptation. Pulsed mode should be used to determine whether or not mitral and tricuspid insufficiency are present. Flow mapping techniques may be employed to estimate the degree of incompetence. Continuous mode should be also be utilized to record the regurgitant flow signal so that the signal intensity may be assessed. Infrequently, a left ventricular-to-right atrial shunt may be detected during the Doppler examination of a primum defect.

Septal Defect Repair

Doppler techniques are a reliable means of evaluating the effects of surgical intervention. In cases of septal defect repair, it is desireable to perform a pre-operative Doppler examination in order to calculate the pulmonary-to-systemic flow ratio. The flow ratio may then be re-calculated after surgery and compared to the pre-operative value.

In ventricular septal defect repair, the patch integrity should be checked using pulsed mode. The sample volume is positioned at the edge of the patch and carefully moved around the periphery while listening for a systolic flow signal. There is often some flow disturbance in the right ventricle immediately after surgery, but this gradually disappears in a successful closure. The persistence of such a flow disturbance may indicate the presence of residual shunting or the presence of a small septal defect close to the repair site. Turbulence in the pulmonary artery may also be recorded if the patch is leaking as a result of the series effect. By calculating the Doppler-derived pulmonary-to-systemic flow ratio, the magnitude of the residual shunt can be estimated.

The same technique is applicable in the evaluation of atrial septal defect repair. The sample volume is moved around the patch periphery while listening for an low intensity systolic flow signal. When an early to mid-systolic flow signal is recorded, the patch integrity should be suspect. Flow across the tricuspd and pulmonary valves should then be examined. If there is significant residual shunting, increased flow velocities may be recorded at the tricuspid and pulmonary orifices.

Patent Ductus Arteriosus

When a patent ductus arteriosus is suspected, Doppler ultrasound provides a rapid means of establishing the diagnosis. Indirect evidence of shunt flow may initially be obtained during the pulsed mode examination of pulmonary flow from the parasternal or subcostal window. Placement of the sample volume slightly downstream from the pulmonary valve may result in the recording of bidirectional flow. The systolic flow velocity may be increased, and the spectral flow pattern appears disturbed. After moving the sample volume further downstream, diastolic flow towards the transducer may be recorded; this represents part of the ductal flow signal.

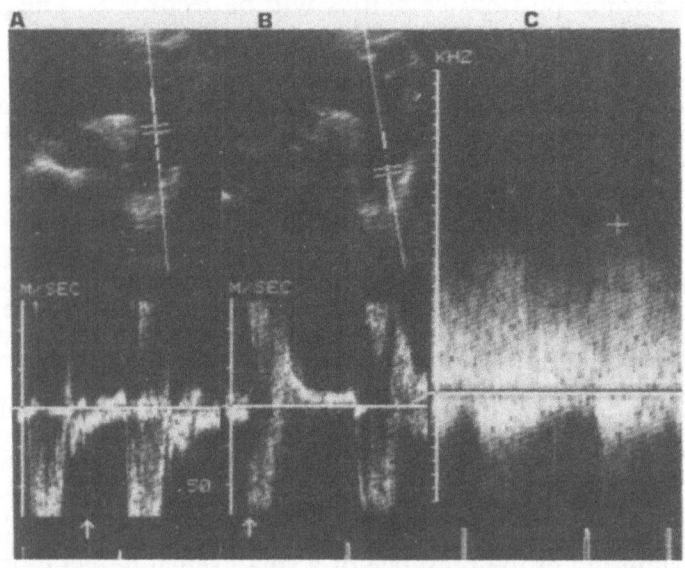

Fig. 6-8. Patent ductus arteriosus. A. Pulsed Doppler recording of flow in the descending aorta proximal to the ductus. The diastolic flow moves way from the transducer at this level. B. Pulsed Doppler recording of the aortic flow distal to the duct; the direction of the diastolic flow has reversed. C. The characteristic ductal flow patttern in the pulmonary artery recorded with continuous mode from the left sternal border. The negative systolic flow represents the pulmonary flow. The continuous flow with a softly delineated envelope represents the ductal shunt flow.

At the level of the pulmonary artery bifurcation, the pulsed mode flow pattern may be heavily aliased in both systole and diastole. Switching to continuous mode allows the examiner to resolve the peak flow velocities and to determine the direction of flow. When a patent ductus arteriosus is present, a characteristic continuous flow into the pulmonary artery is recorded. The negative systolic flow represents the pulmonary flow, while the continous positive flow represents the ductal shunt flow. The ductal flow velocity curve has a fine envelope, and it may be difficult to initially determine the peak flow velocity. By using the appropriate high pass filter setting and aligning the continuous wave beam with the ductal jet, the peak shunt flow velocity can be ascertained.

In the absence of pulmonary hypertension, the maximal ductal flow velocity occurs near end-systole, and is approximately 4.0 m/s. The peak flow velocity can be used to predict the aortic-to-pulmonary pressure gradient by applying the modified Bernoulli equation. If the systolic blood pressure is known, the systolic pulmonary artery pressure (SPA) can be estimated by subtracting the value of the pressure gradient (ΔP) from the value of the systolic blood pressure (SBP):

$$SPA = SBP - \Delta P$$

Good correlations with invasive estimates of systolic pulmonary artery pressure have been reported using this technique (65). An optimal Doppler recording is required in order to successfully estimate the systolic pulmonary artery pressure. If the peak ductal flow velocity has not been recorded, the aortopulmonary pressure gradient will be underestimated. This results in an overestimation of the systolic pulmonary artery pressure.

When examining pulmonary flow with pulsed mode alone, contradicting flow patterns may be infrequently recorded with changes in sample volume position. Usually the ductal jet tends to stream along the lateral wall of the pulmonary artery, and lateral sample volume placement results in the recording of positive diastolic flow. Medial sample volume placement, however, may result in the recording of continuous flow away from the transducer. This flow pattern does not represent right-to-left ductal shunting, but is produced by the deflection of the ductal jet away from the pulmonary valve cusps. A marked flutter of the pulmonary cusps can usually be recorded in these cases.

In the presence of pulmonary hypertension, the ductal flow signal may only be recorded in early diastole, and the peak flow velocity is reduced. The duration of the diastolic ductal flow signal has been shown to have an inverse correlation with the severity of pulmonary hypertension (79). If the sample volume is not optimally positioned however, only a portion of the ductal flow signal will be recorded. The flow duration will therefore be shortened, and the degree of pulmonary hypertension overestimated. Confirmation that the pulmonary artery pressure is elevated can be obtained by recording the flow signal through a ventricular septal defect, if present. If the peak flow velocity through the septal defect is reduced, then the right ventricular systolic pressure and hence the systolic

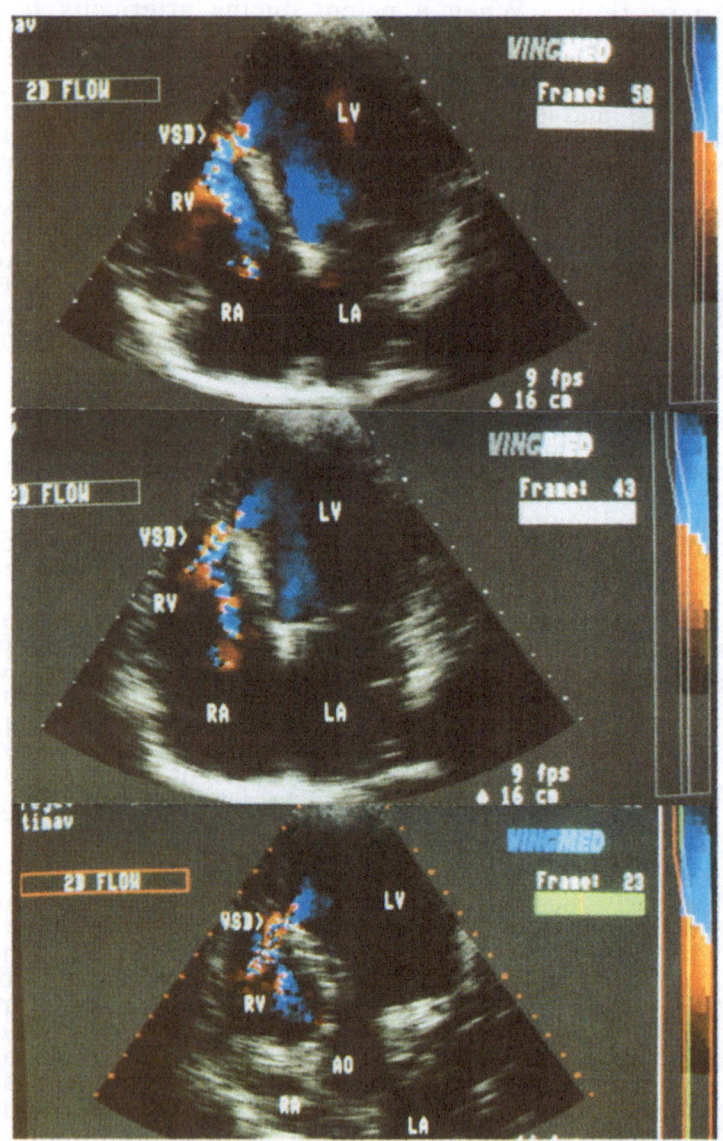

Fig. 6-9. Color flow mapping in ventricular septal defect. Top and center. Flow through a muscular ventricular septal defect is visualized in the apical four chamber view using the red/blue color scheme with variance. The left to right shunt flow is seen as a mosaic pattern in the interventricular septum and right ventricular cavity. The blue flow bolus in the left ventricle is the left ventricular outflow. Bottom. The shunt flow was also visualized using an apical five chamber view.

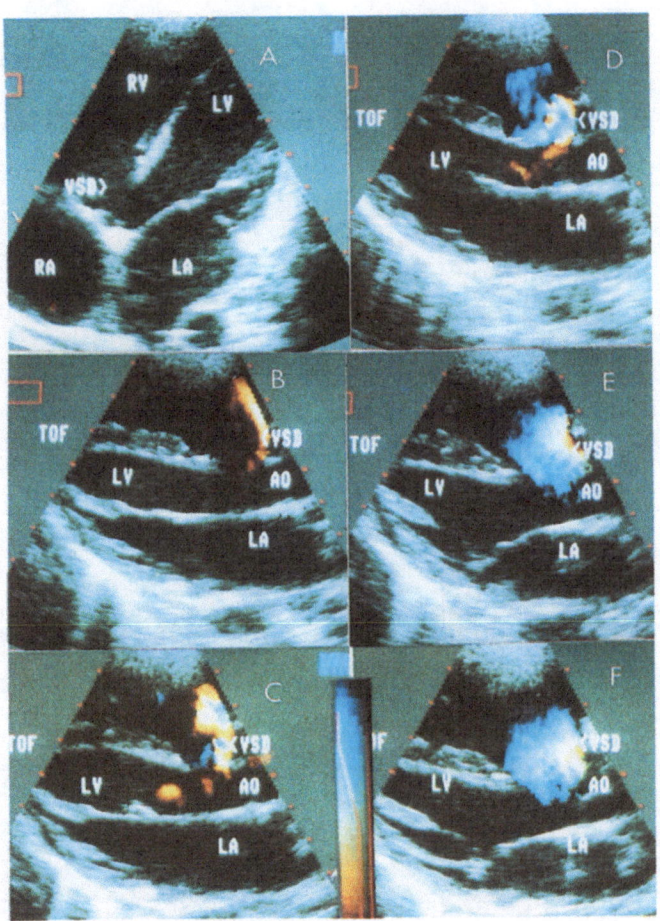

Fig. 6-10. This study was obtained in a 12 year old patient with an uncorrected Tetrology of Fallot using a 5.0 MHz transducer and the rainbow color flow map. Using this color assignment, shades of yellow and orange represent forward flow, while shades of aqua and blue represent reverse flow. A. The large septal defect was demonstrated in the apical 4 chamber view. B.From the left parasternal position, the over-riding septum is demonstrated and the onset of diastolic left to right shunting occurs. C. The core flow velocity has exceeded the Nyquist limit, and aliasing is noted. D. An eddy in the right venticular outflow tract forms later in diastole, as pressure between the ventricles equalizes. E&F. The right to left shunt in systole is visualized in shades of blue from the parasternal long axis view. The core flow velocity has aliased, and is depicted in shades of yellow-orange.

215

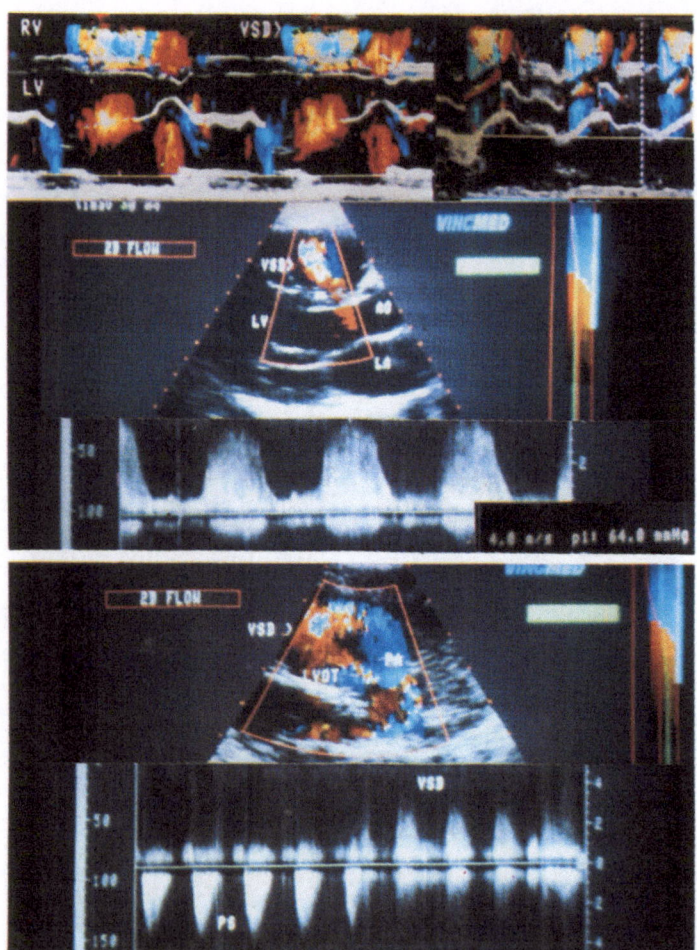

Fig. 6-11. Multimodality asessment of ventricular septal defect and pulmonary stenosis. A. The M-mode recording of the left ventricle shows exaggerated septal motion. B. Color flow display of the ventricular septal defect recorded from the parasternal long axis view. Shades of red indicate positive flow, while shades of blue indicate negative flow. The mosaic pattern represents the shunt flow through the defect. C. Continuous mode recording of flow through the septal defect. The peak flow velocity is 4.0 m/s, and the estimated interventricular gradient is 64 mm Hg. D. Color flow display of right ventricular outflow recorded from a modified short axis view. The shunt flow can be seen streaming into the right ventriuclar outflow tract. The blue flow bolus represents the right ventricular outflow. Distal to the pulmonary valve, a mosaic flow pattern is visualized. This represents the flow distal to the obstructed pulmonary valve. E. Continuous mode sweep from the pulmonary artery flow (negative spectral trace) to the ventricular septal defect flow (positive spectral trace) recorded from the left sternal border. The maximum velocity of pulmonary flow is 3.7 m/s, corresponding to a peak transvalvular gradient of 55 mm Hg. The spectral envelope of the shunt flow is not as clearly recorded as in trace C.

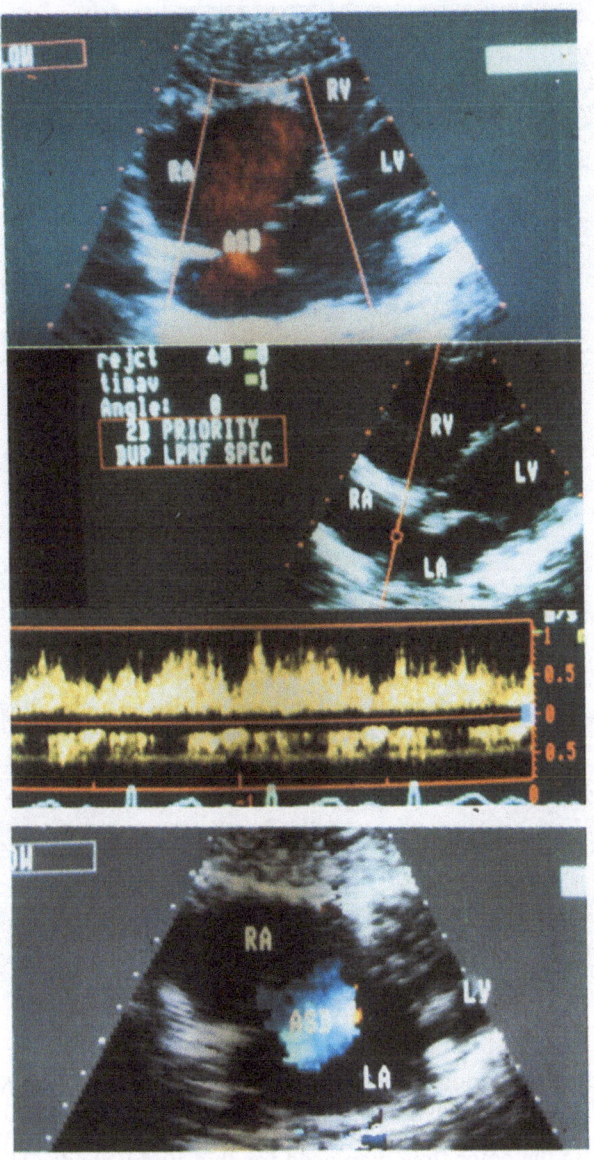

Fig. 6-12. A. Color flow display of flow through an atrial septal defect recorded from the subcostal window. A red flow bolus is seen moving across the interatrial septum, indicating the presence of a left to right shunt. B. Pulsed mode recording of flow through the atrial septal defect in the same patient. The sample volume is positioned in the region of echo dropout. C. Color flow display of flow through an atrial septal defect with right to left shunting. A blue flow bolus is seen crossing the interatrial septum.

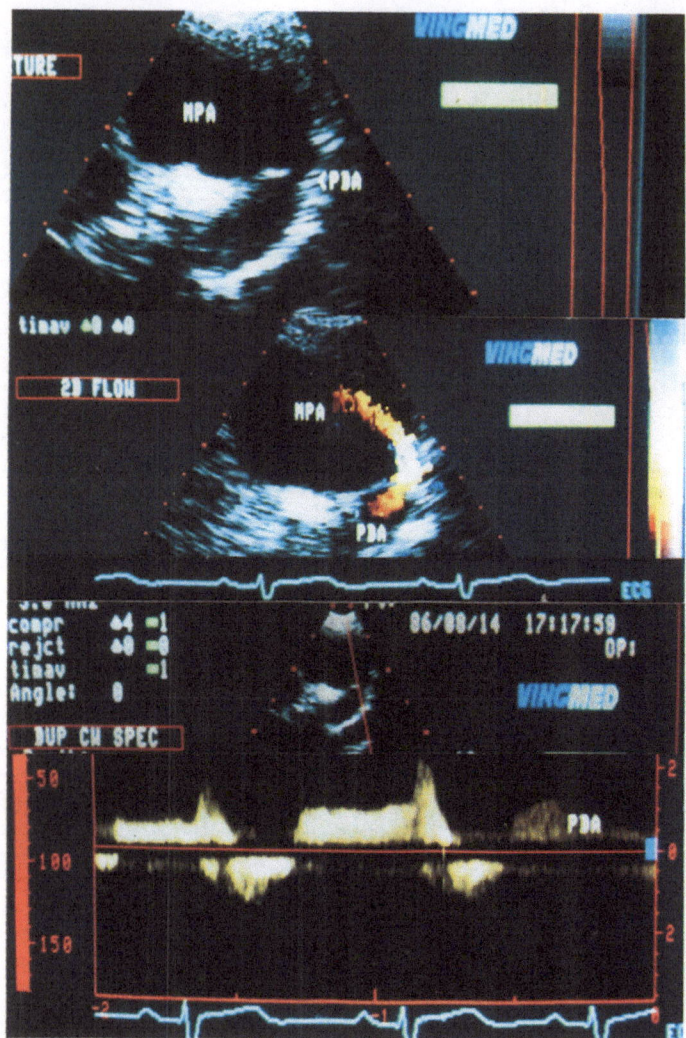

Fig. 6-13. Patent ductus arteriosus and pulmonary hypertension. Top. Modified short axis view of the base of the heart. The patent ductus and the dilated main pulmonary artery are clearly visualized. Middle. An orange-hued flow bolus can be seen streaming into the main pulmonary artery. In the color flow map used for this study, shades of orange and yellow indicate positive flow, whereas shades of blue indicate negative flow. The ductal jet tends to flow along the lateral wall of the main pulmonary artery. Bottom. The continuous mode recording of the flow through the patent ductus arteriosus. The low velocity of the ductal flow indicates the presence of pulmonary hypertension. During isovolumic contraction, the pulmonary artery pressure decreases, resulting in an increased ductal flow velocity before the onset of systole.

218

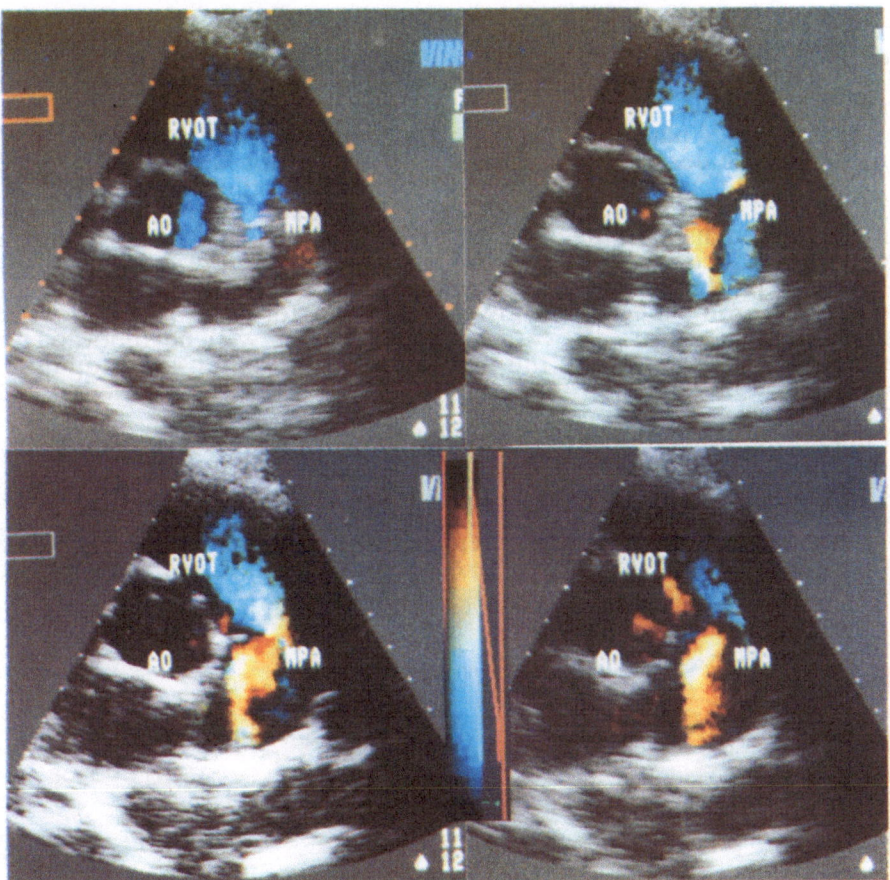

Fig. 6-14. Color flow mapping in pulmonary stenosis. A. In early systole, a dark blue flow bolus is seen in the right ventricular outflow tract. The dark blue hues indicate that the flow is moving at a relatively low velocity. B. A few frames later, the right ventricular outflow has increased in velocity, and the flow bolus is now colored in brighter shades of blue. A bright orange-yellow flow can be seen originating from the pulmonary annulus; this represents the aliased high velocity flow distal to the pulmonary obstruction. C. By mid-systole. the aliased pulmonary jet curves into the main pulmonary artery. D. Towards the end of systole, darker hues are assigned to the right ventricular outflow, indicating a decreased velocity. The edges of the pulmonary flow bolus have a dark orange color, indicating the presence of lower velocities in the jet periphery.

pulmonary artery pressure is elevated. When tricuspid insufficiency is present, the peak velocity of the regurgitant flow signal will also allow one to predict the systolic pulmonary artery pressure by applying the modified Bernoulli equation.

The presence of a patent ductus arteriosus may also be established from flow recordings in the descending aorta obtained from the suprasternal window. Sample volume placement proximal to the level of the ductus results in the recording of diastolic flow away from the transducer. When the sample volume is moved distal to the duct, the diastolic flow is recorded moving away from the transducer. An aortopulmonary septal defect may give rise to similar flow patterns in the descending aorta. The flow patterns in the ascending aorta in such cases, however, will differ from those recorded in patent ductus arteriosus. Reversed diastolic flow will be recorded in the ascending aorta as well as in the descending aorta when a aortopulmonary defect exists. Only low amplitude diastolic forward flow will be recorded in the ascending aorta when a patent ductus arteriosus is present.

To determine the pulmonary output by Doppler techniques, the pulmonary venous return at the mitral orifice should be interrogated (Fig. 6-15). The systemic output may be determined from the systemic venous return measured in the right ventricular outflow tract proximal to the pulmonary valve. The pulmonary-to-sytemic ratio can then be estimated by dividing the output measured at the mitral orifice by the output measured in the right ventricular outflow tract.

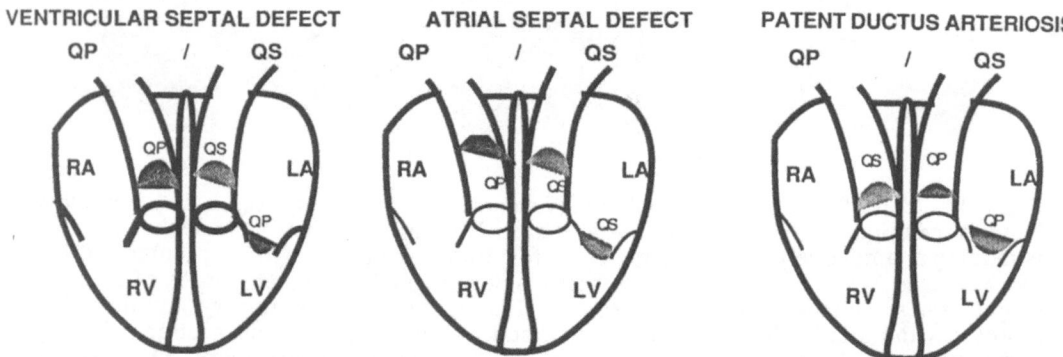

Fig. 6-15. Estimation of the pulmonary (Qp) to systemic (Qs) flow ratio in shunt lesions. Left. In moderate to large ventricular septal defects, the pulmonary flow is measured at the mitral orifice. Center. In moderate to large atrial septal defects, the systemic output can be measured at the aortic or mitral orifice. Right. In patent ductus arteriosus, the pulmonary output is measured at the mitral orifice.

Doppler Flow Imaging in Shunt Lesions

When evaluating shunt lesions, color flow mapping provides a rapid means of determining the presence or absence of shunt flow. Once the presence of a shunt has been established, the spatial orientation of the shunt flow with respect to the transducer position and the anatomical structures allows one to select the optimal imaging window for the conventional Doppler examination.

It may be difficult to rule out the presence of multiple septal defects or apical ventricular septal defects with conventional Doppler techniques, and the conventional Doppler examination can be time-consuming. Color flow analysis in the hands of experienced investigators may reduce the examination time in such cases. Daniels and coworkers have indicated that real time flow imaging facilitates the localization of small muscular and apical setpal defects (62). Special cases such as Eisenmenger's syndrome can be better understood when color flow imaging is combined with conventional Doppler analysis. Bommer et al have utilized color flow analysis to study shunt flow in patients with Eisenmenger's syndrome (13). The direction of systolic septal defect flow was found to be intially left-to-right, and the flow direction reversed during mid-systole. The late systolic right-to-left flow tended to stream into the left ventricular outflow tract and not into the left ventricular cavity. The septal defect flow in diastole was found to be left-to-right as in ventricular septal defect without pulmonary hypertension. The use of a cine-loop format for review of such special cases is helpful when interpreting the real time flow information.

Bi-directional shunting through an atrial septal defect can also be demonstrated with slow motion or cine-loop playback of the recorded atrial shunt flow. However, a high quality video retrieval system is needed in order to prevent image degradation. This is especially true when examining infants and small children because of the rapid heart rates which are encountered.

A variety of flow patterns through a patent ductus arteriosus has been demonstrated with color flow analysis. The optimal transducer alignment for recording the peak velocities in the ductal shunt can be determined from the color flow display. Swannsen and coworkers have indicated that color flow imaging is useful in the differentiation of a constricted ductus arteriosus from the left pulmonary artery in infants (46). The search for a small ductal shunt can be time-consuming when using conventional Doppler modalities. Color flow imaging of the pulmonary flow patterns can greatly facilitate this search, especially when combined with cine-loop playback of the color flow information.

In the future, it is possible that color flow analysis may be employed to directly determine the shunt volume in septal defects. Color images of shunt flow may be interfaced to an image processing computer. Each color flow pixel actually represents a small flow volume owing to the thickness of the sector plane.

The sum of those pixels displaying shunt flow is then the shunt volume of that given frame. However, the number of pixels coding for shunt flow varies considerably from frame to frame and is also dependent upon the sensitivity of the flow imaging mode and the instrument set up. Nevertheless, the severity of shunt lesions may directly be estimated from the real time display if these factors are taken into consideration.

Estimation of the Systolic Pulmonary Artery Pressure

In congenital anomalies, the systolic pulmonary artery pressure can be elevated when there is increased flow in the pulmonary circuit, or when obstruction to pulmonary flow or pulmonary venous return is present. Previously this value could only be estimated at catheterization, but several methods of determining the pulmonary artery pressure with Doppler techniques have been described.

Hatle and coworkers have applied Burstin's method of measuring the interval between pulmonary valve closure and tricuspid valve opening, or Pc-To interval, to estimate the pulmonary artery pressure (6). Burstin's method is based upon the assumption that the Pc-To interval is proportional to the systolic pulmonary artery pressure and inversely proportional to the heart rate. The Pc-To interval can be measured from Doppler traces of pulmonary and tricuspid flow recorded with a simultaneous phonocardiogram. A nomogram is then used to derive the estimated pulmonary artery pressure from the mean Pc-To interval at a given heart rate. Although there are several potential sources of error, a good correlation between the Doppler-derived pulmonary artery pressure and the invasively measured value is possible. When the systolic right atrial pressure is increased, as in moderate to severe tricuspid insufficiency, the systolic pulmonary artery pressure will be underestimated. Underestimation may also occur in the setting of low cardiac output. When atrial fibrillation is present, a larger number of beats must be averaged in order to minimize error when calculating the mean Pc-To interval.

Other investigators have assessed the accuracy of several pulmonary flow parameters in predicting the existence of pulmonary hypertension. The time required to acheive peak pulmonary velocity or acceleration time, and the ratio of acceleration time to right ventricular ejection time have been shown to be inversely related to the pulmonary artery pressure. These time intervals are measured directly from the pulmonary flow velocity curve. The acceleration time is the interval from the beginning of pulmonary flow to the peak of the flow velocity curve. The right ventricular ejction time is the interval from the beginning to the cessation of systolic flow in the pulmonary artery.

Generally, an acceleration time less than 110 ms is indicative of pulmonary hypertension, and a regression equation may be used to estimate the mean pulmonary artery pressure. Perez et al found the value of the acceleration time in normal children to be greater than 115 milliseconds, while the mean ratio of acceleration time to ejection time was 0.43. (11).

In the group of children with pulmonary hypertension, the mean acceleration time was 71 milliseconds, and the mean ratio of acceleration time to ejection time was 0.29. Matsuda and coworkers found that an acceleration time less than 90 ms indicated the presence of a mean pulmonary artery pressure greater than 25 mm Hg (36).

The acceleration time varies with heart rate, and more intervals should be measured to derive the mean acceleration time when the heart rate is not constant. The presence of right ventricular dysfunction will also change the value of the acceleration time. When the pulmonary artery pressure is elevated, retrograde flow or zero flow is frequently recorded in mid- to end-systole, and the determination of the right ventricular ejection time becomes equivocal. Slight changes in sample volume placement may significantly alter the appearance of the pulmonary flow velocity curve, thereby changing the value of the acceleration and ejection times. The presence of eddy currents and valve fluttering can also interfere with the Doppler recording of pulmonary flow. To circumvent these problems, it is possible to measure these time intervals from the flow velocity pattern recorded in the right ventricular outflow tract proximal to the pulmonary valve, as suggested by Kitabatake et al (37).

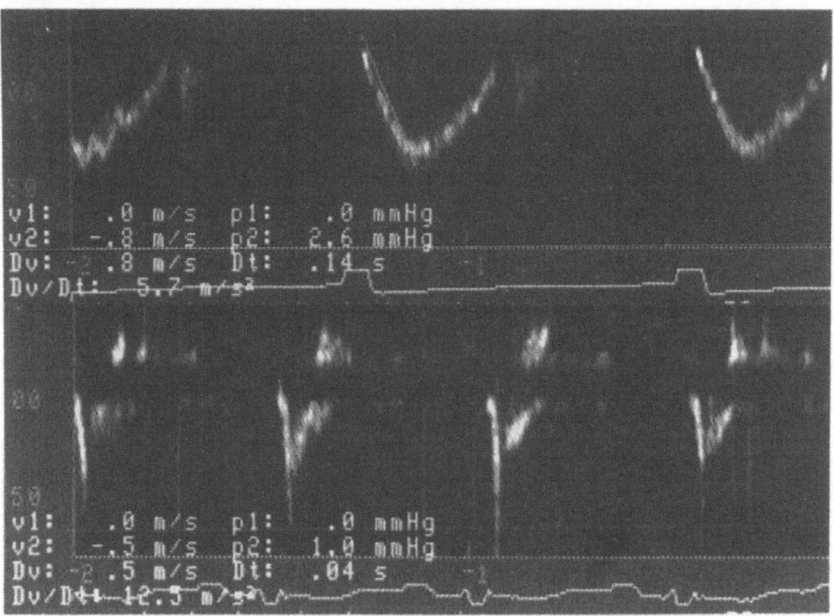

Fig. 6-16. Top. Pulmonary acceleration time in a normal adolescent. The acceleration time is 140 ms. Bottom. An average pulmonary acceleration time of 40 ms was measured in this patient with pulmonary hypertension. Note the reversed direction of flow in mid-systole; the presence of reversed flow makes it difficult to determine the right ventricular ejection time from the spectral trace.

In the presence of tricuspid regurgitation, estimation of the systolic right ventricular pressure and pulmonary artery pressure is possible. The maximum regurgitant flow velocity is substituted into the modified Bernoulli equation to obtain the systolic right ventricular pressure. The right atrial pressure is assumed to be negligible, but it must be taken into account when there is venous distension. When the right atrial pressure is elevated, the value of the right atrial pressure must be added to the calculated gradient to avoid underestimation of the systolic right ventricular pressure and systolic pulmonary artery pressure. In patients with pulmonary insufficiency, one can also determine whether or not the diastolic pressure in the pulmonary artery is increased. A regurgitant flow velocity greater than 1.7 m/s indicates the presence of elevated diastolic pulmonary artery pressure.

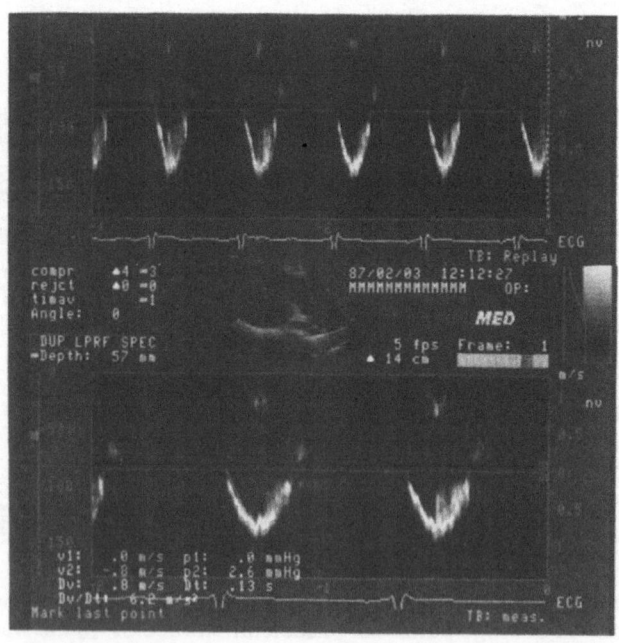

Fig. 6-17. Normal pulmonary flow in a young adult. The pulmonary acceleration time is 130 ms, and the right ventricular ejection time is 265 ms. The acceleration to ejection time ratio is within normal limits .

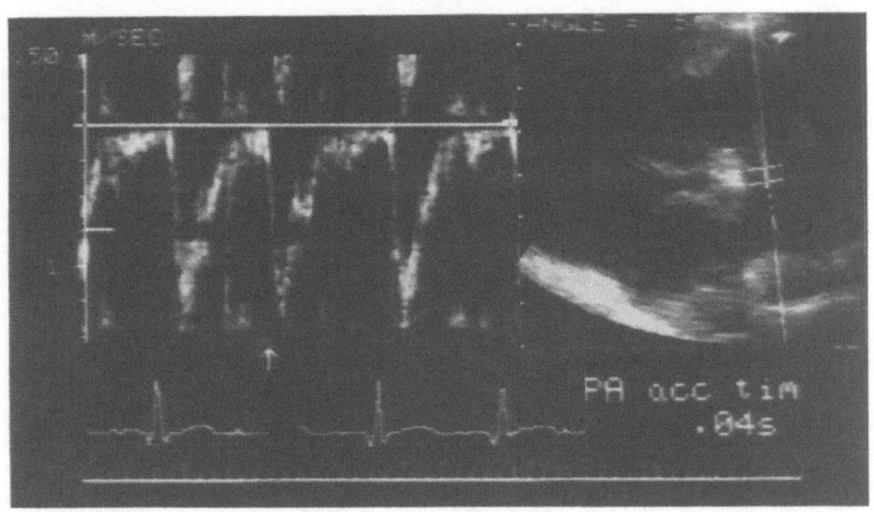

Fig. 6-18. Pulsed mode recording of pulmonary flow in a child with elevated pulmonary artery pressure. The average acceleration time is 40 ms.

Chan and coworkers compared three methods of estimating the pulmonary artery pressure in a group of 50 patients undergoing cardiac catheterization (53). The Pc-To method of predicting the systolic pulmonary artery pressure could not be applied in a large percentage of patients due to the presence of arrhythmia. The pulmonary artery acceleration time was also measured in order to predict the pulmorary artery pressure by a regresion equation. Finally, the peak tricuspid regurgitant velocity was used to estimate the systolic pulmonary artery pressure in those patients with tricuspid insufficiency. They concluded that the tricuspid regurgitation approach to the prediction of the pulmonary flow velocity appeared to be the most useful. The findings of Reidel et al were similar (54). The tricuspid regurgitation approach yielded a reliable estimate of the systolic pulmonary artery pressure, while the ratio of the acceleration time to the right ventricular ejection time was useful in predicting elevated mean pulmonary artery pressure.

The systolic pulmonary artery pressure can also be estimated when some form of aortopulmonary communciation exists, such as a Blalock-Taussig shunt or a patent ductus arteriosus (Fig 6-7). The flow envelope in aortopulmonary shunts is diffuse even when recording from an optimal position, hence underestimation of the peak velocity is a significant source of error. It is essential to obtain a parallel alignment with the flow through these shunts otherwise the peak velocity will be underestimated. Underestimation of the peak flow velocity results in an overestimation of the systolic pulmonary artery pressure. The selection of post-processing compression curves to enhance the spectral flow envelope and the use of a high pass filter greater than 600 Hz will aid in the recording of the low intensity, high velocity shunt flow signals.

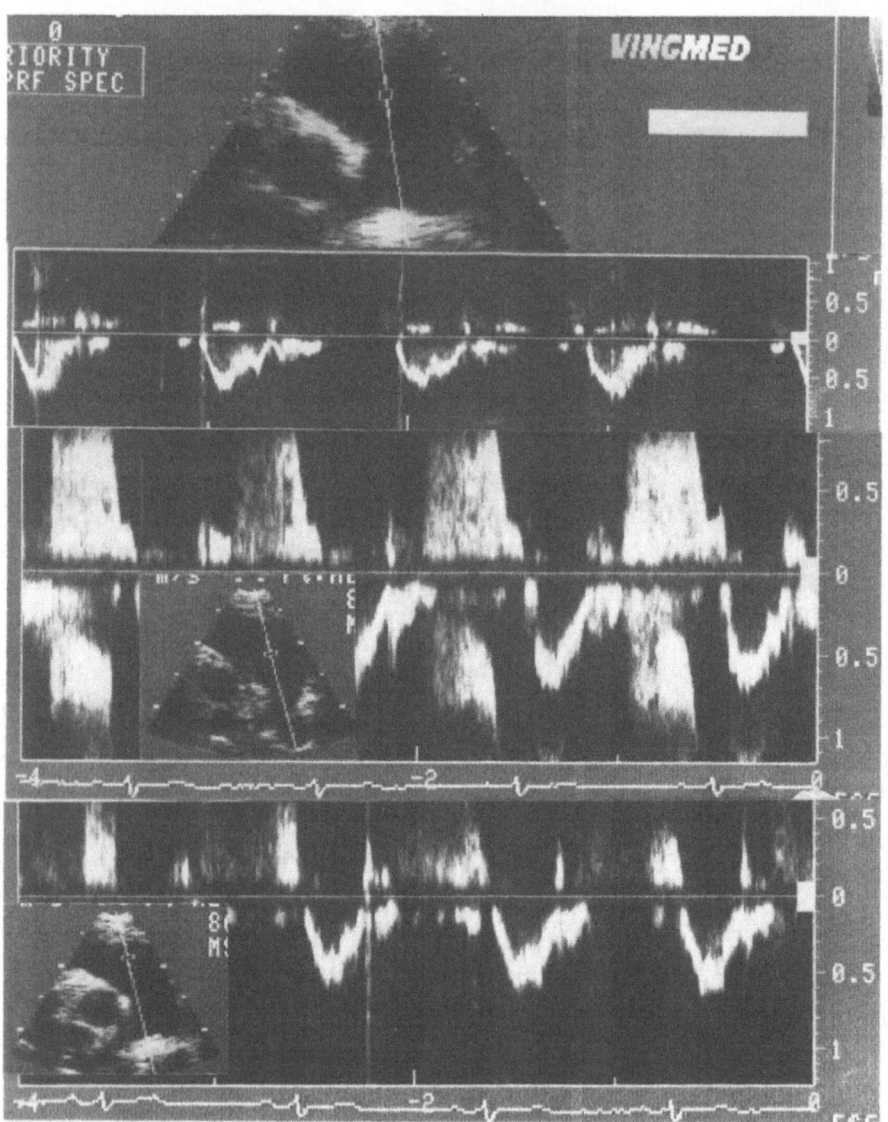

Fig. 6-19. Idiopathic dilatation of the pulmonary artery. Top. Pulsed mode recording of pulmonary flow at the level of the pulmonary valve. As the sample volume is shifted slightly downstream from the valve, a bifid appearance to the pulmonary flow curve is recorded in the second and third beat. Mid-systolic notching of the pulmonary flow curve can be recording in cases of pulmonary hypertension or when there is pulmonary artery dilatation. Middle. Pulsed mode recording of the pulmonary insufficiency in the same patient. Bottom. The sample volume is moved to a distance of 3.0 cm behind the pulmonary valve, and the regurgitant flow signal is still recorded, although its intensity has diminished.

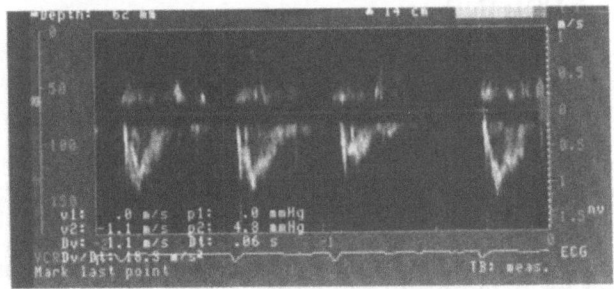

Fig.6-20. The pulmonary artery flow acceleration time will be reduced in the presence of pulmonary artery hypertension. The acceration in this case is 40 ms , while the normal value is greater than 100 ms.

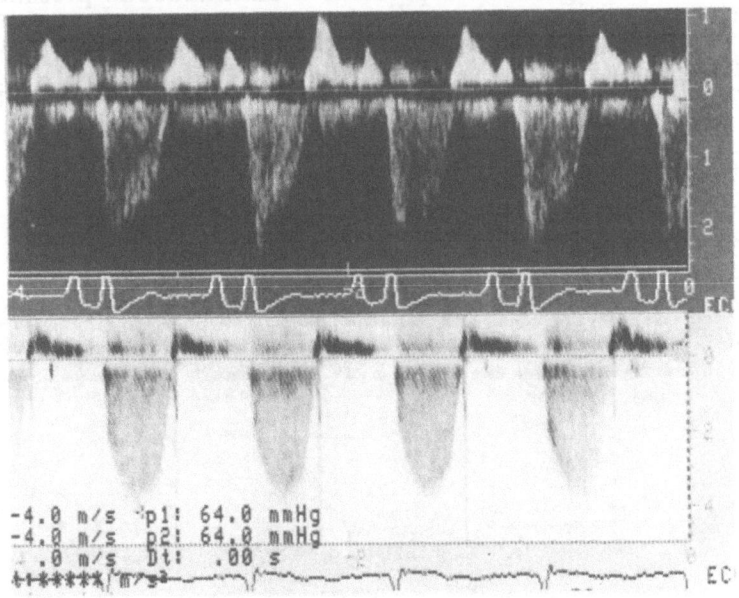

Fig. 6-21. Measurement of the regurgitant peak velocity in patients with tricuspid regurgitation is the most reliable technique for estimating the systolic pulmonary artery pressure. Top. In the presence of physiological tricuspid insufficiency an normal pulmonary artery pressure, the weak signal intensity may cause signal drop out near the peak velocity. Bottom. When the pulmonary artery pressure is elevated and tricuspid insufficiency is present, it is usually possible to record the peak regurgitant velocity if a parallel flow alignment had been acheived. In this case, the systolic pulmonary artery pressure (P2) is estimated to be 64 mm Hg.

OBSTRUCTIVE LESIONS

Aortic Stenosis

Among the forms of aortic obstruction, valvular stenosis most frequently gives rise to symptoms in infancy. The malformed aortic valve may be unicuspid, bicuspid or myxomatous. Usually the unicuspid type will be encountered in cases of critical aortic stenosis. To interrogate the aortic flow, the suprasternal window is most commonly used. The jet in congenital aortic stenosis can be intercepted from the suprasternal position, and jet eccentricity is not a problem as it is in adult aortic stenosis. The continuous wave beam can easily be aligned with the stenotic jet by listening to the audio signal. When the beam-to-flow angle is small, the audio signal has a characteristic high pitch and the spectral envelope is well delineated.

Once an adequate recording of aortic flow has been obtained, the peak velocity may be used to estimate the peak simultaneous pressure gradient by applying the modified Bernoulli equation. Since the peak velocity is sustained in a significant obstruction, the mean Doppler gradient should also be calculated. The Doppler-derived peak gradient represents a simultaneous pressure gradient, while the catheterization peak gradient represents a peak to peak pressure difference. The value of the Doppler-derived peak and mean gradients may vary significantly with the condition of the patient during the ultrasound examination. If the patient is agitated, the calculated gradients will be much higher than those obtained when the patient is sedated (74).

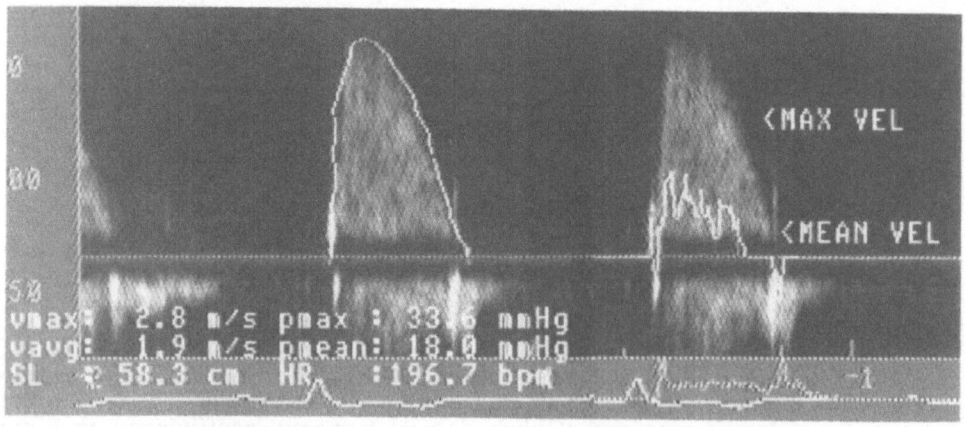

Fig. 6-22. Continuous mode recording from the right parasternal position of flow in the ascending aorta after valvulotomy. The peak and mean gradients are 34 mm Hg and 18 mm Hg, respectively. The analog curves for the mean velocity (MEAN VEL) and the Doppler signal amplitude are also displayed. The spikes for aortic valve opening and closure are clearly indicated in the amplitude trace, which is located above the electrocardiogram.

Patients with bicuspid aortic valves often have a slightly increased aortic flow velocity, or the the value of the peak flow velocity may be within the normal limits during childhood. Fibrotic thickening or calcification of the aortic valve cusps may gradually cause the development of left ventricular outflow obstruction. Increasingly higher aortic flow velocities will be recorded as the valve becomes obstructed.

Doppler techniques may also be used to estimate the residual gradient following valvulotomy, and to assess the degree of insufficiency created by they procedure. The Doppler-derived mean pressure gradient can be compared to the pre-operative value and that obtained at catheterization. A study by Keane and coworkers of aortic valvotomy patients revealed that a high percentage of these patients developed peak systolic gradients greater than 60 mm Hg and had to be re-operated (71). Serial Doppler examinations of post-valvotomy patients are a reliable means of detecting the development of significant outflow obstruction.

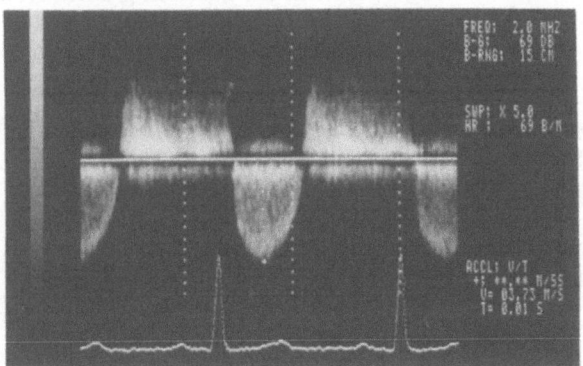

Fig. 6-23 Continuous mode recording of left ventricular outflow in a patient with subvalvular aortic stenosis and insufficiency recorded from the apical window. The maximum velocity was 3.7 m/s. The subvalvular membrane could be seen in the two dimensional image, although the quality of the image was suboptimal.

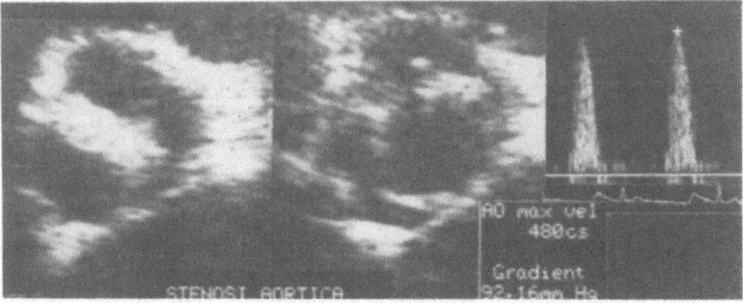

Fig. 6-24. Obstruction of a bicuspid aortic valve. Top. The two dimensional short axis views of the aortic valve demonstrate the presence of extensive cusp thickening. Bottom. Continuous wave Doppler recording of the aortic flow. The peak flow velocity is 4.8 m/s, corresponding to a peak gradient of 92 mm Hg.

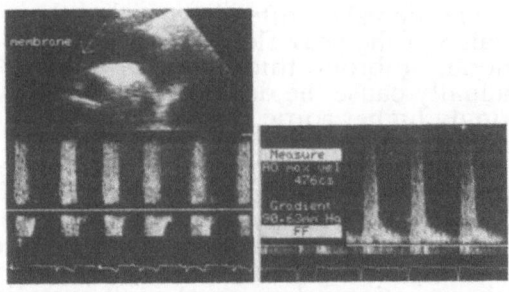

Fig. 6-25. Supravalvular aortic obstruction. Top. The presence of a discrete membrane was demonstrated in the long axis view of the ascending aorta. Middle. The pulsed mode recording of flow in the ascending aorta is heavily aliased at the level of the membrane. Bottom. Continuous mde recording of flow in the ascending aorta from the suprasternal window. The peak flow velocity is 4.8 m/s, corresponding to a peak gradient of 90 mm Hg.

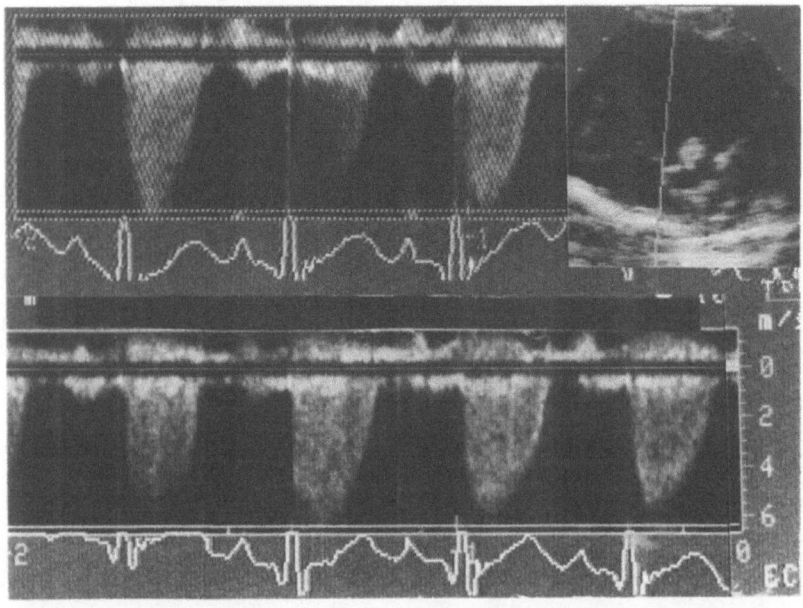

Fig. 6-26 Left ventricular outflow obstruction in an infant with a fibroma. Continuous mode recording of left ventricular outflow. The peak outflow velocity is slightly greater than 6.0 m/s, and the estimated peak outflow gradient is 144 mm Hg. The middle trace was recorded while the infant was moving; note how the flow pattern drops out in the second beat, leaving only the left ventricular outflow signal proximal to the obstruction. The fibroma can be seen as a mass in the left ventricular outflow tract (top).

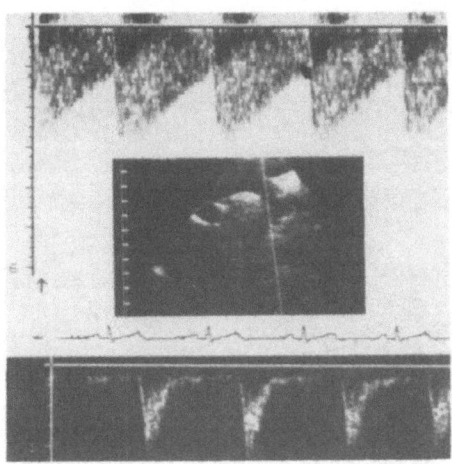

Fig. 6-27. Top. Continuous mode recording of flow in the descending aorta in a patient with coarctation. The peak flow velocity is approximately 2.7 m/s. The black arrow points to the peak velocity in descending aorta proximal to the coarctation. Bottom. Pulsed mode recording of flow in the descending aorta proximal to the coarctation. A peak flow velocity of 1.0 m/s is obtained, corresponding to the peak flow velocity of the superimposed flow in the continuous mode recording.

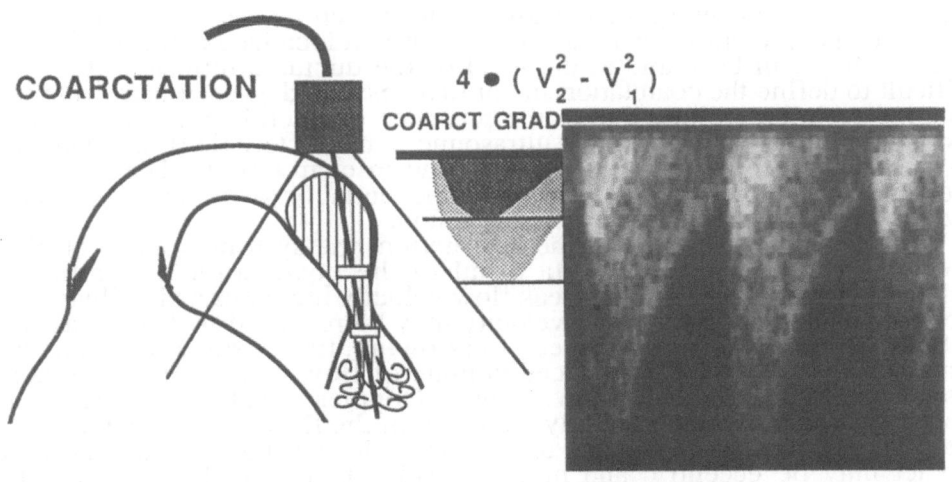

COARCTATION

$$4 \bullet (V_2^2 - V_1^2)$$

COARCT GRAD

Fig. 6-28. To obtain an accurate estimation of the pressure drop across a coarctation one should measure the pressure proximal to the lesion and subtract this from the gradient derived from the peak velocity .

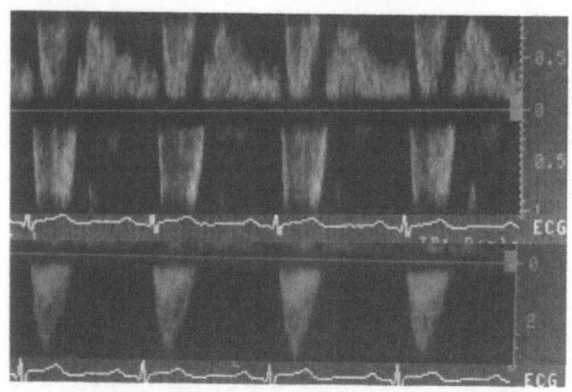

Fig. 6-29. Top. Pulsed mode recording of flow in the descending aorta in a patient with a bicuspid aorta and surgically corrected coarctation. A significant amount of regurgitant flow is recorded in diastole, and the forward flow velocity is increased. Bottom. Continuous mode recording of flow in the descending aorta. The peak velocity distal to the coarctation site is nearly 3.5 m/s, while the peak velocity proximal to the coarctation site is 2.0 m/s. The rapid decrease of the peak distal velocity indicates that there is no significant residual obstruction.

Coarctation of the Aorta

Coarctation of the aorta is a congenital anomaly in which there is an obstruction or narrowing of the distal aortic arch or the descending aorta. Juxtaductal coarctation occurs most frequently; a localized constriction of the aortic lumen can be found at the level of the ductus arteriosus. It may be difficult to define the coarctation site or to assess the degree of narrowing with imaging technique alone due to the presence of lateral resolution artifacts. Using continuous wave Doppler ultrasound, a characteristic flow pattern will be recorded from the suprasternal window in coarctation. The distinctive spectral envelope has been described as exponential or sawtooth in appearance, and the audio signal has a characteristic sound.

With increasing severity of the obstruction, the systolic volume of blood flowing in the descending aorta distal to the coarctation is significantly reduced. At the same time, the peak flow velocity increases and declines more slowly so that a relatively high velocity may be recorded in diastole as well. When there is a significant degree of narrowing, the diastolic flow velocities may exceed 2.0 m/s. The reduced volume of flow distal to the coarctation results in a high velocity but low intensity Doppler signal. Consequently, the peak flow velocity may be faintly recorded on the flow velocity curve. Since the coarctation creates a bending or kinking of the descending limb of the aorta, the jet may be eccentric and hard to track. Occasionally the peak flow velocities in the jet may be more clearly recorded by moving the transducer slightly to the left of the standard suprasternal position.

To calculate the pressure gradient across the coarctation, the peak velocity in the descending aorta must be included in the Bernoulli equation when it exceeds 1.0 m/s.

If the velocity proximal to the coarctation (Vd) is neglected, the gradient (ΔP) will be overestimated. The gradient is calculated as:

$$\Delta P = 4(Vc^2 - Vd^2)$$

where Vc is the peak flow velocity distal to the coarctation. A parallel or nearly parallel alignment of the continuous wave beam to the jet is essential for accurate prediction of the pressure gradient.

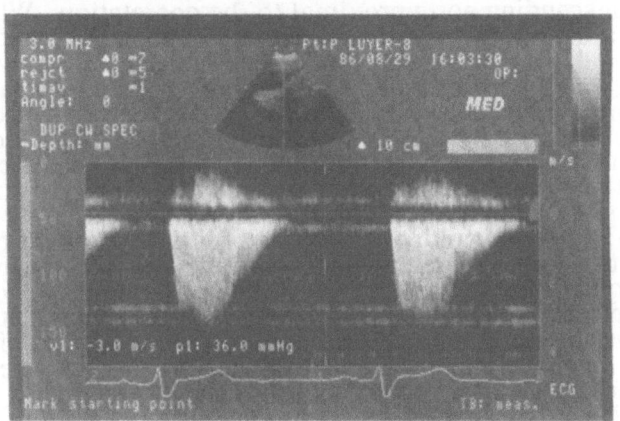

Fig. 6-30 Continuous mode recording in mild coarctation. The peak flow velocity distal to the obstruction is 3.0 m/s and the proximal flow velocity is slightly less than 1.0 m/s. The estimated peak systolic gradient is 32 mm Hg.

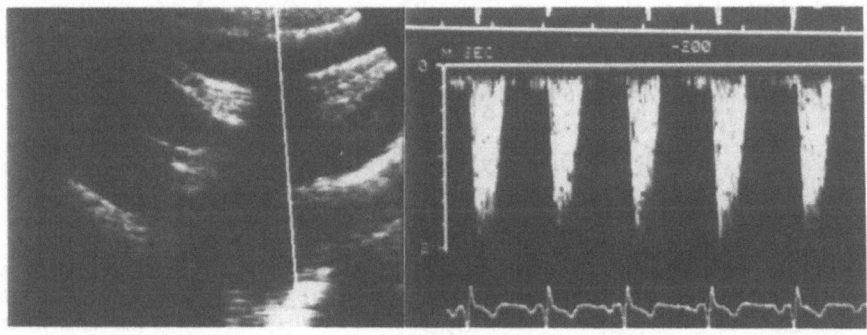

Fig. 6-31 Continuous mode recording in a patient with surgically corrected coarctation. The peak flow velocity is 2.0 m/s, and declines rapidly. Continuous wave Doppler provides an accurate means of post operative follow up in coarctation patients.

233

Because the jet trajectory is unpredictable in coarctation, the jet may bend so acutely that a parallel position to flow can not be acheived even with the use of an independent Doppler transducer. Stevenson et al (55) have demonstrated that the jet angulation is probably responsible for the underestimation of the actual pressure gradient in coarctation. Although the potential for gradient underestimation exists, the Bernoulli equation still allows one to assess the relative severity of the outflow obstruction in patients with coarctation.

The pulsed Doppler examination of flow in the descending aorta indicates the presence of high velocity flow at the level of and downstream from the coarctation site. Pulsed mode should be utilized to obtain Vc, the peak flow velocity in the descending aorta proximal to the coarctation. When flow in the ascending aorta is interrogated, a normal aortic flow pattern is usually recorded in the absence of aortic stenosis. The peak flow velocity in the ascending aorta may be lower than normal due to left ventricular failure.

Aortic isthmus narrowing or infantile coarctation is another form of coarctation characterized by a region of luminal narrowing which may extend from the left subclavian artery to the ductal level. A localized constriction may also exist near the ductus arteriosus. The Doppler examination is performed in the same manner as previously described, and the peak flow velocity may be used to predict the peak pressure gradient existing in the descending aortic limb. A patent ductus arteriosus is frequently associated with infantile coarctation, while it may not be patent in juxtaductal corctation. The ductal lumen serves to widen the effective diameter in the the descending aorta. When the ductus constricts, the hemodynamic effects of the narrowed isthmus lumen become apparent and higher velocities are recorded in the isthmus. Ventricular septal defect is commonly associated with infantile coarctation, and the existence of this lesion should be established or ruled out during the Doppler examination.

Doppler techniques are also helpful in the evaluation of patients with coarctation after surgery. Using pulsed mode, flow in the ascending and descending aorta should be carefully interrogated. In a successful repair, the peak flow velocity in the descending aorta may be moderately increased. This finding may reflect the hyperdynamic state of the left ventricle which is frequently found in such patients (20). The peak flow velocity in the ascending aorta will also be higher than normal in these cases. When a localized significant increase in flow velocity is recorded in the descending aorta, re-coarctation should be suspected.

Right Ventricular Outflow Obstruction

The evaluation of pulmonary stenosis has already been described in the previous chapter, and the decription of pulmonary stenosis here will therefore be brief. In infants and small children, it is generally easier to obtain a good quality continuous mode recording of pulmonary flow from the subcostal window. The peak velocity measured from the subcostal window may actually be greater than that measured from the parasternal window. The jet direction in

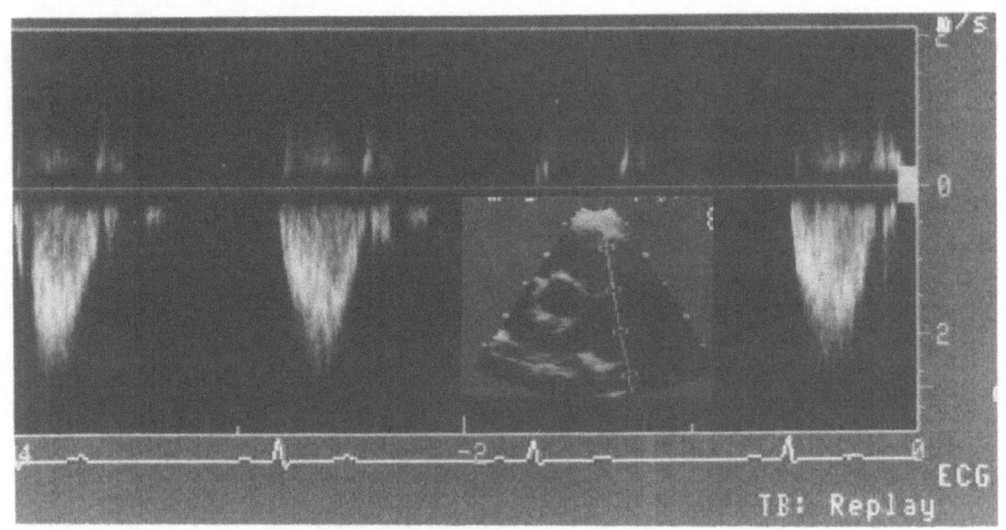

Fig.6-32 . Mild pulmonary stenosis. High pulse repetition frequency mode is used to record the pulmonary flow in this patient with mild pulmonary obstruction. The locations of the four range gates are indicated on the sector image (insert). The maximal velocity is approximately 2.4 m/s, and the estimated peak gradient is 23 mm Hg.

pulmonary stenosis tends to be more variable than the jet direction in congenital aortic stenois, and oblique jets may be encountered. Color flow analysis can be initially used at the beginning of the examination to determine the jet orientation and the optimal transducer position for the continuous mode scan. The peak simultaneous pressure gradient and the mean pressure gradient should be calculated by applying the modified Bernoulli equation. As in aortic stenosis, the peak simultaneous gradient will consistently exceed the peak-to-peak gradient measured at catheterization. However, the difference between the two values is less in cases of right ventricular outflow obstruction (32).

When infundibular and valvular obstruction coexist, the flow through the infundibulum will be superimposed upon the continuous wave recording of pulmonary artery flow (Fig 5-34). The infundibular obstruction represents a dynamic obstruction to flow, and therefore has a late systolic peak velocity. When the peak flow velocity through the infundibulum is increased, it must be included in the calculation of the peak transvalvular gradient. If the increased infundibular flow velocity is excluded from the modified Bernoulli equation, overestimation of the peak transvalvular gradient will occur. The pressure drop across the entire outflow tract can be calculated by substitution of the maximum pulmonary flow velocity into the modified Bernoulli equation.

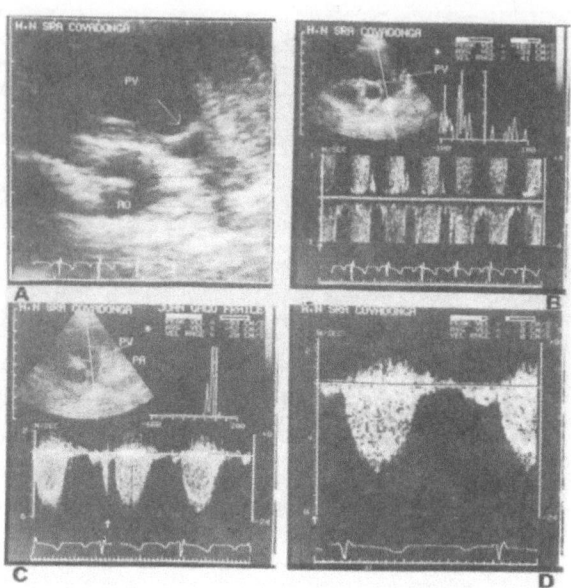

Fig. 6-33. Severe pulmonary stenosis. A. The doming of the pulmonary valve cusps may be clearly seen in this magnified short axis view of the pulmonary artery. B. The pulsed mode recording of pulmonary flow is heavily aliased and the peak velocity can not be ascertained. C. Continuous mode recording of pulmonary flow obtained with the imaging transducer. The maximal flow velocity is 5.0 m/s, corresponding to a predicted peak gradient of 100 mm Hg. D. Continuous mode recording obtained with the independent Doppler transducer. The maximal flow velocity is the same as that recorded in C.

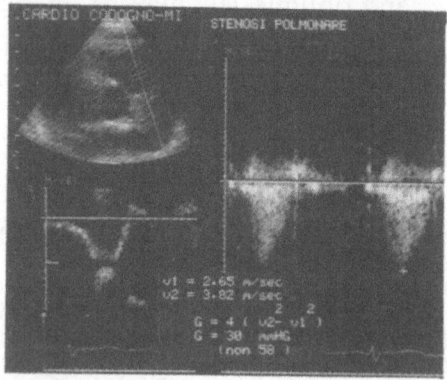

Fig. 6-34. When the infundibular flow velocity is increased, the simplified Bernoulli equation can no longer be applied to estimate the transvalvular gradient. Left. Pulsed Doppler recording of infundibular flow; the peak velocity (v1) is 2.65 m/s. Right continuous mode recording of pulmonary flow with a peak velocity (v2) of 3.8 m/s. The calculated transvalvular gradient id 30 mm Hg, and not 58 mm Hg.

The flow obstruction created by placement of a pulmonary artery band can easily be assessed with continuous wave Doppler ultrasound, and the subcostal window usually provides the narrowest beam-to-flow angle. Calculation of the mean and peak gradient is useful in such cases, since it allows the examiner to determine whether or not the banding procedure has been successful in reducing pulmonary artery flow. If the band is too tight, a high pulmonary flow velocity will be recorded with continuous mode.

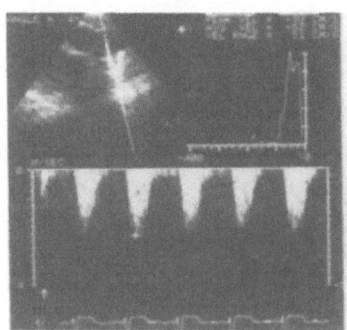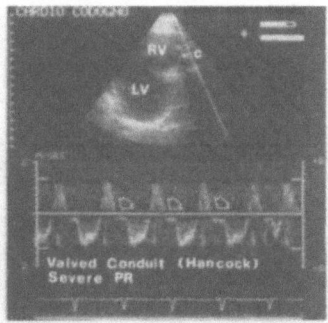

Fig. 6-35. Doppler recordings of conduit flow obtained from a high parasternal position. Left. Continuous mode recording of normal conduit flow in a patient with tricuspid valve atresia. the peak flow velocity is approximately 2.25 m/s, and no regurgitation is detected. Pulsed mode was also used to rule out the presence of heterograft valve incompetence. Right. Pulsed mode recording of severe heterograft valve incompetence in a Hancock conduit. The peak velocity in the regurgitant flow signal declines rapidly, and the regurgitation is no longer recorded at end-diastole (arrows). This finding indicates that equalization of right ventricular and pulmonary artery pressure occurs before end-diastole. (RV = right ventricle, LV = left ventricle, C = conduit, PR = pulmonary regurgitation).

Congenital Mitral Stenosis

Congenital mitral stenosis occurs infrequently as an isolated lesion. The chordae tendinae as well as the mitral leaflets may be abnormal and may insert into two normal papillary muscles or a single fused papillary muscle. The thickened valve does not open as fully as the normal mitral valve; the presence of anomalous chordal attachment further restricts leaflet excursion.

The Doppler evaluation of congenital mitral stenosis is performed from the apical transducer position. Continuous mode should initially be utilized to obtain a parallel alignment to the jet. Either continuous mode or high pulse repetition frequency mode may be employed to record the mitral flow pattern. High pulse repetition frequency mode generally yields an acceptable flow pattern in these cases because the flow velocities are only moderately increased. Calculation of the pressure half time, peak diastolic gradient, and mean gradient is useful in assessing the severity of the inflow obstruction. Often the atrial flow component has the same amplitude or a higher amplitude than the rapid filling component in congential mitral stenosis, but the pressure half time is calculated in the same manner.

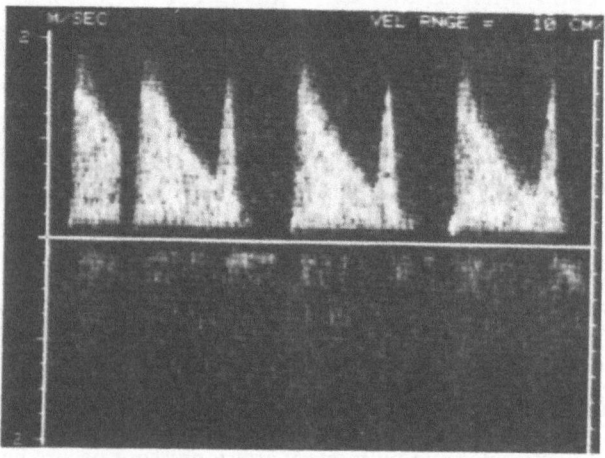

Fig. 6-36. Congenital mitral stenosis. Continuous mode recording of mitral flow from the apical position. The peak flow velocity is approximately 1.8 m/s, and the predicted peak gradient is 13 mm Hg. Note that the atrial flow component has nearly the same amplitude as the rapid filling component.

References

1. Hatle L, Angelsen B. Doppler Ultrasound in Cardiology: Physical Principles and Clinical Applications. Lea & Febiger, Philadelphia, 1982.
2. Walmsley R, Watson H. Clinical Anatomy of the Heart, Churchill Livingstone, New York, 1978.
3. Goldberg S, Allen H, Sahn D. Pediatric and Adolescent Echocardiography: A handbook. Yearbook Medical Publishers, Chicago.
4. Currie P, Hagler D, Seward J, Reeder G, et al. Instantaneous pressure gradient: A simultaneous Doppler and dual catheter correlative study. J AM Coll Cardiol 7;4: 800-806, 1986.
5. Yock P, Popp R. Noninvasive estimation of right ventricular systolic pressure by Doppler ultrasound in patients with tricuspid regurgitation. Circulation 70;4: 657-662, 1984.
6. Hatle L, Angelsen B, Tromsdal A. Noninvasive Estimation of pulmonary artery systolic pressure with Doppler ultrasound. Brit Heart J 45; 2: 157-165, 1982.
7. Hatle L, Brubakk A, Tromsdal A, Angelsen B. Noninvasive assessment of the pressure drop in mitral stenosis by Doppler ultrasound. Brit Heart J 40;131-140, 1978.
8. Teirstein P, Yock P, Popp R. The accuracy of Doppler ultrasound measurements of pressure gradients across irregular, dual and tunnel-like obstructions to blood flow. Circulation 72;577-584, 1985.
9. Stewart WJ, Galvin KA, Gillam LD, et al. Comparison of high pulse repetition frequency and continuous wave Doppler in the assessment of high flow velocity in patients with valvular stenosis and regurgitation. J Am Coll Cardiol 6;565-71,1985.
10. Kitabatake A, Inoue M, Masuyawa T, et al. Noninvasive estimation of pulmonary artery pressure from velocity pattern of right ventricular ejcetion flow by pulsed Doppler technique (abstr) J Am Coll Cardiol 1;657,1983.
11. Perez D, Azancot A, Lamberti A, et al. Hypertension arterielle pulmonaire de l'enfant: Evaluation quantitative par echocardiographie Doppler pulse´. L'information Cardiologique 9;10:820-22, 1985.
12. Gardin J, Burn C, Hughes C, Henry W. Are Doppler aortic flow velocity measurements reproducible? (abstr) Circulation, suppl IV, 62:205, 1981.
13. Bommer W, Rebeck K, Birnbaum S. Two-dimensional color flow imaging of ventricular septal defect in Eisenmenger's syndrome. (abstr) Clin Prog. Electrophysiol and Pacing 4;78, 1986.
14. Smith M, Dawson P, Elion J, et al. Systematic correlation of Doppler aortic gradient with specific catheter pressure measurements in experimental aortic stenosis: Mean Doppler gradient is optimal. (abstr) J Am Coll Cardiol 5;2:402, 1986.
15. Houston A, Sheldon, Simpson I. Assessment of the value of continuous wave Doppler echocardiography in 121 infants and children with congenital heart disease. (abstr) Sixth Symp on echocardiography, 84, 1985.

16. Fisher DC, Sahn DJ, Larsen D, et al. The mitral valve orifice method for noninvasive determination of cardiac output by two-dimensional echo-Doppler: Validation and initial clinical trials. Am J Cardiol 49;932, 1982.
17. Hatle L, Rokseth R. Noninvasive diagnosis and assesment of ventricular septal defect by Doppler ultrasound. Acta Med Scand 47;645, 1981.
18. Redel D, Junck H. Description of the blood velocity profiles inside the human main pulmonary artery with the use of color Doppler echocardiography. (abstr) Int Cong Cardiac Doppler;27, 1985.
19. Sanders SP, Yeager S, Williams RG. Measurement of systemic and pulmonic blood flow and Qp/Qs ratio using echocardiography and Doppler velocimetry. Circulation 66;231, 1982.
20. Vargas-Baron J, Sahn DJ, Valdes-Cruz LM, et al. Quantitation of the ratio of the pulmonary to systemic blood flow in patients with ventricular septal defect by range gated pulsed Doppler echocardipgraphy. Circulation 66;318, 1982.
21. Allen HD, Sahn DJ, Lange L, Goldberg S. Noninvasive assessment of surgical systemic to pulmonary artery shunts by range-gated pulsed Doppler echocardiography. J Pediatrics 94;395-491, 1979.
22. Kronik G. The role of echocardiography for the diagnosis and management of congenital heart disease in adults. (abstr), Int post-graduate course on advances in echocardiography, Davos, 11984.
23. Stevenson JG, Kawabori I, Dooley TK, et al. Pulsed Doppler echocardiographic detection of pulmonary hypertension in patent ductus arteriosus, Circulation 60:355, 1979.
24. Stevenson JG, Kawabori I, Guneroth WG. Pulsed Doppler echocardiographic evaluation of the cyanotic newborn: Identification of the pulmonary artery in transposition of the great arteries. Am J Cardiol 46; 849, 1980.
25. Stevenson JG, Kawabori I. Noninvasive determination of pulmonary to systemic flow ratio by pulsed Doppler echocardiography. Circulation 66;232, 1982.
26. Hatle L, Angelsen BA. Noninvasive assessment of aortic stenosis by Doppler ultrasound. Brit Heart J 43;284-292, 1980.
27. Nimura Y. Pitfall and artifacts in Doppler echocardiography (abstr). Int Congress of Cardiac Doppler, 1985: 108-109.
28. Touche T, De Zuttere D, Nitenberg A, Prasquier R. Quantification des stenoses mitrales par echocardiographie Doppler: Reetalonnage avec le catherisme cardiaque simultané. Information Cardiologique 9;832, 1985.
29. Bommer W, Miller L. Real-time two-dimensional color flow Doppler: Enhanced Doppler flow imaging in the diagnosis of cardiovascular disease (abstr). Am J Cardiol 499;944, 1982.
30. Stamm RB, Martin RP. Quantification of pressure gradients across stenotic valves by Doppler ultrasound. J Am Coll Cardiol 2; 707, 1983.

31. Kecioglu-Draelos Z, Goldberg SJ, Areis J, Sahn DJ. Verification and clinical demonstration of the echo Doppler series effect and vortex shed distance. Circulation 63;1322-24, 1981.
32. Hagler DJ, Currie PJ, Seward J, et al. Doppler assessment of congenital stenotic cardiac lesions: Simultaneous continuous wave Doppler - catheter pressure gradient correlation (abstr). Sixth Symposium on Doppler Echocardiography;85, 1985.
33. Currie PJ, Hagler DJ, Seward JB, et al. Instantaneous Pressure Gradient: A Simultaneous Doppler and Dual Catheter Correlative Study. J Am Coll Cardiol 7;4:800-6, 1986.
34. Marx GR, Allen HD, Goldberg SJ. Doppler Echocardiographic estimation of systolic pulmonary artery pressure in pediatric patients with interventricular communications. J Am Coll Cardiol 6;5:1132-7, 1985.
35. Marx GR, Allen HD, Goldberg SJ. Doppler echocardiographic estimation of systolic pulmonary artery pressure in patients with aortic-pulmonary shunts. J Am Coll Cardiol 7;4:880-5, 1986.
36. Matsuda M, Sekiguchi T, Sugishita Y, et al. Reliability of noninvasive estimation of pulmonary hypertension by pulsed Doppler echocardiography. Br Heart J 56:158-64, 1986.
37. Kitabatake A, Inoue M, Asao M, et al. Noninvasive evaluation of pulmonary hypertension by a pulsed Doppler technique. Circulation 68:302-309, 1983.
38. Cacciapuoti T, Varrichio M, D'Avino M, et al. Noninvasive evaluation of left to right shunts by pulsed Doppler echocardiography. Int J Card 13:1; 57-67, 1986.
39. Sullivan ID, Robinson P, Wyse R, et al. Continuous wave Doppler in the evaluation of complex congenital heart disease in infants and children. Int J Card 13:1; 69-77, 1986.
40. Hatle L. Comment of the impact of ultrasonic Doppler studies. Eur Ht J 6:101-104, 1985.
41. Keren G, Meisner JS, Sherez J, et al. Interrelationship of mid-diastolic mitral valve motion, pulmonary venous flow and transmitral flow. Circulation;1:36-44, 1986.
42. Rein AJJ, Hsieh KS, Elixson M, et al. Cardiac output estimation in the pediatric intensive care unit using continuous wave Doppler: Validation and limitations of the technique. Am Heart J 1986; 113: 97.
43. Dittrich H, Hoit B, Sahn DJ. Spatial patterns of mitral flow in patients with congenital cardiomyopathy determined by real time two dimensional echocardiography and Doppler color flow mapping (abstr). J Am Coll Cardiol 1985; 5: 426.
44. Kosturakis D, Goldberg SJ, Allen HD, LOeber C. Doppler echocardiographic prediction of pulmonary arterial hypertension in congenital heart disease. Am J Cardiol 1984; 53: 1110.
45. Foult GM, Blanchard D, Raoul B, et al. Noninvasive measurement of pulmonary artery pressure by pulsed Doppler echocardiography. Circulation 1980; 62: 366.
46. Swenssen RE, Valdes-Cruz, Sahn DJ, et al. Real time Doppler color flow mapping for detection of patent ductus arteriosus. J Am Coll Cardiol 1986; 8: 1059-65.

47. Skjearpe T, Hegrenaes L, Hatle L. Noninvasive estimation of valve area in patient with aortic stenosis by Doppler ultrasound and two dimensional echocardiography. Circulation 1985; 72: 810-8.

48. Stewart WJ, Galvin KA, Gillam LD, Guyer DE, Weyman AE. Comparison of high pulse repetition and continuous wave Doppler echocardiography in patients with valvular stenosis and regurgitation. J Am Coll Cardiol 1985, 6;3: 565-71.

49. Skjaerpe T, Hegrenaes L, Halfdan I. Cardiac Output. In Doppler Ultrsound in Cardiology, second edition, Lea & Febiger, Philadelphia, 1985 (P 306-320).

50. Valdes-Cruz LM, Horowitz S, Mesel E, et al. A pulsed Doppler echocardiographic method for calculating pulmonary and systemic blood flow in atrial level shunts; Validation studies in animals and initial human experience. Circulation 1984; 69:80-86.

51. Serwer GA, Cougle AG, Ekerd JM, Armstrong B. Factors affecting the use of the Doppler determined time from flow onset to maximal pulmonary flow velocity for measurement of pulmonary artery pressure in children. Am J Cardiol 1986; 58: 352-56.

52. Gardin JM, Yoganathan A, McNillan S, et al. Potential problems in making Doppler pulmonary flow artery measurements: Documentation in a flow model (abstr). Second INt Cong Cardiac Doppler 1986; 119.

53. Chan Kl, Currie PJ, Seward JB, Hagler DJ, et al. Comparison of three Doppler methods in the prediction of pulmonary artery pressure (abstr). J Am Coll Cardiol 1986, 7;2:144A.

54. Riedel M, Dennig K, Rudolph. Comparison of various Doppler echocardiographic methods for the estimation of pulmonary artery pressure (abstr). Int Symp on Doppler Echocard 1986;32.

55. Stevenson JG, French JW, Kawabori I. Doppler estimation of the pressure drop in coarctation of the aorta (abstr). Int Symp on Doppler Echocard 1986;36.

56. Sanders S, MacPherson D, Yeager SB. Tempoeral flow velocity profile in the descending aorta in coarctation. J Am Coll Cardiol 1986, 7:3:603-609.

57. Scneider RR, Steingart, Jurado R, et al. Pulsed echo Doppler measures of cardiac stroke volume in man. Mt Sinai J Med 1982; 49: 391.

58. Redel D, Victor S. Pulsed Doppler echocardiography- A noninvasive method for assessment of pulmonary hypertension. Proc of World Cong Ped Cardiol 1980:290.

59. Serwer GA, Armstrong BE, Anderson PAW. Noninvasive detection of retrograde descending aortic flow in infants using continuous wave Doppler ultrasonongraphy. J Pediatr 1980; 97: 394.

60. Stevenson JG, Kawabori I, Brandestini MA. A twenty month experience comparing pulsed Doppler echocardiography and color-coded digital multigate Doppler for detection of atrioventricular valve regurgitation and its severity. In Echocardiology, edited by Rijsterborgh, The Hague, Martinus Nijhof Pub, 1981 (p 399).

61. Wipperman CF, Redel. The mechanism of mesosystolic notching of the pulmonary valve revealed by Doppler flow imaging (abstr). Circulation 1986; 74 (suppl II): 132.

62. Daniels O, Kapusta L, Hopman JCW. The advantage of two dimensional Doppler flow imaging in the diagnosis: Small ventricular septal defct with left to right shunt (abstr). Int Cong Card Doppler 1986: 113.

63. Daniels O, Hopman JCW, Stelinga, et al. Doppler flow characteristics in the main pulmonary artery and the LA/Ao ratio before and after ductal closure in healthy newborns. Pediatr Cardiol 1982; 3 : 99-104.

64. Kronik G, Slany J, Moesslacher H. Contrast M-mode echocardiography in the diagnosis of atrail septal defects in acyanotic patients. Circulation 1979; 59; 372-78.

65.   Skjaerpe T, Hegrenaes L, Hatle L.   Noninvasive estimation of right ventricular systolic pressure by Doppler ultrasound in ventricular septal defect (abstr). Ultrasonar Bull 1983: 92.

66. Hatle L, Rokseth R. Noninvasive diagnosis and assessment of ventricular septal defect by Doppler ultrasound. Acta Med Scand 1981, 64: 47-56.

67.   Ludomirsky A, Huhta JC, Vick GW, et al.   Color Doppler detection of multiple septal defects. Circulation 1986, 74; 6: 1317-22.

68.   Ortiz E, Robinson Pj, Deanfield JE, et al.   Localization of ventricular septal defects by simultaneous display of superimposed colour Doppler and cross sectional echocardiographic images. Br Heart J 1985, 54: 53.

69.   Light LH.   Implications of aortic blood velocity measurements in children. J Physiol 1978, 285: 17.

70. Horowitz S, Lima CO. Valdes-Cruz LM, et al. Validation of an echo Doppler method for calculating severity of discrete stenotic obstructions in a canine model with a pulmonary artery band. Pediat. Res 1983, 17: 114A.

71. Keane JF, Bernard WF, Nadas AS. Aortic stenosis surgery in infancy. Circulation 1975, 52: 1138.

72. Lima CO, Valdes-Cruz LM, Sahn DJ, et al. An echo-Doppler method for prediction of the severity of left ventricular outflow obstruction. Pediat Res 1983, 17: 180.

73.   Johnson SL, Baker DW, Lute RA, Kawabori I.   Detection of small ventricular septal defects by Doppler flowmeter. Circulation 1974 (suppl III), 50: 142.

74. Stevenson JG, Kawabori I, French JW. Critical importance of sedation when measuring pressure gradients by Doppler (abstr). Circulation 1984 (suppl II), 70: 363.

75. Stewart WJ, Jiang L, Mich R, Pandian N, et al. Variable effects of changes in flow rate through the aortic, pulmonary, and mitral valves on valve area and flow velocity: Impact on quantitiative Doppler flow calculations. J Am Coll Cardiol 1985, 6; 3: 653-62.

INDEX